Workbook for

Paramedic Practice Today : Above and Beyond

Volume 2

Workbook for

Paramedic Practice Today : Above and Beyond

Volume 2

Neil Coker
Robert Vroman, editor

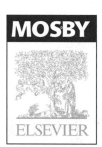

MOSBY

ELSEVIER

11830 Westline Industrial Drive
St. Louis, Missouri 63146

WORKBOOK FOR PARAMEDIC PRACTICE TODAY:
ABOVE AND BEYOND
Volume 2   978-0-323-04378-6
Two-Volume Set   978-0-323-04390-8

ISBN: 978-0-323-04378-6

Executive Editor: Linda Honeycutt
Senior Developmental Editor: Laura Bayless
Publishing Services Manager: Patricia Tannian
Project Manager: Jonathan M. Taylor
Cover Designer: Amy Buxton

Printed in the United States of America

Last digit is the print number: 9   8   7   6   5   4   3   2

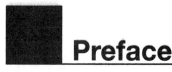

Preface

The workbooks for *Paramedic Practice Today: Above and Beyond* have been developed to aid you in understanding and retaining material presented in the textbook.

There is a workbook chapter for each chapter of the textbook. Textbook objectives and summaries provide you with a quick overview of the key concepts presented in each chapter for convenient review. The workbooks use a variety of question types to aid comprehension, including matching, labeling, short-answer, multiple choice, and case study formats. Matching exercises reinforce key vocabulary and concepts. Labeling exercises provide you with a visual aid in learning core body systems. Short-answer exercises give you an opportunity to explain concepts in your own words and better test your understanding. Multiple-choice test items are established in an educationally sound format. Case studies are used frequently and aid you in putting your knowledge in context. Answers with rationales are provided for you at the back of the book to allow you to check your own work for instant feedback.

For best results, read the corresponding textbook chapter in *Paramedic Practice Today: Above and Beyond* before beginning the workbook chapter. If you have trouble completing these exercises, reread the text chapter and return here to try the workbook chapter again.

Acknowledgments

The editors would like to extend their appreciation to the reviewers who diligently worked on this book.

Jeffrey K. Benes, BS, NREMT-P
Aurora Medical Center
Kenosha, Wisconsin

Kristen Borchelt, NREMT-P
Cincinnati Children's Hospital
Cincinnati, Ohio

Michael Brewer, Med, NREMT-P
University of Mississippi Medical Center
Jackson, Mississippi

Robert Joseph Carter, Flight Paramedic
Center for Emergency Medicine
STAT MedEvac
Pittsburgh, Pennsylvania

Chief Thomas J. Cerbarano, BS, NREMT-P, PPS, CRS
Thomas County Fire Rescue Station 8
Ochlocknee, Georgia

Kevin Thomas Collopy, BA, NREMT-P, WEMT
Bell Ambulance, Inc.
Wilderness Medical Associates
Milwaukee, Wisconsin

Peter Connick, EMT-P
Chatham Fire–Rescue
Chatham, Massachusetts
Cape Cod Community College
Emergency Medical Teaching Services, Inc.
Dennis, Massachusetts

Jon Steven Cooper, NREMT-P
Baltimore City Fire and EMS Academy
Baltimore, Maryland

Elizabeth Criss, RN, Med, MS, CEN, CCRN
University Medical Center
Tucson, Arizona

Jeff Dietrich, BSAS, AAS, NREMT-P, CCP
Greenville Technical College
Greenville, South Carolina

Hunter Elliot, NREMT-P
The Center for Emergency Health Services
Williamsburg, Virginia

Jeffrey S. Force, BA, NREMT-P
Pikes Peak Community College
Penrose–St Francis Health Services
Colorado Springs, Colorado

Fidel Garcia, EMT-P
Professional EMS Education, LLC
EMS Program
Mesa State College
Grand Junction, Colorado

Mark K. Goldstein, BSN, RN, EMT-P
William Beaumont Hospital
Royal Oak, Michigan
Oakland Community College
Auburn Hills, Michigan

Leslie Hernandez, BS, NREMT-P
Bulverde–Spring Branch EMS
LPMH and Associates
Spring Branch, Texas

Terry Horrocks, NREMT-P
Baltimore City Fire Department
Baltimore, Maryland

Robert L. Jackson, Jr., NREMT-P, CCEMTP, BA, MAPS, MAR
Paramedic
University of Missouri Health Care
Columbia, Missouri
Capital Regional Medical Center
Jefferson City, Missouri

Sean Kivlehan, BA, AAS, EMT-P, CIC
St. Vincent's Hospital
New York, New York

Robert Lamey, MSIT, NREMT-P
University of Baltimore (retired)
Baltimore, Maryland

Michael G. Miller, BS, RN, NREMT-P
EMS Education
Creighton University
Omaha, Nebraska

Kirk E. Mittelman, BS, NREMT-P
University of Utah
Salt Lake City, Utah
Mt. Nebo Training Association
Provo, Utah
Lone Peak Fire District
Alpine, Utah

Laraine Moody, MSN, RN, CP NP
Children's Hospital of Michigan
Detroit, Michigan

Greg Mullen, MS, NREMT-P
National EMS Academy
Lafayette, Louisiana

Timothy J. Perkins, BS, EMT-P
Virginia Department of Health
Office of Emergency Services
Richmond, Virginia

Gregg D. Ramirez, BS, EMT-P
Northwest Regional Training Center
Vancouver, Washington

Ken Reardon, Paramedic
Our Lady of Mercy Medical Center
New York, New York

Larry Richmond, AS, NREMT-P, CCEMT-P
Mountain Plains Health Consortium
Fort Meade, South Dakota

Maureen Shanahan, RN, BSN, MN
City College of San Francisco
San Francisco, California

G. Everett Stephens, MD, FAAEM
Department of Emergency Medicine
University of Louisville
Louisville, Kentucky

Contents

35 Obstetrics and Gynecology

READING ASSIGNMENT

Chapter 35, pages 2-31, in *Paramedic Practice Today: Above and Beyond*.

OBJECTIVES

After completing this chapter, you will be able to:
1. Review the anatomic structures and physiology of the female reproductive system.
2. Identify the normal events of the menstrual cycle.
3. Describe how to assess a patient with a gynecologic complaint.
4. Explain how to recognize a gynecologic emergency.
5. Describe the general care for any patient with a gynecologic emergency.
6. Describe the pathophysiology, assessment, and management of specific gynecologic emergencies.
7. Identify the normal events of pregnancy.
8. Describe how to assess an obstetric patient.
9. Describe the procedures for handling complications of pregnancy.
10. Identify the stages of labor and the paramedic's role in each stage.
11. Differentiate normal and abnormal delivery.
12. State indications of an imminent delivery.
13. Identify and describe complications associated with pregnancy and delivery.
14. Explain the use of the contents of an obstetrics kit.
15. Differentiate the management of a patient with predelivery emergencies from a normal delivery.
16. State the steps in the predelivery preparation of the mother.
17. Establish the relation between standard precautions and childbirth.
18. State the steps to assist in the delivery of a new born.
19. Describe the management of the mother after delivery.
20. Discuss the steps in the delivery of the placenta.
21. Describe how to care for the newborn.
22. Describe how and when to cut the umbilical cord.
23. Summarize neonatal resuscitation procedures.
24. Describe the procedures for handling abnormal deliveries and maternal complications of labor.
25. Describe special considerations of a premature baby.
26. Describe special considerations when meconium is present in amniotic fluid or during delivery.

CHAPTER SUMMARY

- The major female reproductive structures include the uterus, ovaries, fallopian tubes, and vagina. During the menstrual cycle, the endometrium is prepared by the hormones estrogen and progesterone to receive a fertilized egg. If the egg is not fertilized, the lining is shed as menstruation.
- Assessment and management of the patient with a gynecologic emergency should include a history that focuses on the chief complaint and specifically addresses vaginal bleeding, abdominal pain, and the possibility of pregnancy. These may be sensitive issues for the patient and you should maintain a caring, professional attitude at all times.
- Most gynecologic problems are not life threatening; however, ectopic pregnancy can kill otherwise healthy women. Any woman with vaginal bleeding and abdominal pain who might be pregnant should be monitored for shock and transported for further evaluation.
- Domestic violence and sexual assault are terrifying for the patient. Your primary responsibility is to keep your patient and yourself safe from further violence. Try to cooperate with law enforcement authorities in collecting evidence whenever possible.
- Pregnancy is a normal event in the human life cycle. When an egg is fertilized, it travels down the fallopian tube and implants in the lining of the uterus. The egg develops into an embryo, which is attached by the umbilical cord to the placenta. The placenta is the organ that exchanges nutrition and toxins for the embryo. After 8 weeks the embryo is called a *fetus*. The normal length of pregnancy is 38 to 40 weeks.
- The enlarging uterus causes physiologic changes unique to pregnancy. Heart rate and respiratory rate

1

increase slightly, and blood pressure decreases slightly. Blood volume is significantly increased. The enlarging uterus can compress major blood vessels in the abdomen to cause supine hypotension syndrome. To avoid this, transport a woman on her left side during the second half of pregnancy.

- An obstetric history should start with the chief complaint and its relation, if any, to the pregnancy. Always ask about the presence of vaginal bleeding, contractions, or abdominal pain. Try to establish the EDC, gravidity, and parity of the patient. If the mother is at least 20 weeks pregnant, listen for fetal heart tones on physical examination of the abdomen.
- Vaginal bleeding and abdominal pain in the first trimester of pregnancy may be signs of a miscarriage or an ectopic pregnancy. Both conditions may cause life-threatening bleeding. Closely monitor these patients for shock and transport as soon as possible.
- Placental abruption and placenta previa are complications of late pregnancy that may cause vaginal bleeding. Previa often is associated with painless, bright red bleeding, whereas abruption may be associated with abdominal pain and a tender uterus. Significant vaginal bleeding is not normal before delivery and should prompt careful monitoring for shock and rapid transport.
- Preeclampsia is a disorder of the second half of pregnancy that may include signs such as hypertension, severe swelling of the extremities, and vomiting and symptoms such as abdominal pain and headaches. The most serious complication of preeclampsia is seizures. Assume that any seizure in pregnancy is caused by preeclampsia and treat with careful airway management, supplemental oxygen, IV access, and prompt transport. The drug of choice for eclamptic seizures is magnesium sulfate.
- Like pregnancy, childbirth is a normal event in the human life cycle and usually progresses without difficulty no matter where it happens. In this country most deliveries occur in hospitals or birthing centers with medical professionals in attendance. If you are called to help with a delivery, reassure the mother, prepare for delivery, assist with the birth, and then monitor the mother and baby closely after delivery. The ABCs apply here as they do in any patient.
- Labor is divided into three stages. The first stage begins with the onset of contractions and ends when the cervix is fully dilated. The second stage is the time from complete dilation of the cervix until the delivery of the infant. The third stage begins after the infant is delivered and ends with delivery of the placenta.
- Some indicators that delivery may be imminent include the sensation of needing to push, rupture of membranes, and contractions longer than 1 minute and closer than 2 to 3 minutes apart. If you suspect delivery is imminent, examine the mother for crowning or perineal bulging.
- If you must deliver the infant outside the hospital, try to find a private and protected place. Remember to use standard precautions, including wearing a gown, gloves, mask, and protective eyewear.
- Supplies for delivery include clean linens, a bulb syringe, umbilical cord clamps, gauze, sponges, scissors, and a container for the placenta.
- Allow the head to deliver in a gradual, controlled manner. Check for the umbilical cord wrapped around the baby's neck and (if present) pull the cord over the baby's head. Immediately suction the infant's nose and mouth before the body delivers. If meconium is present, suction the mouth and nose thoroughly, provide oxygen, and watch for breathing difficulties.
- After the body delivers, dry the baby and cut and clamp the umbilical cord. Assess the baby's ABCs. Stimulate the infant to breatheless, if necessary, and provide oxygen as needed.
- If the placenta delivers, place it in a clean container and transport it to the hospital with mother and infant.
- It is easy to focus on only one of your patients after delivery. Continue to reassess ABCs in both mother and baby and provide support as needed.
- Up to 500 mL of blood loss after delivery is normal and should be expected. If the mother continues to have brisk bleeding, massage the uterus through the abdominal wall and encourage her to breastfeed if possible to slow the bleeding.
- *Preterm delivery* is defined as delivery before the thirty-seventh week of pregnancy. Preterm infants may need more aggressive resuscitation than term infants and are more prone to hypoxia, respiratory distress, and hypothermia. Keep the infant warm and provide ventilatory assistance as needed.
- Abnormal presentations include breech presentation, shoulder dystocia, limb presentation, and cord prolapse. In all these situations placing the mother in a knee-chest position provides the widest possible diameter of the pelvis and may expedite delivery. In the case of cord prolapse, it will help reduce pressure on the cord.
- Fetal demise is a horrific event for the mother. A gentle, supportive demeanor should be maintained at all times. Err on the side of doing everything to aid in the infant's survival.
- Uterine complications of delivery can include inversion or rupture. Both are life-threatening events that require prompt recognition and treatment for shock.
- Pregnant women are at increased risk of pulmonary embolism. Suspect this diagnosis if a woman is short of breath, reporting pleuritic chest pain, and coughing up blood.
- Trauma is the leading cause of death among pregnant women in the United States. The best care for the fetus is good care for the mother. Treat her aggressively, as you would any other trauma victim. Always position a pregnant woman in the left lateral recumbent position when possible. If she requires a backboard, it can be tilted to the left to reduce the risk of supine hypotensive syndrome.

SHORT ANSWER

1. What term is used to describe each of the following situations?

_____ An abortion that occurs naturally
_____ An illegal attempt to cause an abortion
_____ An abortion induced for justifiable medical reasons in an authorized medical setting
_____ A fetus dies at less than 20 weeks and is retained in uterus at least 2 months thereafter
_____ An abortion in which the uterus is unable to expel all of the products of conception

2. Number the following structures in the order the ovum traverses them during the menstrual cycle.

_____ Cervix
_____ Uterus
_____ Fallopian tube
_____ Vagina
_____ Ovary

3. What is mittelschmerz?

4. What is the endometrium? What happens to the endometrium if a fertilized ovum does not implant in it?

5. What are two complications that can develop as a result of an incomplete abortion?

6. What problem should be suspected in any female patient of childbearing age who complains of lower abdominal pain or who presents with a sudden onset of shock with no readily identifiable cause?

7. What is the first question you should *always* ask any female patient who presents with lower abdominal pain?

8. Your patient is a 23-year-old gravida 2, para 1 (G2P1) in the last trimester. She states that when she lies down on her back, she becomes dizzy and "blacks out." If she sits up or rolls onto her side, the symptoms subside. What is her problem and how can this problem be prevented?

9. What is the best position in which to transport a patient who is in late-term pregnancy? Why?

10. What drug is used to prevent seizures in patients with preeclampsia?

11. What precautions should be taken when this drug is administered?

12. What drug will antagonize the toxic effects of this drug?

13. What are the only two situations in which a paramedic may place his or her hand in the vagina of a pregnant woman?

14. Following the delivery of a normal infant, what is your first priority?

15. List the three methods that may be used to control postpartum bleeding.

16. During a breech delivery, what should you do if the infant's head does not deliver within 3 minutes of the body?

17. What is a prolapsed umbilical cord? What should you do if you discover a prolapsed cord when you examine a patient?

_____

_____

_____

_____

18. During a delivery, an infant's upper shoulder will not deliver because it is caught under the mother's pubic bone. What should be done to assist in the delivery?

_____

_____

_____

_____

19. Why should the placenta be transported to the hospital with the mother and infant?

_____

_____

_____

_____

20. If an infant is born still enclosed in the amniotic sac, what should you do?

_____

_____

_____

_____

21. A patient in labor states that she feels as though she needs to move her bowels. When you examine her, you notice that the vaginal area is beginning to bulge outward. In what stage of labor is the patient?

_____

_____

_____

_____

22. What are Braxton Hicks contractions? How can Braxton Hicks contractions be distinguished from true labor?

_____

_____

_____

_____

23. What is a shoulder dystocia? How is shoulder dystocia managed?

_____

_____

_____

_____

24. What is the most common cause of an inverted uterus? If this problem occurs, how should you manage the patient?

_____

_____

_____

_____

25. An infant presents with what appears to be a loop of umbilical cord around the neck. How would you manage this problem?

_____

_____

_____

_____

26. During a delivery, you discover that the infant's arm is protruding from the vagina. What is this problem called? How should you manage this situation?

_____

_____

_____

_____

27. List two possible causes of pulmonary embolism in pregnant patients.

_____

_____

28. A patient states that her last normal menstrual period was May 12, 2008. Predict her estimated date of confinement.

_____

_____

_____

29. What is the relationship of the height of the uterine fundus to the length of pregnancy?

_____

_____

_____

30. What is a tocolytic agent? Why are beta-adrenergic agents such as ritodrine or terbutaline effective tocolytic agents?

_____

_____

_____

4

MULTIPLE CHOICE

1. You are assisting with a vaginal delivery. The infant's head has been delivered and the mouth and nose suctioned. To deliver the anterior shoulder, you should gently _____.
   A. guide the infant's head downward
   B. guide the infant's head upward
   C. lift the infant's head to a transverse position
   D. pull on the infant's head

2. The second stage of labor _____.
   A. begins with full cervical dilation and ends with the infant's delivery
   B. begins with the expulsion of a mucous plug
   C. begins with the onset of the first contraction and ends with the delivery of the placenta
   D. usually lasts 8 to 12 hours in the primigravida patient

3. At approximately 20 weeks, the fundus may be located at the level of the _____.
   A. fifth thoracic vertebra
   B. symphysis pubis
   C. umbilicus
   D. xiphoid process

4. You are called to transfer a 24-year-old G1P0 at 25 weeks' gestation from your local hospital to a maternal-fetal special care unit 1 hour away. The patient's physician has just given her 0.25 mg of terbutaline by Sub-Q injection. Terbutaline has been given because it will _____.
   A. dilate the mother's airways, improving oxygenation of the fetus
   B. dilate placental blood vessels, improving fetal oxygenation
   C. promote lung maturation with early onset of surfactant production
   D. relax uterine smooth muscle, interrupting preterm labor

5. You are transporting a 22-year-old G2P1 with a diagnosis of preeclampsia. She is receiving magnesium sulfate via continuous IV infusion at 1 g/hr. En route, she begins to complain of weakness and extreme thirst. Her skin becomes flushed. Her pulse rate slows, and she becomes hypotensive. What drug will reverse these symptoms?
   A. Atropine
   B. Calcium
   C. Dopamine
   D. Epinephrine

6. A 28-year-old G2P1 has been in active labor for about 12 hours. On examination, you discover the infant's arm is extending from the vagina. You should _____.
   A. handle the delivery in the same manner as a normal delivery
   B. hold the infant in the vagina until you reach the hospital
   C. insert a gloved hand into the vagina and reposition the infant for delivery
   D. transport to the hospital immediately

7. A 17-year-old female in the seventh month of her first pregnancy complains of a severe headache, spots before her eyes, and upper abdominal pain. Edema of the face, feet, and hands is present. Vital signs are BP—160/110 mm Hg; P—112 beats/min bounding; R—22 breaths/min shallow, regular. The patient is in immediate danger of having a _____.
   A. cerebrovascular accident
   B. myocardial infarction
   C. seizure
   D. spontaneous pneumothorax

8. A 23-year-old female who is in active labor complains that she needs to use the bathroom. The vaginal area is bulging outward and the top of the infant's head is visible. In what stage of labor is the patient?
   A. Crowning
   B. First
   C. Second
   D. Third

9. A 23-year-old female complains of sharp pain in the right lower quadrant of her abdomen that began suddenly 10 minutes ago. She says her last menstrual period was about 8 weeks ago and that she has had a small amount of vaginal bleeding for 2 days. She is weak, pale, and sweating heavily. Vital signs (supine) are: BP—106/70 mm Hg; P—118 beats/min weak, regular; R—26 breaths/min shallow, regular. Vital signs (sitting) are: BP—90/50 mm Hg; P—122 beats/min, thready; R—28 breaths/min shallow, regular. The patient probably has what problem?
   A. Acute appendicitis
   B. Ruptured ectopic pregnancy
   C. Spontaneous abortion
   D. Uterine rupture

10. A 26-year-old female in the last trimester of her pregnancy complains of a sudden onset of dizziness, weakness, and severe, constant abdominal pain. She is pale and diaphoretic. Palpation of the abdomen reveals a "rock hard" uterus. A small amount of vaginal bleeding is present. The patient has what problem?
    A. Abruptio placentae
    B. Placenta previa
    C. Spontaneous abortion
    D. Uterine rupture

11. A 24-year-old female in the last trimester of her first pregnancy complains of a sudden onset of heavy, painless vaginal bleeding. She is confused and anxious. Her skin is pale, cool, and clammy. Palpation of her abdomen reveals what seems to be a normal pregnant uterus. The patient has what problem?
    A. Abruptio placentae
    B. Placenta previa
    C. Spontaneous abortion
    D. Uterine rupture

12. A 24-year-old female complains of pain in the left lower quadrant of her abdomen associated with nausea and vomiting. She says the pain began about 1 week after her last menstrual period and has been associated with moderate greenish-yellow vaginal discharge. What is the most likely cause of her problem?
    A. Pelvic inflammatory disease
    B. Placenta previa
    C. Ruptured ectopic pregnancy
    D. Spontaneous abortion

13. What should you do during a breech delivery if the infant's head does not deliver within 3 minutes of the body?
    A. Give high-concentration oxygen and push on the mother's abdomen to speed delivery.
    B. Give high-concentration oxygen to the mother and transport immediately.
    C. Pull on the infant's legs while massaging the mother's abdomen to speed delivery.
    D. Push the vaginal wall away from the infant's nose and mouth to form an airway and transport immediately.

14. What is your first priority following the birth of an infant?
    A. Clamp and cut the umbilical cord.
    B. Deliver the placenta.
    C. Ensure the infant's airway and breathing are adequate.
    D. Treat the mother for blood loss.

15. If an infant is born still enclosed in the amniotic sac, what should you do?
    A. Cut the umbilical cord.
    B. Proceed with the delivery in the normal manner because the sac will rapidly deteriorate.
    C. Puncture or tear the sac and remove it from around the infant.
    D. Transport immediately code 3.

16. What are the only times a paramedic may insert his or her hand into the vagina of a pregnant patient?
    A. Cephalic presentation and prolapsed umbilical cord
    B. Limb presentation and prolapsed umbilical cord
    C. Placenta previa and breech birth
    D. Prolapsed umbilical cord and breech birth

17. The placenta should be transported to the hospital so it can _____.
    A. be disposed of properly
    B. be examined to ensure all of it has been expelled
    C. be weighed before disposal
    D. continue to provide oxygen to the infant

18. What is the first stage of labor?
    A. The period during which contractions are 2 to 4 minutes apart
    B. The period from delivery of the infant until delivery of the placenta
    C. The period from full dilation of the cervix until the infant is delivered
    D. The period from the onset of contractions until the cervix is fully dilated

19. What should you do if heavy or excessive bleeding is present following delivery?
    A. Pack the vagina with sterile gauze.
    B. Raise the lower extremities and give oxygen.
    C. Raise the lower extremities, give oxygen, and gently massage the lower abdomen.
    D. Treat for shock and avoid massaging the lower abdomen.

20. If the placenta has not delivered soon after the infant, what should you do?
    A. Aggressively massage the lower abdomen to promote delivery of the placenta.
    B. Apply a cold pack to the lower abdomen to promote delivery of the placenta.
    C. Pull on the cord to speed delivery of the placenta.
    D. Transport without delay.

21. The area between the vagina and the anus is the _____.
    A. patella
    B. perineum
    C. peritoneum
    D. pleura

22. Your patient is a 22-year-old female who is 8 months' pregnant and who was on the "down" escalator at a shopping mall. When the escalator suddenly stopped, the patient fell approximately 15 ft to the bottom of the escalator. She is awake and alert, complaining of pain in her lower back, right wrist, and right ankle. Her skin is warm and dry. Radial pulses are present, strong, and regular. How should the spine board be positioned when this patient is transported?
    A. So the patient is tilted toward her left side
    B. So the patient is tilted toward her right side
    C. With the patient's head slightly elevated
    D. With the patient's lower extremities slightly elevated

23. When vital signs are taken on the patient in the previous question, you would anticipate that pregnancy would result in her _____.
    A. heart rate being faster and blood pressure being higher
    B. heart rate being faster and blood pressure being lower
    C. heart rate being slower and blood pressure being higher
    D. heart rate being slower and blood pressure being lower

24. Management of the patient in the previous question should include _____.
    A. assisted ventilations with a bag-mask device
    B. humidified oxygen via nasal cannula
    C. oxygen via nonrebreather mask
    D. ventilation with an oxygen-powered ventilation device (demand valve)

Case one

A 24-year-old female in the last trimester of her first pregnancy complains of a sudden onset of heavy, painless vaginal bleeding. She is not oriented to place and time. Her respirations are rapid and shallow. The patient's skin is pale, cool, and moist. Radial pulses are absent. The carotid pulse is weak and regular. Vital signs are P—128 beats/min weak, regular; R—26 breaths/min shallow, regular; BP—76/50 mm Hg. Palpation of the abdomen reveals what seems to be a normal pregnant uterus.

1. From what problem is the patient suffering?

2. How would you manage this patient?

When you reach the hospital, the emergency department physician (a moonlighting psychiatry resident) wants to perform a vaginal examination.

3. What should you tell the physician about the risks of performing a vaginal examination in a patient with this problem?

Case two

A 36-year-old G4P3 is in the seventh month of her pregnancy. She complains of a sudden onset of dizziness and weakness associated with severe, constant abdominal pain. She is pale and diaphoretic. Radial pulses are weak and rapid. The uterus is tender to palpation and is "rock-hard." A small amount of vaginal bleeding is present. Vital signs are: BP—84/68 mm Hg; P—126 beats/min weak, regular; R—22 breaths/min shallow, regular. The patient has a history of chronic, essential hypertension controlled with diet and diuretics.

1. From what problem is the patient suffering?

2. What is the cause of the patient's dizziness and weakness?

3. What is the cause of the tachycardia, hypotension, pallor, and diaphoresis?

4. Why is the patient's uterus tender and "rock-hard"?

5. How are the patient's age and multiparity associated with this problem?

6. How is the patient's underlying hypertension associated with this problem?

_____
_____
_____
_____

7. How would you manage this patient?

_____
_____
_____
_____

Case three

A 23-year-old female complains of sudden "sharp" pain in her left lower abdominal quadrant. She is restless and anxious. Her respirations are rapid and shallow. The patient's radial pulses are rapid and weak. Her skin is pale, cool, and diaphoretic. The patient's last menstrual period was approximately 8 weeks ago. She thought at first that she might be pregnant; then she began to experience a small amount of vaginal bleeding during the last 2 days. The patient uses an intrauterine device (IUD) for contraception. Vital signs are: BP—102/82 mm Hg; P—118 beats/min weak, regular; R—22 breaths/min shallow, regular.

1. What problem probably is present?

_____

2. Where in the female reproductive tract is this problem most likely to occur? Why?

_____
_____
_____
_____

3. Why has the patient been experiencing a small amount of vaginal bleeding over the last couple of days?

_____
_____
_____
_____

4. Is the patient's use of an IUD relevant to her current problem? Why?

_____
_____
_____
_____

5. What is the principal complication associated with this problem?

_____

When the patient is moved from a supine to a sitting position, her vital signs are: BP—88/68 mm Hg; P—132 beats/min, thready; R—26 breaths/min shallow, regular. She complains of feeling as though she is "going to pass out."

6. What problem do these changes in the vital signs suggest?

_____

7. What term is used to describe these changes?

   _____

8. How would you manage this patient?

   _____
   _____
   _____
   _____

36 Neonatology

READING ASSIGNMENT

Chapter 36, pages 32-71, in *Paramedic Practice Today: Above and Beyond*.

OBJECTIVES

After completing this chapter, you will be able to:
1. Define the terms *newborn, newly born,* and *neonate*.
2. Discuss antepartum and intrapartum factors associated with an increased risk for neonatal resuscitation.
3. Identify the factors that lead to premature birth and low birth weight newborns.
4. Discuss the assessment findings associated with primary and secondary apnea in the neonate.
5. Discuss pulmonary perfusion and asphyxia.
6. Describe the etiology, epidemiology, history, and physical findings for the following congenital anomalies:
   - Tracheoesophageal fistula
   - Diaphragmatic hernia
   - Choanal atresia
   - Pierre Robin sequence
   - Meningomyelocele
   - Cleft lip and palate
   - Omphalocele
7. With the patient history and physical examination findings, develop a treatment plan for newborns with the following conditions:
   - Tracheoesophageal fistula
   - Diaphragmatic hernia
   - Choanal atresia
   - Pierre Robin sequence
   - Meningomyelocele
   - Cleft lip and palate
   - Omphalocele
8. Discuss the indications, necessary equipment, technique, and assessment of the newborn's response for the following interventions:
   - Blow-by oxygen delivery
   - Ventilatory assistance
   - Orogastric tube insertion
   - Chest compressions
   - Tracheal intubation
   - Vascular access
   - Needle chest decompression
9. Identify the primary signs used for evaluating a newborn during resuscitation.
10. Discuss the initial steps in and formulate a treatment plan for providing initial care to a newborn, including transport guidelines.
11. Identify the appropriate use of the Apgar score in caring for a newborn.
12. Calculate the Apgar score for various newborn situations.
13. Describe the etiology, epidemiology, history, and physical findings for newborn cardiac arrest.
14. Develop a treatment plan for a newborn in cardiac arrest.
15. Discuss the signs of hypovolemia in a newborn.
16. Discuss the treatment plan to stabilize the neonate after cardiac arrest.
17. Describe the etiology, epidemiology, history, and physical findings for the following conditions:
    - Meconium aspiration
    - Apnea
    - Bradycardia
    - Prematurity
    - Respiratory distress or cyanosis
    - Seizures
    - Fever
    - Hypothermia
    - Hypoglycemia
    - Vomiting
    - Diarrhea
    - Birth injury
18. With the patient history and physical examination findings, develop a treatment plan (including transport destination) for newborns with the following conditions:
    - Meconium aspiration
    - Apnea
    - Bradycardia
    - Prematurity
    - Respiratory distress or cyanosis
    - Seizures
    - Fever
    - Hypothermia
    - Hypoglycemia
    - Vomiting
    - Diarrhea
    - Birth injury
19. Discuss the effects of maternal narcotic use on the newborn and formulate a treatment plan for the newborn with narcotic depression.

CHAPTER SUMMARY

- Although fewer than 10% of newborns require emergency care, you must always be prepared for newborn resuscitation when assisting with a delivery.
- Some conditions increase the likelihood that resuscitation will be necessary.
- In most cases, drying, warming, and suctioning are sufficient to cause a newborn to breathe effectively and may be the only resuscitative measures needed. If additional care is required, you must know how to manage a newborn's airway, assist ventilations, perform chest compressions, establish vascular access, and give medications.
- You must be aware of the capabilities of the hospitals in your area to determine the most appropriate destination for healthy and high-risk newborns.
- Although your care will be focused on the newborn, remember to explain what you are doing to family members as you provide care.

SHORT ANSWER

1. Complete the following chart.

	0	1	2
Appearance			
Pulse			
Grimace			
Activity			
Respirations			

2. List the sequence of steps in the management of a distressed neonate included in the inverted pyramid.

3. Immediately following the delivery of an infant, what should be your first priorities?

4. Why do infants and small children require special precautions to prevent them from becoming cold?

5. What is the principal sign that should guide the resuscitation of a newborn?

6. How is supplemental oxygen administered to a newborn infant?

7. What is the function of pulmonary surfactant?

8. At approximately what point in gestation does pulmonary surfactant begin to be produced?

9. What intervention is required for infants born before this point in gestation?

10. When should a newborn infant's ventilations be assisted with a bag-mask device?

11. When should chest compressions be performed on a newborn infant?

12. What is the rate of chest compressions used for a newborn infant?

13. What is the ratio of chest compressions to ventilations used for a newborn infant?

14. Describe three ways to obtain a heart rate measurement on a newborn.

15. What is meconium?

_____
_____
_____
_____

16. If a newborn presents with particulate staining of the amniotic fluid with meconium, what determines the actions you should take?

_____
_____
_____
_____

17. What is acrocyanosis?

_____
_____
_____
_____

18. What is the best location on the newborn's body for evaluating for the presence of central cyanosis?

_____
_____
_____
_____

19. How is vascular access in a newborn infant most easily achieved?

_____
_____
_____
_____

20. What is the initial drug of choice for management of bradycardia in a newborn? If this drug is not effective, what is the second-line drug?

_____
_____
_____
_____

21. What is a meningomyelocele?

_____
_____
_____
_____

22. How should a meningomyelocele be managed?

_____
_____
_____
_____

23. What is an omphalocele?

_____
_____
_____
_____

24. How should an omphalocele be managed?

_____
_____
_____
_____

MULTIPLE CHOICE

1. A neonate is an infant from the time of birth to _____.
   A. 24 hours of age
   B. 1 month of age
   C. 1 week of age
   D. 3 months of age

2. *Newborn* or *newly born infant* is a term used to describe a neonate _____.
   A. before delivery of the placenta
   B. during the first few hours of life
   C. until it is discharged from the hospital
   D. until the umbilical cord has been cut

3. A newborn infant's respiratory rate should be _____.
   A. 12 to 20 breaths/min
   B. 20 to 30 breaths/min
   C. 40 to 60 breaths/min
   D. 60 to 80 breaths/min

4. At 1230 hours, you are dispatched to the maternity store at a local mall where you find a woman in active labor. Examination reveals the baby's head is crowning. When you deliver the infant, it is covered with a greenish-black material. The infant is gasping without moving air. What should you do?
   A. Give oxygen by blow-by and transport.
   B. Intubate the trachea and apply direct suction to the ET tube.
   C. Position the infant head down and stimulate breathing by rubbing its back.
   D. Ventilate the lungs immediately with a bag-mask and high-concentration oxygen.

5. While delivering a baby, you note the amniotic fluid contains a substance resembling dark pea soup. Following delivery, the baby immediately begins to breathe, is actively moving its extremities, and has a heart rate of 140 beats/min. Cyanosis of the hands and feet is present. What should you do?
   A. Dry the infant thoroughly and wrap in warm blankets.
   B. Give oxygen by blow-by.
   C. Perform endotracheal intubation using the endotracheal tube as a suction catheter.
   D. Ventilate the lungs with 100% oxygen using a bag-mask.

6. The first-line medication for newborn resuscitations is _____.
   A. atropine
   B. epinephrine
   C. fluid
   D. oxygen

7. *Acrocyanosis* refers to a _____.
   A. bluish discoloration of the peripheral extremities
   B. bluish discoloration of the trunk
   C. gray-ashen color of the skin
   D. nonblanching skin rash

8. Which of the following statements about skin color in a newborn immediately after birth is correct?
   A. Both central cyanosis and cyanosis of the extremities are abnormal.
   B. Both cyanosis of the extremities and central cyanosis are common and normal.
   C. Central cyanosis is common, but cyanosis of the extremities is abnormal.
   D. Cyanosis of the extremities is common, but central cyanosis is abnormal.

9. You have just assisted in the delivery of an infant born at 34 weeks' gestation. The infant is small and limp and has obvious central cyanosis. After warming, drying, and stimulating, the infant makes weak flexing extremity movements. Respirations are 10 breaths/minute and gasping. There is no grimace when the infant's airway is suctioned. The pulse rate is 78 beats/min. Your next step will be to _____.
   A. administer blow-by oxygen for 30 seconds
   B. administer epinephrine
   C. begin bag-mask ventilation
   D. begin chest compressions

10. If there is no improvement after your treatment of the patient in the previous question, what is the 1-minute Apgar score?
    A. 0
    B. 2
    C. 3
    D. 4

11. What is the first priority following the birth of an infant?
    A. Clamping and cutting the umbilical cord
    B. Controlling maternal blood loss
    C. Delivering the placenta
    D. Ensuring that the infant's airway and breathing are adequate

12. If an infant does not cry or breathe within 30 seconds after birth, what should you do first?
    A. Blow oxygen at 5 L/min onto the mouth and nose.
    B. Hold the infant upside down and slap it on the buttocks.
    C. Hold the infant lower than the placenta.
    D. Stimulate the infant by tapping the soles of its feet or rubbing its back.

13. The need for intervention with ventilation and CPR in a newborn is determined by _____.
    A. a 1-minute Apgar score of 0 to 3
    B. a 1-minute Apgar score of 4 to 6
    C. a 1-minute Apgar score of 5 to 8
    D. apnea and insufficient pulse rate after stimulation, suction, and oxygen

14. If a newborn's heart rate is less than 100 beats/min, what should you do?
    A. Give oxygen by blow-by for 30 seconds and then reevaluate the heart rate.
    B. Immediately begin chest compressions and bag-mask ventilation.
    C. Ventilate the lungs with a bag-mask and oxygen for 30 seconds and then reevaluate the heart rate.
    D. Ventilate the lungs with a bag-mask and oxygen if the infant's respirations are slow or gasping.

15. A newborn infant has adequate respirations and heart rate, but its arms and legs are cyanotic. What should you do?
    A. Artificially ventilate the lungs for 30 seconds and reevaluate skin color.
    B. Begin chest compressions.
    C. Give oxygen by blow-by and observe for improvement.
    D. Immediately begin chest compressions with artificial ventilation.

16. You are delivering the infant of an 18-year-old female who has been living in a shelter for the homeless. Her speech is slurred, and she is drowsy and apathetic. You notice needle tracks on her arms. She admits to "shooting up" with heroin 2 hours ago to relieve the pain of labor. Which of the following statements best describes the way you should deal with this situation?
    A. Naloxone should be given by IV push to the mother immediately to avoid serious respiratory depression in the newborn.
    B. The infant probably will develop respiratory depression following delivery and should receive naloxone as quickly as possible to reverse this problem.
    C. The infant probably will not suffer significant problems because narcotics do not cross the placental barrier easily.
    D. The infant probably will suffer respiratory depression following delivery but should not be given naloxone because a withdrawal reaction might occur.

17. You have delivered the baby of a woman who has a history of diabetes mellitus. At about 30-minutes postpartum you should check the infant's blood glucose level because _____.
    A. a decreased blood glucose level at this time will help predict whether the infant will also have diabetes.
    B. an elevated blood glucose level at this time will help predict whether the infant will also have diabetes.
    C. it is at risk for developing hyperglycemia
    D. it is at risk for developing hypoglycemia

18. A female infant you have just delivered is in severe respiratory distress. Central cyanosis unresponsive to bag-mask ventilation is present. Physical examination reveals a small, flat abdomen; absent breath sounds over the left lung field; and displacement of the heart sounds to the right. What problem do you suspect?
    A. Diaphragmatic hernia
    B. Meconium aspiration
    C. Meningomyelocele
    D. Omphalocele

19. Appropriate management for the infant in the previous question would include positioning her head and thorax_____.
    A. higher than her abdomen and feet, avoiding placement of a nasogastric or orogastric tube, ventilating with a bag-mask, and preparing to intubate
    B. higher than her abdomen and feet, placing a nasogastric or orogastric tube, and withholding further bag-mask ventilation until an endotracheal tube is placed
    C. higher than her abdomen and feet, placing a nasogastric or orogastric tube, ventilating with a bag-mask, and preparing to intubate
    D. lower than her abdomen and feet, placing a nasogastric or orogastric tube, and withholding further bag-mask ventilation until an endotracheal tube is placed

20. Determine the Apgar score for the following infant. Appearance: completely cyanotic; pulse: below 100 beats/min; grimace: frowns when stimulated; activity: limp; respirations: slow, irregular.
    A. 1
    B. 3
    C. 5
    D. 7

21. Appropriate methods for stimulating a newborn include _____.
    A. flicking the soles of the feet and gently rubbing the back
    B. flicking the soles of the feet and slapping the buttocks
    C. vigorous rubbing and flicking the soles of the feet
    D. vigorous rubbing and slapping the buttocks

22. Which statement about "milking" or stripping the umbilical cord following delivery is correct?
    A. It is contraindicated because it decreases blood viscosity and causes hypovolemia.
    B. It is contraindicated because it produces polycythemia and increases blood viscosity.
    C. It is indicated because it corrects hypovolemia from blood loss during delivery.
    D. It is indicated because it increases the newborn's red cell mass and improves oxygenation.

23. Chest compressions should be performed on a newborn if the heart rate is _____.
    A. between 60 and 80 beats/min but not increasing with assisted ventilations and supplemental oxygen
    B. between 80 and 100 beats/min and central cyanosis is present
    C. less than 60 beats/min
    D. less than 60 beats/min or between 60 and 80 beats/min if the heart rate is not increasing with assisted ventilations and supplemental oxygen

24. Which of the following best describes the correct technique for giving chest compressions and ventilations to a newborn infant?
    A. Rate 100 breaths/min; compression to ventilation ratio 3 to 1
    B. Rate 120 breaths/min; compression to ventilation ratio 3 to 1
    C. Rate 120 breaths/min; compression to ventilation ratio 5 to 1
    D. Rate 180 breaths/min; compression to ventilation ratio 5 to 1

25. A premature newborn is an infant born before _____.
    A. 28 weeks' gestation or with a weight of less than 0.5 kg
    B. 32 weeks' gestation or with a weight of less than 0.6 kg
    C. 37 weeks' gestation or with a weight of less than 2.2 kg
    D. 40 weeks' gestation or with a weight of less than 2.2 kg

26. A newborn suspected of being hypovolemic should be given _____.
    A. 10 mL/kg of Ringer's lactate or normal saline
    B. 10 mL/kg of D_5LR or D_5NS
    C. 20 mL/kg of D_5W
    D. 20 mL/kg of Ringer's lactate or normal saline

27. Fever in a neonate _____.
    A. is not a cause for concern unless the infant is sweating heavily
    B. is not a problem, because the immune system is immature and neonates frequently develop minor infections
    C. should be considered a sign of a life-threatening infection until proven otherwise
    D. should be treated by using cold packs to lower the core temperature

28. When you suction a newborn's airway you should _____.
    A. squeeze the suction bulb after placing it into the infant's mouth
    B. suction the mouth first so there is nothing there to aspirate if the infant gasps when the nose is suctioned
    C. suction the nose first because infants are obligate nasal breathers
    D. suction the nose first so there is nothing there to aspirate if the infant gasps when the mouth is suctioned

Case one

A 38-year-old female is 26 weeks' pregnant. This is her fourth pregnancy. She previously has delivered three healthy infants at term with no complications. She complains of a sudden onset of severe abdominal pain. Her skin is cool, pale, and diaphoretic. Radial pulses are absent. The carotid pulse is rapid and thready. Capillary refill is longer than 2 seconds. Respirations are rapid and shallow. Palpation of the abdomen reveals a rigid, tender uterus. There is no obvious vaginal bleeding.

As you continue en route to the hospital, the patient suddenly discharges a large amount of fluid from her vagina. The fluid is bloody and is mixed with a dark green, particulate material.

1. What is this dark green material called?

   _____

2. What does it indicate about the condition of the fetus?

   _____

3. Given the estimated gestational age of the fetus, what immediate complication should you anticipate after delivery?

   _____
   _____
   _____
   _____

4. What action should you be prepared to take?

   _____

The patient progresses to active labor and within 10 minutes gives birth. The infant is flaccid with no spontaneous movement and has no apparent respiratory effort. The pulse rate is 40 beats/minute and weak. Central cyanosis is present. You estimate the infant's weight at 1 kg. No obvious congenital deformities are present.

5. What should you do?

   _____
   _____

6. Thirty seconds after beginning treatment, the infant's heart rate is 48 beats/minute. What should you do now?

   _____
   _____

7. Thirty seconds later, the heart rate rises to 88 beats/minute. What should you do now?

   _____
   _____

The infant's heart rate continues to rise steadily. The infant remains flaccid with no spontaneous movement. She is pale and peripheral pulses are weak.

8. What is the most likely cause of these signs and symptoms?

   _____
   _____

9. How should this problem be managed?

   _____
   _____

10. What other cause(s) for these signs and symptoms should be considered?

_____

_____

Case two

A 36-week-old, female infant weighing 5 lb, 9 oz, has been delivered vaginally. The infant is limp, is taking slow, gasping respirations, and has cyanotic extremities.

1. What should be your initial step in managing this patient?

_____

_____

_____

_____

2. Why is it important to dry neonates well and keep them in a warm environment?

_____

_____

3. If the patient does not respond to the initial steps of neonatal resuscitation, what should you do?

_____

_____

4. Where is the most reliable location on a neonate to check for central cyanosis?

_____

5. When should a neonate receive bag-mask ventilation?

_____

6. Once bag-mask ventilation is begun, what physical assessment finding guides further resuscitation?

_____

_____

7. How can a pulse rate measurement be obtained on a newborn?

_____

After 1 minute of bag-mask ventilation, the infant has a heart rate of 46 beats/min.

8. What are the parameters for beginning chest compressions on a distressed neonate?

_____

_____

9. Why are chest compressions performed on neonates even though a pulse is present?

_____

_____

10. At what rate should chest compressions be performed on a neonate?

_____

11. What is the depth of compression that should be used?

_____

12. What compression to ventilation ratio should be used with neonates?

_____

After 1 minute of chest compressions, the infant's heart rate is 56 beats/min.

13. What procedure should be performed at this point?

_____

_____

The infant continues to have a heart rate of 56 beats/min. You decide that it is time to administer medication.

14. What is the first medication that should be given to this patient?

_____

15. What routes are available for administration of this drug?

_____

16. What dose is used when this drug is given intravenously to a newborn?

_____

17. What dose is used when this drug is given endotracheally to a newborn?

_____

18. What is the easiest way to obtain vascular access in a newborn?

_____

19. What are the indications for giving fluid volume replacement to a newborn infant?

_____

20. What formula should be used to calculate the appropriate volume of fluid?

_____

21. Under what circumstances should glucose be given to a distressed newborn?

_____

22. If administration of glucose is indicated, what concentration should be used? Why?

_____

_____

23. What is the neonatal dose of glucose?

_____

24. Under what circumstances should naloxone be given to a newborn?

_____

_____

25. What is the neonatal dose of naloxone?

_____

26. If you suspect that the infant's mother is a narcotics abuser, should the neonate receive naloxone? Why or why not?

_____

_____

37 Pediatrics

READING ASSIGNMENT

Chapter 37, pages 72-134, in *Paramedic Practice Today: Above and Beyond.*

OBJECTIVES

After completing this chapter, you will be able to:

1. Describe Emergency Medical Services for Children and discuss how an integrated system can affect patient outcome.
2. Identify methods and mechanisms that prevent injuries and discuss the paramedic's role in the reduction of infant and childhood morbidity and mortality from acute illness and injury.
3. Describe techniques for successful assessment and treatment of infants and children.
4. Identify typical age-related vital signs and the appropriate equipment used to obtain pediatric vital signs.
5. Identify common responses of families to acute illness and injury of an infant or child and techniques for successful interaction.
6. Determine appropriate airway adjuncts and ventilation devices for infants and children and complications of improper use of these devices.
7. Discuss appropriate tracheal intubation equipment for infants and children.
8. Identify complications of an improper tracheal intubation procedure in infants and children.
9. List the indications for gastric decompression for infants and children.
10. Discuss age-appropriate vascular access sites and necessary equipment for infants and children.
11. Identify complications of vascular access for infants and children.
12. Discuss appropriate transport guidelines for infants and children.
13. Discuss appropriate receiving facilities for low- and high-risk infants and children.
14. Differentiate upper airway obstruction from lower airway disease.
15. Define respiratory distress, failure, and arrest and describe the general approach to the treatment of a child with each of these conditions.
16. Describe the etiology, epidemiology, history, and physical findings of croup, epiglottitis, and bacterial tracheitis.
17. By using the patient history and physical examination findings, develop a treatment plan for a patient who has croup, epiglottitis, or bacterial tracheitis.
18. Describe the etiology, epidemiology, history, and physical findings of asthma, bronchiolitis, and pneumonia.
19. By using the patient history and physical examination findings, develop a treatment plan for a patient who has asthma, bronchiolitis, or pneumonia.
20. Describe the etiology, epidemiology, history, and physical findings of shock in infants and children.
21. By using the patient history and physical examination findings, develop a treatment plan for a patient in shock.
22. Identify the major classifications of pediatric cardiac rhythms.
23. Describe the etiology, epidemiology, history, and physical findings of cardiac dysrhythmias in infants and children.
24. By using the patient history and physical examination findings, develop a treatment plan for a patient who has a cardiac dysrhythmia.
25. Discuss the primary causes of cardiopulmonary arrest in infants and children.
26. Describe the primary causes of altered mental status in infants and children.
27. Describe the etiology, epidemiology, history, and physical findings of neurologic emergencies in infants and children.
28. By using the patient history and physical examination findings, develop a treatment plan for a patient who has a neurologic emergency.
29. Identify common lethal mechanisms of injury in infants and children.
30. Discuss anatomic features of children that predispose or protect them from certain injuries.
31. Describe the pathophysiology, assessment, and treatment of infants and children with trauma.
32. Describe aspects of infant and children airway management affected by potential cervical spine injury.
33. Identify infant and child trauma patients who require spinal immobilization.
34. Discuss fluid management and shock treatment for infant and child trauma patients.
35. Determine when pain management and sedation are appropriate for infants and children.
36. Define *child abuse* and *child neglect*.

37. Define *sudden infant death syndrome* and describe its etiology, epidemiology, history, and physical findings.
38. Discuss the parent and caregiver responses to the death of an infant or child.
39. Identify appropriate parameters for performing infant and child cardiopulmonary resuscitation.
40. Define *children with special healthcare needs* and *technology assistance*.
41. Discuss the unique assessment and treatment considerations for a child with special healthcare needs.

CHAPTER SUMMARY

- The emergency medical services for children (EMSC) program works to make sure that the entire spectrum of emergency services, including primary prevention of illness and injury, acute care, and rehabilitation, is provided to children and adolescents as well as adults.
- Children are at high risk for many injuries that can lead to death or disability. Predictable injuries stem from a dangerous situation or risky behavior.
- The pediatric chain of survival represents a sequential series of events to assess, support, or restore effective ventilation and circulation to the infant or child in respiratory or cardiopulmonary arrest. The sequence consists of four important steps: prevention of illness or injury, early CPR, early EMS activation, and early advanced life support. The importance of prevention is reflected in the links of the chain.
- The PAT is a useful tool for quickly determining if a child is "sick" or "not sick." Three main areas are assessed: appearance, (work of) breathing, and circulation.
- Determine a child's CUPS status after completing the initial assessment and giving appropriate care for life-threatening emergencies. The CUPS assessment scale classifies patients as *c*ritical, *u*nstable, *p*otentially unstable, or *s*table. The CUPS assessment also can be used to help determine the speed of transport and the facility to which the child should be transported if a choice is available.
- Allow an ill child to assume a position of comfort. When suctioning, avoid hypoxia and upper airway stimulation. When giving oxygen, use a nonrebreather mask if possible. If the child will not tolerate a nonrebreather mask, use blow-by oxygen. If a child requires transport to the hospital, decide if the patient requires transport by ground ambulance with or without lights and sirens or air ambulance. Do not delay transport to perform procedures that can be done en route.
- Use age-appropriate words and phrases when talking to a child. Keep the child warm and allow him or her to have a favorite toy or blanket if possible.

- Be sure appropriate basic life support care is performed before advanced life support care. If you must perform ongoing care that requires a flat surface, such as bag-mask ventilation or CPR, place the child on a spine board or stretcher. Transport children with less serious conditions who do not require spine board stabilization and ongoing care with a restraint device (such as a child safety seat) appropriate for size and age. Properly secure safety seats in the ambulance. Parents riding along with the patient should use seat belts or other restraints.
- Categories of respiratory compromise include upper airway obstruction and lower airway disease. A foreign body may block the upper or lower airways. Conditions that may cause upper airway obstruction include croup, epiglottitis, and bacterial tracheitis. Conditions that may cause lower airway disease include asthma, bronchiolitis, and pneumonia.
- Perfusion is the circulation of blood through an organ or a part of the body. Perfusion delivers oxygen and other nutrients to the cells of all organ systems and removes waste products. Shock (hypoperfusion) is the inadequate circulation of blood through an organ or a part of the body. The initial signs of shock may be subtle in an infant or child. The effectiveness of compensatory mechanisms largely depends on the child's previous cardiac and pulmonary health. The presence of hypotension differentiates compensated shock from decompensated shock. Hypotension is a late sign of cardiovascular compromise in an infant or child. In the pediatric patient, the progression from compensated to decompensated shock occurs suddenly and rapidly. When decompensation occurs, cardiopulmonary arrest may be imminent.
- In the pediatric patient, dysrhythmias are divided into four broad categories based on heart rate: normal for age, slower than normal for age (bradycardia), faster than normal for age (tachycardia), or absent or pulseless (cardiac arrest). In children dysrhythmias are treated only if they compromise cardiac output or have the potential for deteriorating into a lethal rhythm. Although disorders of heart rate and rhythm are uncommon in infants and children, when they do occur they most often are because of hypoxia secondary to respiratory arrest and asphyxia.
- In infants and children tachycardia is present if the heart rate is faster than the upper limit of normal for the patient's age. Tachycardia may represent either a normal compensatory response to the need for increased cardiac output or oxygen delivery or an unstable dysrhythmia. If an infant or child is symptomatic because of bradycardia, initial treatment is directed at assessment of the airway and breathing rather than giving epinephrine, atropine, or other drugs. This is because problems with adequate oxygenation and ventilation are more common in children than cardiac causes of bradycardia.

- In adults, sudden nontraumatic cardiac arrests usually are the result of underlying cardiac disease. In children, cardiac arrest usually is the result of respiratory failure or shock that progresses to cardiopulmonary failure with profound hypoxemia and acidosis and eventually cardiopulmonary arrest.
- A child with altered mental status displays changes in personality, behavior, or responsiveness inappropriate for age. The child may appear agitated, combative, sleepy, withdrawn, slow to respond, or completely unresponsive. The most common causes of altered mental status in the pediatric patient are hypoxia, head trauma, seizures, infection, hypoglycemia, and drug or alcohol ingestion.
- Most pediatric seizures are provoked by disorders that begin outside the brain, such as high fever, infection, syncope, head trauma, hypoxia, toxins, or dysrhythmias. A febrile seizure is a generalized seizure that occurs with fever in childhood between the ages of 3 months and 5 years (most occur between ages 6 and 18 months).
- Meningitis is an inflammation of the meninges, the membranes covering the brain and spinal cord. Viral meningitis (also called *aseptic meningitis*) is the most common type. Meningitis also can be caused by infections with several types of bacteria or fungi.
- Most cases of pediatric toxic exposure are unintentional, occur in the home, and involve only a single substance. Children younger than 6 years are at the greatest risk for unintentional poisoning.
- Blunt trauma is the most common mechanism of serious injury in the pediatric patient. Falls are the single most common cause of injury in children. Among children 5 to 9 years of age, pedestrian injuries are the most common cause of death from trauma. Children younger than 5 years are at risk of being run over in the driveway. Penetrating trauma is less common in young children but is becoming an increasing problem in adolescents, particularly in urban areas.
- Children can have spinal nerve injury without damage to the vertebrae, a condition called SCIWORA. Although spinal cord and spinal column injuries are uncommon in the pediatric patient, children younger than 8 years tend to sustain injury to the upper (C1 and C2) cervical spine region.
- In children chest trauma is associated with a high mortality rate. The greater elasticity and flexibility of the chest wall in children makes rib and sternum fractures less common than in adults; however, force is more easily transmitted to the underlying lung tissues, resulting in pulmonary contusion, pneumothorax, or hemothorax.
- In children abdominal trauma is the third leading cause of traumatic death after head and thoracic injuries. It is the most common cause of unrecognized fatal injury in children. The spleen is the most frequently injured abdominal organ during blunt trauma. The liver is the second most commonly injured solid organ in the pediatric patient with blunt abdominal trauma but the most common cause of lethal hemorrhage.

- In a submersion incident, a child's signs and symptoms may vary from no symptoms to cardiac arrest depending on the type and duration of submersion. All submersion victims should be transported to the hospital for evaluation and observation, even those who appear to have recovered fully.
- Methods for assessing pain in the pediatric patient vary according to the age of the child. Use an age-appropriate pain rating scale. The same scale should be used consistently by all persons caring for the child. A good assessment tool to use is the Wong-Baker Faces pain rating scale. This scale combines three scales in one: facial expressions, numbers, and words. The scale consists of six cartoon faces ranging from a smiling face depicting "no hurt" to a tearful, sad face illustrating "worst hurt."
- Child maltreatment includes intentional physical abuse or neglect, emotional abuse or neglect, and sexual abuse of children, usually by adults. Child abuse is unlikely if the child's story is volunteered without hesitation and matches that of the caregiver. Determining the difference between an intentional injury and an accident often is difficult.
- SIDS is the sudden and unexpected death of an infant that remains unexplained after a thorough case investigation, including performance of a complete autopsy, examination of the death scene, and review of the clinical history. Most SIDS deaths occur during the first 6 months of life, most between the ages of 2 and 4 months.
- Children with special healthcare needs are those who have or are at risk for chronic physical, developmental, behavioral, or emotional conditions that require use of health and related services of a type and amount not usually required by typically developing children. Children reliant on technology are a subgroup of children with special healthcare needs that depend on medical devices for their survival. Equipment failure may result in a medical emergency.

SHORT ANSWER

1. Complete the chart to compare and contrast asthma and bronchiolitis in each category.

	Asthma	Bronchiolitis
Age group affected		
History of allergies		
History of low-grade fever		

2. Complete the chart to compare and contrast croup and epiglottitis in each category.

	Croup	Epiglottitis
Etiology (bacterial or viral)		
Age groups affected		
Speed of onset		
Pain on swallowing		
Presence of drooling		
Fever		

21

3. What is the most common form of shock in pediatric patients?

_____

_____

_____

4. What is a fontanel?

_____

_____

_____

5. What change occurs in the fontanelles of a dehydrated infant?

_____

_____

_____

_____

6. What is status asthmaticus?

_____

_____

_____

_____

7. How is a patient with status asthmaticus managed?

_____

_____

_____

_____

8. Why should skin turgor be checked in patients who are having an asthma attack?

_____

_____

_____

9. Why is it important to determine the medications taken by an asthmatic patient before beginning any therapy?

_____

_____

_____

_____

10. Why should oxygen be humidified when it is administered to an asthma patient?

_____

_____

_____

_____

11. What is the prehospital treatment for croup?

_____

_____

_____

_____

12. What is the principal danger facing a patient with epiglottitis?

_____

_____

_____

_____

13. What is SIDS?

_____

_____

_____

14. What is the most common cause of cardiac arrest in children?

_____

_____

_____

15. What is the principal cause of death from seizures?

_____

_____

_____

16. What is status epilepticus?

_____

_____

_____

17. What is the drug of choice for managing status epilepticus in the prehospital setting?

_____

_____

_____

18. How is hypovolemic shock corrected in pediatric patients? Why is this technique used?

_____

_____

_____

19. How is the proper size of endotracheal tube selected for pediatric patients?

_____

_____

20. Why are uncuffed endotracheal tubes used on infants and children younger than 8 years old?

_____

_____

_____

21. How is the proper paddle size for defibrillation or cardioversion of a pediatric patient selected?

_____

_____

_____

_____

22. What is the suggested initial setting for defibrillation of pediatric patients? What energy is used on subsequent shocks?

_____

_____

_____

_____

23. What is the minimum dose of atropine for pediatric patients? Why?

_____

_____

_____

_____

24. What three routes are available for drug administration to children during cardiopulmonary arrest?

_____

_____

_____

_____

25. What drug is always used first in the management of symptomatic bradycardia in pediatric patients?

_____

_____

_____

_____

26. What is the IV dose of epinephrine in pediatric cardiac arrest?

_____

_____

_____

_____

27. What is the endotracheal dose of epinephrine in pediatric cardiac arrest?

_____

_____

_____

_____

MULTIPLE CHOICE

1. Children and infants who are burned are more likely to suffer significant fluid loss than adults because _____.
   A. crying increases fluid loss
   B. IVs usually cannot be run fast enough to keep up with volume loss
   C. pediatric patients need more fluid than adults when they are healthy
   D. the body surface area of pediatric patients is larger in proportion to body volume

2. A 4-month-old infant has been vomiting and having watery diarrhea for 2 days. The baby's lips and oral mucosa are dry, and his fontanelle is sunken. Extremities are cold to the elbows and knees. Capillary refill time is 5 seconds. The ECG monitor shows a narrow complex tachycardia with a rate of 200 beats/min. Management of this patient should include _____.
   A. infusion of 20 mL/kg of isotonic crystalloid
   B. blood glucose level determination
   C. infusion of 20 mL/kg of isotonic crystalloid and blood glucose level determination
   D. cardioversion at 0.5 to 1.0 J/kg

3. The peak incidence for SIDS is in which age group?
   A. 1 to 6 months
   B. 6 to 9 months
   C. 9 to 12 months
   D. Less than 1 month

4. "Jitteriness" and trembling in a pediatric patient with hypoglycemia are caused by the body's activation of the _____.
   A. parasympathetic nervous system, resulting in the liver storing additional glycogen
   B. parasympathetic nervous system, resulting in the pancreas secreting additional insulin
   C. sympathetic nervous system, resulting in the liver releasing additional glucose
   D. sympathetic nervous system, resulting in the pancreas secreting additional glucagon

5. You are dispatched to an elementary school for an 8-year-old, 26-kg male with a history of diabetes. You find the boy confused, diaphoretic, and tachycardic. When you attempt to measure his blood glucose level, the glucometer malfunctions. The most appropriate therapy following management of the ABCs and obtaining IV access is to give oxygen and _____.
   A. administer $D_{10}W$ at a dose of 1 to 2 mL/kg
   B. administer $D_{25}W$ at a dose of 1 to 2 mL/kg
   C. give $D_{25}W$ at a dose of 2 to 4 mL/kg
   D. rapidly transport the child to a children's hospital

6. In children, cardiac output is most dependent upon _____.
   A. blood pressure
   B. heart rate
   C. peripheral vascular resistance
   D. stroke volume

23

7. The first-line medication for all pediatric resuscitations is _____.
   A. atropine
   B. epinephrine
   C. fluid
   D. oxygen

8. Which of the following groups of signs and symptoms would be most typical of a patient with epiglottitis?
   A. Expiratory stridor, coughing, rales, and cyanosis
   B. Expiratory wheezing, rales, coughing, high fever
   C. Inspiratory stridor, "seal bark" cough, low-grade fever, and orthopnea
   D. Inspiratory stridor, pain on swallowing, high fever, and drooling

9. Common nontraumatic causes of shock in the pediatric patient include _____.
   A. anaphylaxis and volume depletion
   B. sepsis and anaphylaxis
   C. sepsis and volume depletion
   D. sepsis, volume depletion, and AV blocks

10. Late signs of shock in the pediatric patient include _____.
   A. bradycardia, hypotension, and pallor
   B. hypotension and bradycardia
   C. hypotension, bradycardia, and tachypnea
   D. tachypnea and pallor

11. What is the most common cardiac dysrhythmia in pediatric patients?
   A. Asystole
   B. Sinus bradycardia
   C. Sinus tachycardia
   D. Ventricular fibrillation

12. In what age group is croup most common?
   A. 4 years to 7 years
   B. 6 months to 6 years
   C. Older than 7 years
   D. Newborn to 1 year

13. Management of a child with croup and mild to moderate respiratory difficulty would include blow-by oxygen and _____.
   A. subcutaneous epinephrine
   B. nebulized saline and nebulized racemic epinephrine
   C. subcutaneous epinephrine and nebulized saline
   D. subcutaneous epinephrine, nebulized saline, and nebulized racemic epinephrine

14. The leading cause of death in children and young adults is _____.
   A. foreign body airway obstruction
   B. poisoning
   C. sepsis
   D. trauma

15. Which of the following is the most likely initial skin color finding in a child with compensated shock?
   A. Cyanosis
   B. Mottled
   C. Pallor
   D. Red and/or flushed

16. In which of the following pediatric patients is surgical cricothyrotomy indicated?
   A. A 4 year old with an obstructed airway that does not respond to abdominal thrusts
   B. A 6 year old with severe trauma to the face with moderate bleeding
   C. A 12 year old who is coughing because of a suspected obstructed airway
   D. A 14 year old with an obstructed airway who does not respond to abdominal thrusts

17. You respond to a home where an infant was reportedly choking on a toy. You arrive to find the 1-year-old infant unconscious, unresponsive, and apneic. The baby is being ventilated by a first responder volunteer EMT who arrived 2 minutes before you and is using a bag-mask device with 100% oxygen. The ventilations are producing adequate chest rise. Your initial assessment reveals absent respirations and a pulse rate of 50 beats/min. Your next step to perform or direct to be performed is _____.
   A. begin chest compressions
   B. intubate
   C. obtain IV access and administer atropine
   D. obtain IV access and administer epinephrine

18. A previously healthy 5-year-old child is brought to your EMS station because she suddenly became lethargic and pale. There is no history of vomiting, diarrhea, fever, or trauma. Your initial assessment reveals a rapid, narrow complex tachycardia at a rate greater than 200 beats/min. This ECG should be considered _____.
   A. atrial flutter
   B. sinus tachycardia
   C. supraventricular tachycardia
   D. ventricular tachycardia

19. In which age group is fever the most common cause of seizures?
   A. Newborn to 4 years old
   B. 3 months to 5 years old
   C. 6 months to 10 years old
   D. 2 years to 6 years old

20. Which of the following are likely findings in a pediatric patient with early septic shock?
   A. Tachycardia with bounding pulses and slow capillary refill
   B. Tachycardia with bounding pulses; warm, flushed skin; slow capillary refill
   C. Tachycardia with bounding pulses; warm, flushed skin; slow capillary refill; and irritability
   D. Warm, flushed skin; slow capillary refill; and irritability

21. You respond to a residence for a 3-year-old child experiencing respiratory difficulty with inspiratory stridor and retractions. He had a runny nose and slight fever last night before going to bed. The patient also has a "barking" cough. You should suspect that this child has _____.
    A. bronchiolitis
    B. croup
    C. epiglottitis
    D. foreign body airway obstruction

22. Observations of a child made from across the room before initial contact should include _____.
    A. muscle tone, interaction, skin color, respiratory effort and rate
    B. muscle tone, skin color, capillary refill, respiratory rate
    C. respiratory effort, capillary refill, skin color, muscle tone
    D. respiratory effort, muscle tone, skin color, airway

23. A 6-year-old male developed severe respiratory distress with inspiratory stridor about 20 minutes ago. His mother tells you he "seemed to be perfectly healthy" until about 4 hours earlier when he began to complain of a severe sore throat. The patient is sitting on the side of the bed leaning forward with his neck slightly extended. Respiratory distress with accessory muscle use and intercostal retractions is present. The child is drooling profusely. When he tries to talk, his voice sounds "muffled." He is suffering from a life-threatening emergency because he may experience _____.
    A. airway obstruction
    B. cardiac dysrhythmias
    C. respiratory arrest
    D. seizures

24. A 3-year-old male awakened about 15 minutes ago with respiratory distress and stridor. He is sitting upright in bed. Accessory muscle use and intercostal retractions are present, but drooling is absent. The lips and nailbeds are cyanotic. The patient coughs frequently, producing a sound similar to a seal's bark. When he attempts to talk, his voice is very hoarse. The patient's mother tells you that he has had a "cold" with a low-grade fever for "2 or 3 days." The treatment for this patient would include _____.
    A. humidified oxygen and nebulized racemic epinephrine
    B. intubation and high-concentration oxygen
    C. systemic therapy with 1:1000 epinephrine
    D. systemic therapy with terbutaline

25. A 3-month-old infant suddenly developed cyanosis and expiratory wheezing. Retractions and nasal flaring with a respiratory rate of 80 breaths/min are present. The patient appears to be conscious but is restless and "jittery." The patient's mother reports he has had a mild "cold" with a cough for 2 or 3 days. The patient has a low-grade fever. There is no family history of asthma or allergies. The initial treatment would be _____.
    A. endotracheal intubation and assisted ventilation
    B. epinephrine 1:1000 Sub-Q
    C. humidified oxygen
    D. nebulized racemic epinephrine

26. Which of the following combinations of laryngoscope blades and endotracheal tubes should be used when intubating a 2-year-old child?
    A. McIntosh blade; cuffed tube
    B. McIntosh blade; uncuffed tube
    C. Miller blade; cuffed tube
    D. Miller blade; uncuffed tube

27. You respond to a near drowning. A 2-year-old child fell into a swimming pool with a submersion time of 2 minutes. The child is unresponsive, cyanotic, apneic, and pulseless. A firefighter is performing CPR. You are able to place an endotracheal tube easily, but vascular access has not yet been obtained. The ECG shows a sinus bradycardia at 30 beats/min. What should you do?
    A. Give 0.01 mg/kg epinephrine 1:10,000 down the endotracheal tube.
    B. Give 0.02 mg/kg atropine down the endotracheal tube.
    C. Give 0.1 mg/kg epinephrine 1:1000 down the endotracheal tube.
    D. Start an intraosseous line immediately.

Case one

A 3-month-old infant suddenly developed cyanosis and expiratory wheezing. Retractions and nasal flaring are present with a respiratory rate of 80 breaths/min. The infant appears to be conscious, but is restless and jittery. The patient's mother reports that he has had a mild "cold" with a cough for 2 or 3 days. He also has had a low-grade fever. There is no family history of asthma or allergies, but a 6-year-old sibling has had symptoms of a "cold" for about 5 days.

1. What is the patient's problem?
   _____

2. What microorganism usually is responsible for this problem?
   _____

3. What is the relationship between the sibling's cold and the patient's problem?
   _____

4. Why is the patient wheezing?
   _____

5. How would you manage this patient?
   _____
   _____
   _____
   _____

Case two

You are called to see a 6-month-old infant. The mother's chief complaint is that the child has been irritable for the last few days, does not feed well, sweats when he attempts to take the bottle, and turns "funny colors" when he feeds. Physical examination reveals an infant that is awake and fussy. Respirations are 40 breaths/min. The skin is pink, but the distal extremities are cool. Capillary refill is 2 seconds. Radial pulses are palpable but are too rapid to count. The patient's ECG is shown here:

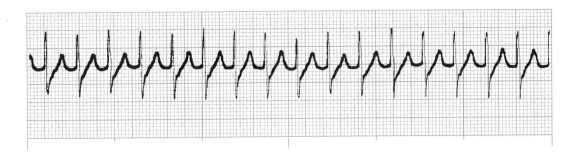

1. What dysrhythmia is present?
   _____

2. Is the rhythm too fast, too slow, or absent?
   _____

3. Is the patient stable or unstable?
   _____

4. What accounts for the sweating and color changes when the patient attempts to feed?
   _____

5. How would you manage this patient?

_____

_____

_____

_____

Case three

You respond to a mottled, cyanotic 3-month-old, 5-kg infant who responds only to painful stimuli. Pulses are too rapid to count and thready proximally. There are no distal pulses in the upper or lower extremities. The distal extremities are cold. Capillary refill is 5 seconds. Respirations are labored at 66 breaths/min. The patient's ECG is shown below.

1. What dysrhythmia is present?

_____

2. Why are the patient's cardiac output and blood pressure decreased?

_____

3. Why are the patient's respirations rapid and labored?

_____

4. Is this patient stable or unstable?

_____

5. How would you manage this patient?

_____

_____

_____

_____

Case four

You are called to evaluate a 15-month-old infant with a 3-day history of diarrhea. Mom reports that the child refused the bottle this morning. He is sleepy and lethargic today.

1. Could this patient be in shock?

_____

2. What additional information do we need?

_____

_____

On initial observation, you note a lethargic child sitting in his mother's lap. Respirations are 46 breaths/min, shallow, and unlabored. Pulse is 178 beats/min, weak, and regular. Blood pressure is 90 mm Hg by palpation. The extremities are cool with mottled skin. Skin turgor is poor. The oral mucous membranes are dry. Temperature is 38° C. Breath sounds are present, equal, and clear bilaterally.

3. Is this patient in shock?

_____

4. What signs and symptoms suggest the patient is in shock?

_____

_____

5. From what type of shock is this patient suffering? What clinical findings suggest this mechanism?

_____

_____

_____

_____

6. Is this compensated or decompensated shock?

_____

7. What would be your approach to this patient?

_____

_____

_____

_____

When you attempt to start an IV, all attempts fail.

8. What would you do now?

_____

_____

_____

_____

9. How do you know this method of obtaining vascular access has been successful?

_____

_____

_____

_____

10. When vascular access is achieved, what fluid would you give?

_____

11. How much would you give?

_____

The patient's blood gases are pH—7.20, $PaCO_2$—20.

12. What is the patient's acid-base status?

_____

13. How should you manage this acid-base imbalance?

_____

_____

_____

_____

Case five

You respond to a report of a near drowning. A 4-year-old male fell into a swimming pool with a submersion time of 2 minutes. The child is unresponsive, cyanotic, apneic, and pulseless. A firefighter who responded is performing CPR. The patient's ECG follows.

1. What dysrhythmia is present?

   _____

2. At what rate should chest compressions be performed?

   _____

3. How deeply should the sternum be compressed?

   _____

4. When you attempt to endotracheally intubate this patient, what technique should you use? Why?

   _____
   _____
   _____
   _____

   You are able to place an endotracheal tube easily, but have not yet been able to obtain vascular access.

5. What medication should you give to this patient?

   _____

6. What route should you use?

   _____

7. What dose should you give?

   _____

Case six

The patient is an 11-month-old female who ingested six 0.25-mg digoxin tablets about 2 hours ago. She is awake and alert. Pulse is 50 beats/min strong, regular. Respirations are 30 breaths/min regular, unlabored. Capillary refill is less than 2 seconds. The patient's skin is pink and warm. Blood pressure is 90 mm Hg by palpation. The patient's ECG follows.

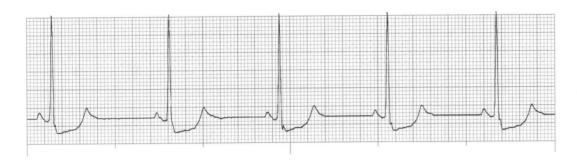

1. What dysrhythmia is present?

   _____

2. What effects can be anticipated from ingestion of a toxic dose of digitalis?

   _____
   _____
   _____
   _____

3. Is the patient's dysrhythmia consistent with the anticipated effects of a digitalis ingestion?

   _____
   _____
   _____
   _____

4. Is this patient stable or unstable?

   _____

5. How do you account for this?

   _____
   _____
   _____
   _____

6. How would you manage this patient?

   _____
   _____
   _____
   _____

Case seven

A 6-year-old boy was the front-seat passenger in a vehicle involved in a rollover accident. The child was not restrained. The child is pulseless and apneic with contusions on the anterior chest and open fractures of both femurs. Chest compressions are being performed and the patient's lungs are being ventilated with 100% oxygen via bag-mask device. The patient's ECG follows.

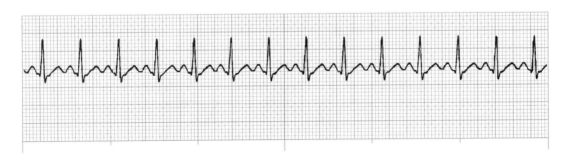

1. What is the patient's rhythm?

   _____

2. Since the patient is unconscious, pulseless, and apneic, what is this clinical situation called?

   _____

3. List five possible causes of this clinical situation.

   _____
   _____
   _____
   _____
   _____

4. After an IV has been established, what is the first medication that should be given?

   _____

5. What is the initial dose of this medication?

   _____

6. What is the repeat dose of this medication?

   _____

Case eight

A 7-month-old child is pulseless and apneic. CPR is in progress. The patient's lungs are being ventilated with 100% oxygen via bag-mask device. The ECG follows.

1. What is the patient's rhythm?

   _____

2. Is this a common dysrhythmia in pediatric cardiac arrest? Why or why not?

   _____

3. When this rhythm occurs in pediatric cardiac arrest what problems should be suspected?

   _____

4. How would you select the proper defibrillator paddle size for this patient?

   _____

5. If your defibrillator paddles are too large, how should you defibrillate this patient?

   _____

6. What is the initial energy setting for defibrillation of a pediatric patient?

   _____

7. What is the energy setting for all subsequent shocks?

_____

8. How do you select the proper size endotracheal tube for this patient?

_____

9. When you intubate an infant or small child, where should you listen for breath sounds? Why?

_____

After intubating this patient you hear breath sounds in both lung fields and over the epigastrium.

10. What has happened?

_____

_____

11. What should you do?

_____

_____

The patient has been successfully intubated. However, IV access has not yet been obtained.

12. What drug can be given at this point?

_____

13. Why is this drug beneficial in cardiac arrest?

_____

14. By what route can this drug be given?

_____

15. What are the initial and repeat doses of the drug when it is given by this route?

_____

Case nine

You are called to see a 9-month-old male who has "stopped breathing." The mother's boyfriend is babysitting and states that the infant fell off the couch. The baby currently is lying in a crib. The child is lethargic and is breathing slowly at a rate of 8 breaths/min. The child's skin is warm and capillary refill is brisk. Heart rate is 140 beats/min. The left pupil is dilated and fixed. The right pupil is in mid-position and reacts sluggishly. Linear bruises are present on both upper arms.

1. What problem accounts for the patient's unequal pupils and slow respirations?

_____

2. What mechanism of injury is suggested by the linear bruises on the patient's upper arms?

_____

_____

3. What aspects of this situation lead you to believe the boyfriend is not telling the truth?

_____

_____

4. How would you manage this patient?

_____

_____

5. How would you deal with the underlying cause of the situation?

_____
_____

Case ten

A 6-year-old male became ill about 3 hours ago and is complaining of a severe sore throat. He is sitting upright in bed, crying, and noticeably drooling. His mother says that he will not eat or drink because he says it hurts too much to swallow. The patient appears to be very frightened. Vital signs are: BP—128/92 mm Hg; P—118 beats/min strong, regular; R—30 breaths/min shallow, stridulous. The patient's temperature by tympanic thermometer is 104° F.

1. What problem do you suspect is present?

_____

2. What type of microorganism typically causes this disease?

_____

3. Why are children from ages 4 to 7 particularly susceptible to this problem?

_____
_____

4. What is the greatest immediate danger facing this patient?

_____
_____

5. How should this patient be managed?

_____
_____
_____
_____

6. The incidence of this disease in the pediatric population seems to be declining. What probably accounts for this phenomenon?

_____
_____

Case eleven

A call is received at 0130 hours for a "sick child." When you arrive, a distraught mother tells you that her 6-year-old son is "having fits." The patient has been ill for the last 3 days with an upper respiratory tract infection. Approximately 30 minutes ago, he began having generalized tonic-clonic seizures. He has had three episodes of seizure activity so far. You find the child apparently asleep on his bed. He is difficult to arouse. As you examine him, his eyes suddenly open and deviate sharply to the right. He rapidly develops another tonic-clonic seizure.

1. Do you suspect that this patient's problem may be febrile seizures? Why or why not?

_____
_____

2. What are probable causes for this child's seizures?

_____
_____

3. What term is used to describe recurrent seizures without an intervening period of consciousness?

_____

4. Should you check this patient's blood glucose level? Why or why not?

   _____

5. What medication should you use to manage this patient's seizures?

   _____

6. What side effects should you anticipate when this medication is given?

   _____

38 Geriatrics

Chapter 38, pages 135-168, in *Paramedic Practice Today: Above and Beyond.*

OBJECTIVES

After completing this chapter, you will be able to:

1. Discuss population demographics demonstrating the rise in the elderly population in the United States.
2. Discuss issues facing society concerning the elderly.
3. Discuss society's view of aging and the social, financial, and ethical issues facing the elderly.
4. Assess the various living environments of elderly patients.
5. Describe the local resources available to assist the elderly and create strategies to refer at-risk patients to appropriate community services.
6. Discuss common emotional and psychological reactions to aging, including causes and manifestations.
7. Compare pharmacokinetics in elderly patients versus younger adults.
8. Discuss drug distribution, metabolism, and excretion in the elderly patient.
9. Discuss the impact of polypharmacy and medication noncompliance on patient assessment and management.
10. Discuss medication issues of the elderly, including polypharmacy, dosing errors, and increased drug sensitivity.
11. Discuss the problems with mobility in the elderly and develop strategies to prevent falls.
12. Discuss how problems with sensation affect communication and patient assessment.
13. Discuss problems with continence and elimination and develop communication strategies to provide psychological support.
14. Apply the pathophysiology of multisystem failure to the assessment and management of medical conditions in the elderly patient.
15. Discuss factors that may complicate assessment of the elderly patient.
16. Describe principles to use when assessing and communicating with an elderly patient.
17. Compare the assessment of an elderly patient versus a young patient.
18. Discuss common complaints of the elderly.
19. Discuss the normal and abnormal age-related changes of the pulmonary system.
20. Describe the epidemiology of pulmonary diseases in the elderly, including incidence, morbidity and mortality rates, risk factors, and prevention strategies for patients with pneumonia, chronic obstructive pulmonary disease, and pulmonary embolism.
21. Compare the pathophysiology of pulmonary diseases in the elderly versus younger adults, including pneumonia, chronic obstructive pulmonary disease, and pulmonary embolism.
22. Discuss the assessment of the elderly patient with pulmonary complaints, including pneumonia, chronic obstructive pulmonary disease, and pulmonary embolism.
23. Identify the need for intervention and transport of the elderly patient with pulmonary complaints.
24. Develop a treatment and management plan for the elderly patient with pulmonary complaints, including pneumonia, chronic obstructive pulmonary disease, and pulmonary embolism.
25. Discuss the normal and abnormal cardiovascular system changes with age.
26. Describe the epidemiology for cardiovascular diseases in the elderly, including incidence, morbidity and mortality rates, risk factors, and prevention strategies for patients with myocardial infarction, heart failure, dysrhythmias, aneurysm, and hypertension.
27. Compare the pathophysiology of cardiovascular diseases in the elderly versus younger adults, including myocardial infarction, heart failure, dysrhythmias, aneurysm, and hypertension.
28. Discuss assessment of the elderly patient with complaints related to the cardiovascular system, including myocardial infarction, heart failure, dysrhythmias, aneurysm, and hypertension.
29. Identify the need for intervention and transportation of the elderly patient with cardiovascular complaints.
30. Develop a treatment and management plan for the elderly patient with cardiovascular complaints, including myocardial infarction, heart failure, dysrhythmias, aneurism, and hypertension.
31. Discuss the normal and abnormal age-related changes of the nervous system.
32. Describe the epidemiology of nervous system diseases in the elderly, including incidence, morbidity and mortality rates, risk factors, and prevention strategies for patients with cerebral vascular disease, delirium, dementia, Alzheimer's disease, and Parkinson's disease.

33. Compare the pathophysiology of nervous system diseases in the elderly versus younger adults, including cerebral vascular disease, delirium, dementia, Alzheimer's disease, and Parkinson's disease.

34. Discuss the assessment of the elderly patient with complaints related to the nervous system, including cerebral vascular disease, delirium, dementia, Alzheimer's disease, and Parkinson's disease.

35. Identify the need for intervention and transportation of the patient with complaints related to the nervous system.

36. Develop a treatment and management plan for the elderly patient with complaints related to the nervous system, including cerebral vascular disease, delirium, dementia, Alzheimer's disease, and Parkinson's disease.

37. Discuss the normal and abnormal age-related changes of the endocrine system.

38. Describe the epidemiology for endocrine diseases in the elderly, including incidence, morbidity and mortality rates, risk factors, and prevention strategies for patients with diabetes and thyroid diseases.

39. Compare the pathophysiology of diabetes and thyroid diseases in the elderly versus a younger adults.

40. Discuss the assessment of the elderly patient with complaints related to the endocrine system, including diabetes and thyroid diseases.

41. Identify the need for intervention and transportation of the patient with endocrine problems.

42. Develop a treatment and management plan of the elderly patient with endocrine problems, including diabetes and thyroid diseases.

43. Discuss the normal and abnormal age-related changes of the gastrointestinal system.

44. Discuss assessment of the elderly patient with complaints related to the gastrointestinal system.

45. Identify the need for intervention and transportation of the patient with gastrointestinal complaints.

46. Develop and execute a treatment and management plan of the elderly patient with gastrointestinal problems.

47. Discuss the assessment and management of an elderly patient with gastrointestinal hemorrhage and bowel obstruction.

48. Compare the pathophysiology of gastrointestinal hemorrhage and bowel obstruction in the elderly versus younger adults.

49. Discuss the normal and abnormal age-related psychiatric changes.

50. Describe the epidemiology of depression and suicide in the elderly, including incidence, morbidity and mortality rates, risk factors, and prevention strategies.

51. Compare the psychiatry of depression and suicide in the elderly versus younger adults.

52. Discuss the assessment of the elderly patient with psychiatric complaints, including depression and suicide.

53. Identify the need for intervention and transport of the elderly psychiatric patient.

54. Develop a treatment and management plan of the elderly psychiatric patient pertinent to depression and suicide.

55. Discuss the normal and abnormal age-related changes of the integumentary system.

56. Describe the epidemiology of pressure ulcers in the elderly, including incidence, morbidity and mortality rates, risk factors, and prevention strategies.

57. Compare the pathophysiology of pressure ulcers in the elderly versus younger adults.

58. Discuss the assessment of the elderly patient with complaints related to the integumentary system, including pressure ulcers.

59. Identify the need for intervention and transportation of the patient with complaints related to the integumentary system.

60. Develop a treatment and management plan for the elderly patient with complaints related to the integumentary system, including pressure ulcers.

61. Discuss the normal and abnormal age-related changes of the musculoskeletal system.

62. Describe the epidemiology for osteoarthritis and osteoporosis, including incidence, morbidity and mortality rates, risk factors, and prevention strategies.

63. Compare the pathophysiology of osteoarthritis and osteoporosis in the elderly versus younger adults.

64. Discuss the assessment of the elderly patient with complaints related to the musculoskeletal system, including osteoarthritis and osteoporosis.

65. Identify the need for intervention and transportation of the patient with musculoskeletal complaints.

66. Develop a treatment and management plan of the elderly patient with musculoskeletal complaints, including osteoarthritis and osteoporosis.

67. Discuss the normal and abnormal age-related changes relevant to toxicology.

68. Discuss the assessment of the elderly patient with complaints related to toxicology.

69. Identify the need for intervention and transportation of the patient with toxicologic problems.

70. Develop and execute a treatment and management plan for the elderly patient with toxicologic problems.

71. Describe the epidemiology of drug toxicology in the elderly, including the incidence, morbidity and mortality rates, risk factors, and prevention strategies. toxicology.

72. Compare the pathophysiology of drug toxicity in the elderly versus younger adults.

73. Discuss the use and effects of commonly prescribed drugs for the elderly patient.

74. Discuss the assessment findings common in elderly patients with drug toxicity.
75. Discuss the management and considerations when treating an elderly patient with drug toxicity.
76. Describe the epidemiology for drug and alcohol abuse in the elderly, including incidence, morbidity and mortality rates, risk factors, and prevention strategies.
77. Compare the pathophysiology of drug and alcohol abuse in the elderly versus younger adults.
78. Discuss the assessment findings common in elderly patients with drug and alcohol abuse.
79. Discuss the management and considerations when treating an elderly patient with drug and alcohol abuse.
80. Discuss the normal and abnormal age-related changes of thermoregulation.
81. Discuss the assessment of the elderly patient with complaints related to thermoregulation.
82. Identify the need for intervention and transportation of the patient with environmental considerations.
83. Develop and execute a treatment and management plan for the elderly patient with environmental considerations.
84. Compare the pathophysiology of hypothermia and hyperthermia in the elderly versus younger adults.
85. Discuss the assessment findings and management plan for elderly patients with hypothermia and hyperthermia.
86. Describe the epidemiology of trauma in the elderly, including incidence, morbidity and mortality rates, risk factors, and prevention strategies for patients with orthopedic injuries, burns, and head injuries.
87. Compare the pathophysiology of trauma in the elderly versus younger adults, including orthopedic injuries, burns, and head injuries.
88. Discuss the assessment findings common in elderly patients with traumatic injuries, including orthopedic injuries, burns, and head injuries.
89. Discuss the management and considerations when treating an elderly patient with traumatic injuries, including orthopedic injuries, burns, and head injuries.
90. Identify the need for intervention and transport of the elderly patient with trauma.

CHAPTER SUMMARY

- The elderly population accounts for a significant number (34%) of all EMS responses.
- Most elderly people live independently. When illness makes independent living impossible, some seniors are able to afford live-in nursing help or assisted living situations. Nursing home care usually is covered by Medicare, and many elderly people live in nursing homes in the end stages of life because of severe disability.
- Power of attorney of healthcare and living wills are becoming more prevalent. Unless a clear advance directive is present, however, prehospital providers should provide aggressive care to all elderly people.
- Changes in drug distribution, decreased drug metabolism, decreased drug excretion, and polypharmacy make adverse drug reactions a common reason for illness in the elderly.
- Make an accurate list of medications the patient is taking or bring the actual bottles of medications with the patient to ensure an accurate medication history. Many elderly people are not able to recall all the medications they are taking.
- Many factors contribute to the increased risk of falling in elderly people. Among these are vision changes, brain diseases, dementia, musculoskeletal disorders, and medication side effects.
- Presbyopia, cataracts, and glaucoma can cause visual impairment in the elderly and subsequent functional decline.
- Most older patients are able to hear normal conversation. Those with hearing loss often are able to function well with hearing aids. Make sure hearing aids are in place before questioning elderly patients with hearing loss.
- Incontinence is never a result of normal aging. Fecal and urinary incontinence can be caused by severe illness, such as spinal cord compression, and can cause skin breakdown and infection.
- Assessment of an elderly patient must be done carefully because the elderly often process information slower and need a longer time to provide a history.
- Chest pain and shortness of breath are two common presentations for elderly patients and can be caused by numerous illnesses. Every elderly patient with one of these two symptoms should be treated as if he or she has a serious emergency.
- Resuscitation of elderly patients should be done in the same manner as for younger patients and just as aggressively.
- Elderly patients often are most comfortable while sitting or with extra padding. Transport in the position of comfort for most older patients except when splinting an injury or when spinal precautions are needed.
- The aging process causes decreased strength in respiratory muscles, decreased ability of oxygen to cross into the bloodstream, and increased bronchoconstriction.
- The lung examination is unreliable in determining a cause for shortness of breath. A history of chronic obstructive pulmonary disease (COPD) or heart failure should guide initial treatment of shortness of breath in a patient with one of these diagnoses.
- The cardiovascular system of elderly patients is prone to hypertension and coronary artery disease and loses its ability to respond to physiologic stress.
- Coronary artery disease, thoracic and abdominal aneurysms, congestive heart failure, and dysrhythmias are more common in older patients and can be life

threatening. Maintain a high level of suspicion for elderly patients regarding cardiovascular emergencies.

- Slight psychomotor slowing is expected in aging, but severe memory deficits and changes in cognition are not normal.
- Acute weakness or change in level of consciousness in an elderly person must be considered an intracranial emergency and necessitates rapid transport because hospital treatment often is time dependent.
- Dementia is a chronic memory problem with long-term declines in intellectual functioning (e.g., Alzheimer's disease); delirium usually is an acute, often reversible, process that produces decreased cognition and level of consciousness.
- Consider hyperglycemia and hypoglycemia in any elderly patient with a history of diabetes or neurologic change. Blood glucose testing should be routine to identify these glucose abnormalities quickly.
- Abdominal and GI emergencies usually present atypically in the elderly, with diminished or vague symptoms. Twenty-four percent of elderly patients with acute abdominal pain in the ED require surgery.
- In suspected toxicologic emergencies, obtaining an accurate history and additional information is the most important part of finding a diagnosis.
- Beta-blocker medications are used for hypertension, to control dysrhythmias, or to decrease oxygen demand of the heart tissue. These medications block the ability of the heart to respond to stress by increasing heart rate and contractility.
- Diuretics cause water to be excreted by the kidneys. Adverse reactions include electrolyte abnormalities and dehydration.
- Digoxin is used in congestive heart failure (CHF) to increase contractility of the heart or control the rate of atrial fibrillation. Digoxin can easily reach a toxic level and cause many different cardiac dysrhythmias.
- Warfarin is used in many elderly people to prevent blood clot formation. Some indications for its use are atrial fibrillation, history of blood clots, and artificial heart valves. Patients taking warfarin are at increased risk of bleeding.
- Chemical dependency is present in up to 10% of the elderly population. Alcohol accounts for most of this dependency and should be addressed in elderly people in whom it is suspected.
- Decreased muscle mass for shivering and thinner skin for insulation put the elderly at risk for hypothermia.
- Hyperthermia is more prevalent in elderly people because of fewer sweat glands, medication side effects, and a decreased ability to seek a cooler environment.
- Depression is underrecognized in the elderly population; the elderly also complete suicide more frequently.
- Older patients have thin skin, which is more susceptible to infection, breakdown, and injury from trauma.
- OA affects 80% of patients older than 60 years and causes significant pain and difficulty with mobility.

- Osteoporosis is the most common bone disease in the United States and is characterized by loss of bone density, causing an increased risk of fracture.
- Traumatic injury carries an increased mortality rate in the elderly compared with younger patients. Falls are the most common cause of trauma in the elderly population.
- Older patients have decreased brain volume, which allows blood to accumulate in the skull after head injury without immediate neurologic deficits. Significant intracranial bleeding may not be symptomatic until days after the trauma.

SHORT ANSWER

1. What effect does aging have on dermal blood supply and thickness? How does this affect wound healing? How does this affect severity of burn injuries in the elderly?

_____

_____

_____

_____

2. What effect does aging have on bone resorption? Which gender is particularly affected? What effect does this have in victims of sudden deceleration trauma?

_____

_____

_____

_____

3. What effect does aging have on respiratory reserve capacity? What effect does this have on the ability of older patients to compensate for chest trauma or acute respiratory disease such as pulmonary embolism, spontaneous pneumothorax, or pneumonia?

_____

_____

_____

_____

4. What effect does aging have on myocardial reserve capacity? What effect does this have on volume resuscitation of the older trauma patient?

_____

_____

_____

_____

5. What effect does aging have on the peripheral blood vessels? What effect does this have on the older patient's ability to compensate for volume loss? What effect does this have on the older patient's ability to tolerate hot or cold environments?

_____

_____

_____

_____

6. What effect does aging have on the kidneys? What effect does this have on the response of the patient to drugs? What effect does this have on the response of the patient to fluid therapy for hypo-volemia?

_____

_____

_____

_____

7. During your assessment of an older person, you determine that skin turgor on the back of the hand is decreased. Is this change necessarily the result of volume depletion? Where can you check skin turgor in an older person to more reliably determine if it is decreased?

_____

_____

_____

_____

8. A nursing home patient is found to have severe pedal edema. On examination, no other signs or symptoms of right-sided heart failure are detected. He reportedly spends 12 to 14 hours a day sitting in front of the television with his feet in a dependent position. What is a possible mechanism for his pedal edema?

_____

_____

_____

_____

9. What is a silent MI? Why are the elderly prone to having silent MIs? What other group of patients tend to have silent MIs?

_____

_____

_____

_____

10. What effect does aging have on the size of the brain relative to the size of the cranial cavity? What effect does this produce regarding the on set of signs and symptoms from a subdural hematoma?

_____

_____

_____

_____

11. A patient is receiving beta-blocker therapy. What effect does this have on your ability to detect the early signs of shock? Why?

_____

_____

_____

_____

12. A patient who is receiving diuretic therapy is at particular risk for developing what electrolyte imbalance? What complication can result from this electrolyte imbalance?

_____

_____

_____

_____

13. What effect does aging have on hepatic blood flow and on the ability of the liver to metabolize drugs? What change does this effect dictate for the dosing of most drugs?

_____

_____

_____

_____

MULTIPLE CHOICE

1. The geriatric patient who is experiencing a silent MI is most likely to present with _____.
   A. dyspnea or abdominal pain
   B. diaphoresis or tachycardia
   C. neck pain or bradycardia
   D. atrial fibrillation or dyspnea

2. In the United States, the most common cause of dementia among older persons is _____.
   A. Parkinson's disease
   B. Alzheimer's disease
   C. multiinfarct dementia
   D. depression

3. The most common psychiatric disorder among geriatric patients is _____.
   A. schizophrenia
   B. paranoia
   C. depression
   D. posttraumatic stress disorder

4. When you are assessing or managing an older patient, you should _____.
   A. talk louder than normal since most of the elderly have difficulty hearing
   B. use physical contact to compensate for loss of sight or hearing
   C. call the patient "dear" or "honey" to show you care
   D. separate the patient from friends and family as soon as possible to reduce anxiety

5. Special problems that may be encountered when dealing with geriatric patients may include _____.
   A. lowered pain thresholds
   B. decreased thirst with a tendency to develop volume overload
   C. increased susceptibility to general deterioration as a result of illness
   D. increased sensitivity of taste and smell, resulting an a tendency to become easily nauseated

6. Your patient is an 80-year-old male who has been confined to bed for several weeks. The patient has a long history of alcohol abuse. He suffered an acute anterior MI 2 years ago. His ankles and feet are grossly edematous. His neck veins are flat when he is placed in a semisitting position. The lung fields are clear, and there is no apparent abdominal distention. You notice that the head of the patient's bed is elevated, placing his feet in a dependent position. The edema of his ankles and feet probably is a result of _____.
   A. prolonged immobility and the positioning of his lower extremities
   B. right-sided heart failure resulting in high hydrostatic pressures in the systemic circulation
   C. liver disease that has caused low plasma oncotic pressures
   D. left-sided heart failure resulting in high hydrostatic pressures in the systemic circulation

7. Your patient is a 90-year-old female who has been experiencing episodes of nocturnal confusion for several weeks. She has a history of hypertension and has had three acute MIs during the past 2 years. She takes metoprolol, hydrochlorothiazide, and a potassium supplement for management of her high blood pressure. She also takes sertraline (Zoloft) to manage depression. During the physical examination, you notice a number of large, translucent blisters on her lower legs. These blisters are most likely the result of _____.
   A. an allergic reaction to one of her antihypertensive medications
   B. toxic effects caused by the antidepressant medication
   C. increased hydrostatic pressure caused by right-sided CHF
   D. degenerative effects of the aging process on the skin of the lower extremities

8. Acute etiologies that may be mistaken for "senile dementia" include _____.
   A. subdural hematomas, Huntington's disease, or brain tumors
   B. drug overdoses, medication interactions, or electrolyte imbalances
   C. CNS infections, electrolyte imbalances, or Parkinson's disease
   D. subdural hematomas, medication interactions, or Alzheimer's disease

9. Patients taking diuretics are at risk for developing which of the following electrolyte imbalances?
   A. Hypocalcemia
   B. Hypokalemia
   C. Hypercalcemia
   D. Hyperkalemia

10. Which combination of signs and symptoms would be most suggestive of an acute myocardial infarction in a geriatric patient?
   A. Extreme weakness, syncope, malaise, jaundice
   B. Syncope, loss of bladder and bowel control, confusion, stiff neck, headache
   C. Extreme weakness, syncope, loss of bladder and bowel control, malaise
   D. Extreme weakness, syncope, confusion, stiff neck, headache, jaundice

11. A 78-year-old woman drove her car into a utility pole while attempting to avoid a dog that had run into the street. She is awake and alert, and is complaining of pain in her right ankle. The right ankle is swollen and deformed. When you palpate a radial pulse, you notice that the cardiac rhythm is irregular. You apply a monitor and observe the rhythm below. The patient's skin is warm and dry. Her respirations are 18 breaths/min and regular. Blood pressure is 130/76 mm Hg. She tells you she takes a pill to "thin her blood." You see the ECG shown below. The most appropriate action would be to _____.

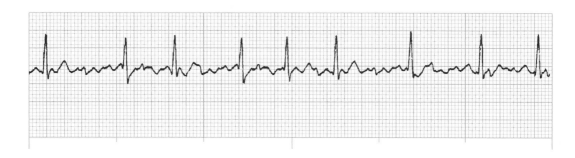

A. administer high-concentration oxygen, start an IV, and give adenosine 6 mg IV push
B. ask the patient to perform a vagal maneuver
C. give oxygen by nonrebreather mask, start an IV, and administer 2.5 mg of diltiazem slow IV push
D. splint the injured ankle; apply a cervical collar, spine board, and head blocks; and transport

12. An 82-year-old male stumbled and fell. He is sitting on the curb, complaining of pain in his left knee. When you examine the area, you notice that his pants are torn and there is a skin abrasion. He is awake and alert. His skin is warm and dry. Because he reports a history of "heart trouble," you attach monitoring leads. You see the ECG shown below. His blood pressure is 146/92 mm Hg. The most appropriate action would be to _____.

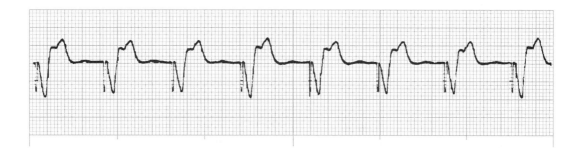

A. administer high-concentration oxygen, start an IV, and administer atropine 0.5 mg IV push
B. give oxygen by nonrebreather mask, establish an IV, and give lidocaine 1 mg/kg IV push
C. administer oxygen at 12 to 15 L/min, start an IV, and attach the external pacemaker as a precautionary measure
D. dress and bandage the abrasion, ask about tetanus prophylaxis, and determine whether transport is desired

13. This is the ECG of a 72-year-old male complaining of nausea and seeing yellow-green halos around lights. He has a history of an acute MI 3 years ago. He reports taking a "water pill" and a "little white pill that's supposed to strengthen my heart." He is awake, alert, and oriented. Breath sounds are present and equal bilaterally with a few crackles audible in the lung bases. His skin is warm and dry. Radial pulses are present, strong and regular. Capillary refill is 2 seconds. Mild (1+) pedal edema is present. What is the dysrhythmia?

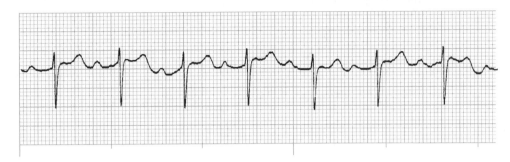

A. Normal sinus rhythm
B. Sinus bradycardia
C. Sinus dysrhythmia
D. Sinus rhythm with first-degree AV block

14. The patient in the previous question should be monitored closely because he is at risk of developing _____.
A. junctional tachycardia
B. nonparoxysmal atrial tachycardia with 2 to 1 AV block
C. sinus bradycardia
D. second- or third-degree AV block

15. The most likely underlying cause for the problem affecting the patient in the previous question is _____.
A. silent acute MI
B. digitalis toxicity
C. hypokalemia
D. hypoxia secondary to pulmonary edema

CASE STUDIES

Case one

A 73-year-old male called for help because he fell while trying to get up from a chair. He says that about 20 minutes ago, he developed pain in his lower back that radiated to his left leg. The pain was accompanied by a strong sensation of needing to move his bowels. When he tried to stand, he discovered that his legs were weak and numb. The pain in his back is continuing to worsen. The patient thinks he broke his back when he fell. His wife thinks he has had a stroke. The patient has had high blood pressure for about 15 years. He is 6 feet 2 inches tall and weighs in excess of 300 pounds. He smokes two packs of cigarettes per day. His doctor has told him he has poor circulation to his legs. His skin is pale, cool, and diaphoretic. Vital signs are: BP—102/60 mm Hg; P—120 beats/min weak, regular; R—18 breaths/min shallow, regular. Breath sounds are present and equal bilaterally. The abdomen is soft and nontender. The lower abdomen is mottled. The patient's legs show no spontaneous movement or withdrawal to pain. They are cold and mottled. The femoral pulses are very weak bilaterally. There are no pedal pulses. The patient's back is not tender to palpation.

1. What is your differential diagnosis of this patient?

_____

_____

_____

_____

Chapter **38** **Geriatrics**

2. Could he have a lumbar spine fracture with spinal cord injury?

_____

3. Could he be having a stroke?

_____

4. Why are the patient's lower extremities mottled and his blood pressure low?

_____
_____
_____
_____

5. Why does he have back pain that radiates to his left leg?

_____
_____
_____
_____

6. Why does he not have abdominal pain?

_____
_____
_____
_____

7. How would you manage this patient?

_____
_____
_____
_____

Case two

A 73-year-old man with a history of prostate cancer experienced sudden severe pain in his lower back accompanied by pain radiating to both lower extremities. He is now experiencing weakness and paresthesias in both lower extremities. He is lying in bed.

1. What problem do you suspect?

_____

2. How would you manage this patient?

_____
_____
_____
_____

Case three

An 82-year-old female has vague complaints of feeling weak and fatigued. She has a long history of diabetes and poorly controlled chronic essential hypertension. She takes a host of medications for her problems but cannot remember which ones she took today. Vital signs are: BP—136/88 mm Hg; P—58 beats/min weak, regular; R—22 breaths/min shallow, regular. Blood glucose level is 150 mg/dL. During your physical examination, you find pedal and pretibial edema and fine bibasilar crackles. Her ECG is as follows:

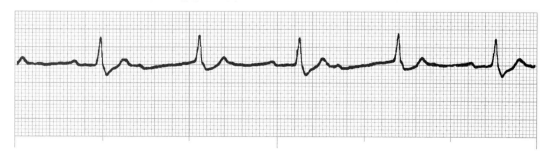

1. What can account for the peripheral edema and the crackles?

_____
_____
_____
_____

2. What problem(s) could account for the complaints of weakness and fatigue?

_____
_____
_____
_____

3. Given the patient's age and history of long-standing diabetes, what problem must be considered?

_____
_____
_____
_____

4. Why is this problem common in patients with diabetes or in the elderly?

_____
_____
_____
_____

5. How would you manage this patient?

_____
_____
_____
_____

Case four

You are called to see a 73-year-old female who has been experiencing episodes of weakness and dizziness. You place the patient on oxygen by nonrebreather mask and attach the monitoring leads. While you continue to interview the patient, she suddenly complains of feeling light-headed and weak. You look at the monitor and see the following rhythm:

1. What is the patient's cardiac rhythm?

_____

2. What is the name of the problem being experienced by the patient?

_____

3. How should you manage this patient?

_____
_____
_____
_____

Case five

A 63-year-old female has a history of weakness and shortness of breath that have increased gradually over 3 days. She denies any history of heart or lung disease. Her only past medical history has been severe osteoarthritis, for which she has been taking "a lot of aspirin." Vital signs are: BP—162/92 mm Hg; P—108 beats/min regular; R—24 breaths/min shallow, regular.

1. What problem(s) do you suspect?

   _____
   _____
   _____
   _____

2. What questions might you ask to help confirm your suspicion?

   _____
   _____
   _____
   _____

39 Abuse and Assault

READING ASSIGNMENT

Chapter 39, pages 169-191, in *Paramedic Practice Today: Above and Beyond*.

OBJECTIVES

After completing this chapter, you will be able to:
1. Discuss the incidence of abuse and assault.
2. Describe the categories of abuse.
3. Discuss examples of intimate partner abuse.
4. Describe characteristics of a person in an abusive relationship.
5. Describe the cycle of violence.
6. Outline techniques for detection of potential violent crime scenes.
7. Describe priorities for crew safety and crime scene awareness.
8. Discuss the assessment and management of the abused patient.
9. Discuss the documentation requirements associated with abuse and assault.
10. Discuss the legal aspects associated with abuse and assault situations.
11. Discuss community resources available to assist victims of abuse or assault.
12. Discuss examples of child abuse and neglect (maltreatment).
13. Identify types of child abuse.
14. Discuss examples of elder abuse.
15. Identify types of elder abuse.
16. Discuss examples of sexual assault.
17. Discuss the assessment and management of a sexual assault patient.
18. Discuss evidence preservation and evidence collection at a crime scene.

CHAPTER SUMMARY

- Domestic violence is a tragedy that affects many members of the community every day. It is an epidemic in the United States. A concerted effort from healthcare professionals, social services, the media, and the legal system working together is necessary to begin to end domestic violence in our society. Domestic violence is everyone's problem. The next victim could be someone close to you.
- Interpersonal (intimate) violence may affect the life of every person, either personally or peripherally.
- One in four women will be in an abusive relationship sometime in her life.
- Violence can take many forms: psychological, verbal, physical, and sexual.
- Violence can affect any age, sex, socioeconomic level, ethnicity, or educational level.
- The elderly and children are the most vulnerable population for unidentified and unresolved abuse.
- Safety is the primary priority at violent crime scenes, and every caution must be used to protect the crew members.
- Reporting requirements vary from state to state regarding the type of abuse or assault. You must be aware of the reporting requirements in your jurisdiction.
- Exact and detailed documentation is essential for all abuse and assault cases.
- Every crime scene needs to be preserved for evidence collection, working collabortively with law enforcement.

SHORT ANSWER/ESSAY

1. List 10 generic risk factors for intimate partner abuse.

_____
_____
_____
_____
_____
_____
_____
_____
_____
_____

2. List common characteristics of abused partners.

_____
_____
_____
_____

3. Describe the approach to a battered patient that is most likely to be effective.

_____
_____
_____
_____

4. List seven factors responsible for the increased incidence of elder abuse.

_____
_____
_____
_____
_____
_____
_____

5. Describe the two major classifications of elder abuse.

_____
_____

6. Define *child abuse*.

_____
_____
_____
_____

7. List common characteristics of child abusers.

_____
_____
_____
_____

8. List eight common behavioral cues indicating that a child may be a victim of abuse.

_____
_____
_____
_____
_____
_____
_____
_____

9. Describe specific and distinct injuries you would expect to find in an abused child.

_____
_____
_____
_____

10. What is shaken baby syndrome?

_____
_____
_____
_____

11. List eight indicators of child neglect.

_____
_____
_____
_____
_____
_____
_____
_____

12. Describe the approach to a victim of sexual assault that is most likely to be effective.

_____
_____
_____
_____

13. Discuss strategies for evidence protection and maintenance of the chain of custody when managing a victim of sexual assault.

_____
_____
_____
_____

MULTIPLE CHOICE

1. Which of the following statements about elder abuse is true?
   A. Elders who are wealthy are more likely to be abused than those who have limited resources.
   B. Institutional abuse may indicate acts of omission, such as failing to address hygiene adequately.
   C. Grandchildren are more likely than any other relatives to be elder abusers.
   D. The incidence of abuse is expected to decrease over the next 20 to 30 years.

2. Which of the following is commonly a factor in cases of abuse being unreported?
   A. The belief that the abuser will change
   B. Unwillingness of victims to cooperate with authorities
   C. Victim's fear of prosecution
   D. Victim's inability to identify their attackers

3. Which of the following behaviors may be construed as abusive?
   A. Insisting that a high school senior work a weekend job to earn money toward her college education
   B. Isolated instances of corporal punishment
   C. Placing a parent or grandparent in nursing care when the burdens of extended care become unmanageable
   D. Withholding of medication from a child who refuses to finish eating dinner

4. Which of the following strategies is best in cases of suspected abuse?
   A. Advise caregivers of their right to silence and notify the police.
   B. Ask caregivers how they possibly could do something so terrible to such an innocent child.
   C. Attempt to trick caregivers into telling you the truth by asking frequent, repetitive questions about the incident.
   D. Provide a safe environment, while nonjudgmentally attempting to obtain details of the event.

5. Which of the following statements about injury patterns in child abuse is correct?
   A. Abdominal injuries account for more than 80% of all child abuse injuries.
   B. Fractures are the second most common injuries in child abuse.
   C. Intentional scald injuries are characterized by "splash burns."
   D. Rib fractures are common in children and usually do not indicate child abuse.

6. Which of the following characteristics is most likely to indicate an abused child?
   A. Apprehension and/or constant alertness for danger
   B. Open display of emotions
   C. Overdependence on parents or caregivers
   D. Self-sufficiency and independence

7. Which of the following guidelines for treating victims of domestic violence is true?
   A. EMS should only report confirmed cases of abuse.
   B. In rape cases, encourage the victim to clean and urinate to lessen the chances of an STD or unwanted pregnancy.
   C. Preservation of the chain of evidence may include placing paper bags over the victim's hands and collecting removed clothing for investigation.
   D. Thorough documentation is prohibited as it may violate the victim's right to privacy.

8. If you suspect child abuse, what should you do?
   A. Attempt to get the parents to confess to child abuse.
   B. Keep your suspicions to yourself since you could be sued if you are wrong.
   C. Privately report your suspicions to the emergency department staff.
   D. Tell the parents you are going to have them investigated for child abuse.

9. A child with socklike burns on his feet _____.
   A. is considered to have a burn of moderate severity
   B. may be a victim of child abuse
   C. probably had scalding water fall on his legs and feet while his socks and shoes were on
   D. should have the injured areas covered with moist dressings

CASE STUDIES

You respond to a home for a sick child. Upon arrival, you find a 6-month-old child in the arms of a teenage girl. She states she is the mother and that the baby is acting "funny" and has not wanted to eat since this morning. The baby girl appears to be awake but not responding appropriately to her surroundings. The infant makes no attempt to cry when removed from the mother's arms for examination. You find the baby to appear healthy. She is dressed appropriately for the season and does not feel hot. When questioned, the mother states that before she left for work that morning the baby took her usual 6 oz of formula and was cooing and playful. When she returned home the child was in her crib and did not respond to her voice or touch. Upon further questioning, you discover that the infant had been in the care of the mother's boyfriend. The boyfriend denies anything happening during the day. The mother seems genuinely concerned about the health and welfare of the baby and begins to cry. A brief physical examination reveals no unusual bruises or other signs of abuse. The infant is flaccid. Her eyes are open, she withdraws to pain, and has no verbal response. Vitals signs are: P—100 beats/min, R—50 breaths/min, capillary refill >2 seconds; glucose—86 mg/dL.

1. List your single most likely diagnosis.

   _____

2. What are the factors that lead you to suspect this diagnosis?

   _____
   _____
   _____
   _____

3. Describe your management of this situation.

_____
_____
_____
_____
_____
_____
_____

40 Patients with Special Challenges

READING ASSIGNMENT

Chapter 40, pages 192-221, in *Paramedic Practice Today: Above and Beyond.*

OBJECTIVES

After completing this chapter, you will be able to:
1. Describe the various etiologies and types of hearing impairments.
2. Recognize the patient with a hearing impairment.
3. Anticipate accommodations that may be needed to manage the patient with a hearing impairment.
4. Describe the various etiologies of visual impairments.
5. Recognize the patient with a visual impairment.
6. Anticipate accommodations that may be needed to manage the patient with a visual impairment.
7. Describe the various etiologies and types of speech impairments.
8. Recognize the patient with a speech impairment.
9. Anticipate accommodations that may be needed in order to properly manage the patient with a speech impairment.
10. Describe the various etiologies of obesity.
11. Anticipate accommodations that may be needed to manage the patient with obesity.
12. Describe paraplegia/quadriplegia.
13. Anticipate accommodations that may be needed to manage the patient with paraplegia/quadriplegia.
14. Define *mental illness*.
15. Describe the various etiologies of mental illness.
16. Recognize the presenting signs of the various mental illnesses.
17. Anticipate accommodations that may be needed to manage the patient with a mental illness.
18. Define the term *developmentally disabled*.
19. Recognize the patient with a developmental disability.
20. Anticipate accommodations that may be needed to manage the patient with a developmental disability.
21. Describe Down syndrome.
22. Recognize the patient with Down syndrome.
23. Anticipate accommodations that may be needed to manage the patient with Down syndrome.
24. Describe the various etiologies of emotional impairment.
25. Recognize the patient with emotional impairment.
26. Anticipate accommodations that may be needed to manage the patient with emotional impairment.
27. Define *emotional/mental impairment* (EMI).
28. Recognize the patient with an emotional or mental impairment.
29. Anticipate accommodations that may be needed to manage the patient with an emotional or mental impairment.
30. Describe the following diseases/illnesses:
    - Arthritis
    - Cancer
    - Cerebral palsy
    - Cystic fibrosis
    - Multiple sclerosis
    - Muscular dystrophy
    - Myasthenia gravis
    - Poliomyelitis
    - Spina bifida
    - Patients with a previous head injury
31. Identify the possible presenting sign(s) for the following diseases/illnesses:
    - Arthritis
    - Cancer
    - Cerebral palsy
    - Cystic fibrosis
    - Multiple sclerosis
    - Muscular dystrophy
    - Myasthenia gravis
    - Poliomyelitis
    - Spina bifida
    - Patients with a previous head injury
32. Anticipate accommodations that may be needed in order to properly manage the following patients:
    - Arthritis
    - Cancer
    - Cerebral palsy
    - Cystic fibrosis
    - Multiple sclerosis
    - Muscular dystrophy
    - Myasthenia gravis
    - Poliomyelitis
    - Spina bifida
    - Patients with a previous head injury
33. Define *cultural diversity*.
34. Recognize a patient who is culturally diverse.
35. Anticipate accommodations that may be needed to manage a patient who is culturally diverse.
36. Identify a patient who is terminally ill.
37. Anticipate accommodations that may be needed to manage a patient who is terminally ill.
38. Identify a patient with a communicable disease.

39. Recognize the presenting signs of a patient with a communicable disease.
40. Anticipate accommodations that may be needed to manage a patient with a communicable disease.
41. Recognize sign(s) of financial impairments.
42. Anticipate accommodations that may be needed to manage the patient with a financial impairment.

CHAPTER SUMMARY

- Many people now survive life-threatening illness and injury. Therefore individuals with special challenges are present in the community and require additional attention when an emergency occurs.
- Accommodations that may be necessary for a patient with a hearing impairment include retrieving the patient's hearing aid, providing paper and pen to aid in communication, and speaking in clear view of the patient.
- When caring for a patient with a visual impairment, retrieve visual aids and describe all patient care procedures before performing them.
- Allow extra time for obtaining the history of a patient with a speech impairment. If appropriate, provide aids such as a pen and paper to assist in communication.
- When caring for a patient who is obese, use appropriately sized diagnostic devices. Secure additional staff members, if needed, to move the patient for ambulance transport.
- Patients with paraplegia or quadriplegia often will require additional staff to assist with moving special equipment to prepare for ambulance transport.
- Once rapport and trust have been established with a patient who has mental illness, care for physical ailments should proceed in the standard manner.
- If the patient has a developmental disability, take extra time to explain what is being done even if it seems that the person does not understand you. Use terminology that is appropriate to the patient's level of ability. Allow more time for the assessment, patient care, and preparation for transport.
- The difficulty in assessing patients with emotional impairments is distinguishing between symptoms produced by stress and those caused by serious medical illness.
- Physical injury and disease may result in pathologic conditions that require special assessment and management skills. Solicit information about the patient's current medications and typical level of functioning in the history.
- *Diversity* refers to differences of any kind such as race, class, religion, gender, sexual preference, personal habitat, and physical or mental ability. Good healthcare depends on sensitivity toward these differences.
- If the patient has a physical disability, gather information about the circumstances or special equipment involved.

Minimize exposure when assessing and treating the patient.

- Often, calls involving the care of a patient with a terminal illness will be emotionally charged encounters that require a great deal of empathy and compassion for the patient and his or her loved ones.
- Some infectious diseases will take a toll on the emotional well-being of affected patients, their families, and loved ones. Be sensitive to the psychological needs of these patients and their families.
- Financial challenges can deprive a patient of basic healthcare services. These patients may be reluctant to seek care for illness or injury.
- If the patient uses specialized equipment, provide reassurance to the patient and family. Make every effort to visit this person before an emergency to get a better understanding of the equipment and why it is being used.
- Pay special attention to family members, and provide support as necessary. Rely on them as a resource, and trust what they tell you. Allow siblings or other family members to assist whenever possible.
- In general, be aware of people with special challenges in the community. Use the appropriate guidelines when interacting with these individuals.

SHORT ANSWER

1. What is cystic fibrosis?
   _____
   _____
   _____
   _____

2. What is the most likely problem associated with cystic fibrosis that EMS personnel would have to manage?
   _____

3. Do all patients with cerebral palsy suffer from developmental delays in cognitive function? How should this affect your interaction with these patients?
   _____
   _____
   _____
   _____

4. If a visually impaired person is accompanied by a guide dog, how should you manage the animal when its owner needs transport to the hospital?
   _____
   _____
   _____
   _____

5. You discover that your patient is visually impaired. Describe three accommodations that you can make to help in your treatment of this patient.

_____

_____

_____

6. As you approach the scene of a motor vehicle crash, an excited female runs up to you and begins to speak. She has a pronounced fluency disorder. List three accommodations that you can make to help communicate with this patient.

_____

_____

_____

7. What is myasthenia gravis?

_____

_____

_____

_____

8. What is the life threat that can be associated with myasthenia gravis? This is referred to as a *myasthenic crisis*.

_____

_____

_____

_____

9. What is postpolio syndrome and whom does it affect?

_____

_____

_____

_____

10. Describe the clinical presentation of a patient with postpolio syndrome.

_____

_____

_____

_____

11. Your elderly female patient is in severe respiratory distress, yet is refusing to go to the hospital because of financial concerns. She states that she cannot pay for the ambulance or the emergency department. What is your response to her?

_____

_____

_____

_____

12. What is Gowers' sign, and what does it indicate?

_____

_____

_____

_____

13. What is apraxia?

_____

_____

_____

_____

MULTIPLE CHOICE

1. A 36-year-old female slipped on some water in her kitchen and suffered a possible fracture or dislocation of her right ankle. The patient is blind secondary to a previous head injury. She lives alone and is aided by a guide dog. Because the patient needs to be transported to the hospital for further care, what is the most appropriate action for handling her guide dog?
   A. Call Animal Control to take custody of the dog, because pets are not your concern.
   B. Have the dog accompany the patient to the hospital.
   C. Leave the dog plenty of water and food, because this injury will require a lengthy hospitalization.
   D. Tell the patient a friend should bring the dog to the hospital.

2. Which of the following is a common etiology of conductive deafness in children?
   A. Labyrinthitis
   B. Otitis externa
   C. Otitis interna
   D. Otitis media

3. Tinnitus is associated with _____.
   A. acetaminophen toxicity and conductive deafness
   B. acetaminophen toxicity and sensorineural deafness
   C. aspirin toxicity and conductive deafness
   D. aspirin toxicity and sensorineural deafness

4. When speaking to your hearing-impaired patient, it is best to _____.
   A. exaggerate gestures in order to hold their attention
   B. face their family member when speaking so they can relay all communications
   C. speak slowly and in a normal voice
   D. speak slowly and loudly

5. Which of the following is the best way to communicate effectively with a hearing-impaired patient?
   A. Continually adjust the patient's hearing aid throughout transport.
   B. Delay transport until a certified interpreter arrives.
   C. Exaggerate facial expressions and lip movements.
   D. Quickly and concisely write questions on a note pad.

6. A 60-year-old female called 9-1-1 because she fell and was unable to get up. Your general impression is that she is awake and alert, is in no obvious distress, and weighs more than 375 lb. She apologizes for calling you and states that her knees gave out when she was walking up the back stairs from outside. She was able to crawl into the kitchen to use the phone. Her husband

Chapter **40 Patients with Special Challenges**

is disabled and cannot lift her. She denies injury but says she needs help to get up. Which of the following is the most appropriate care plan for this patient?
  A. Do your best to assist her to a chair and have a release for nontransport signed.
  B. Perform an assessment before moving her, even though she denies injury.
  C. Since the patient is not injured and since she chose to gain excessive weight, it is not your responsibility to help her since you may hurt yourself trying.
  D. Tell her she needs permanent weight loss while you are waiting for the fire department to respond to assist you with lifting.

7. Your patient responds to questions with incomprehensible speech but will confirm answers appropriately with gestures. The patient's presentation is most indicative of _____.
  A. cognitive aphasia
  B. expressive (motor) aphasia
  C. global aphasia
  D. receptive (sensory) aphasia

8. A developmental disability can best be defined as _____.
  A. a genetic disability in which there is adequate brain development but extensive cerebellar atrophy.
  B. a genetic predisposition to cerebral atrophy.
  C. an acquired predisposition to cerebellar disease.
  D. impaired or insufficient brain development that prevents learning at the usual rate.

9. Which type of arthritis is most often encountered in the prehospital environment?
  A. Juvenile rheumatoid
  B. Osteoarthritis
  C. Rheumatoid
  D. Uremic (gouty)

10. Asymmetric muscle weakness and a reduced size of the affected limb are findings consistent with _____.
  A. multiple sclerosis
  B. myasthenia gravis
  C. postpoliomyelitis syndrome
  D. spina bifida

11. You are called to the home of a child with cerebral palsy. He depends on a ventilator, and the home health aide tells you his tracheostomy tube has malfunctioned. He appears to be in respiratory distress with audible stridor. The initial management of this patient would be to _____.
  A. assess the tracheostomy tube for possible obstruction
  B. remove the tracheostomy tube and replace it with an endotracheal tube
  C. remove the tracheostomy tube and suction the stoma
  D. ventilate the lungs using a bag-mask device

CASE STUDY

You are called to the home of a 12-year-old boy with altered mental status. A home healthcare nurse greets you at the door and tells you the child, who is developmentally delayed, has been agitated, screaming, and vomiting for the past 6 hours, and now is difficult to arouse. She says he has a ventriculoperitoneal shunt. The patient is breathing about 40 times per minute in a Cheyne-Stokes pattern. His heart rate is 62 beats/min with full peripheral pulses. Blood pressure is 148/86 mm Hg. His pupils are equal and sluggishly reactive. He responds only to painful stimuli.

1. What problem do you suspect?

   _____

2. How should you manage the patient?

   _____
   _____
   _____
   _____
   _____
   _____

41 Social Issues

READING ASSIGNMENT

Chapter 41, pages 222-229, in *Paramedic Practice Today: Above and Beyond*.

OBJECTIVES

After completing this chapter, you will be able to:
1. Discuss the effect of cultural differences when rendering patient care.
2. Define *codependency* and explain its effect on patient care.
3. Discuss the impact poverty has on EMS operations.
4. Discuss the financial burdens placed on patients unable to pay for services as well as on society.
5. Understand the impact of homelessness in the United States as it relates to prehospital care.
6. Understand common chronic mental and physiologic illnesses associated with the homeless.

CHAPTER SUMMARY

- Paramedics must possess knowledge of key social issues and understand how those issues could affect treatment.
- Patient populations vary by locale but may include people with ethnic origins and/or religious beliefs unfamiliar to the paramedic. You should become familiar with the values and traditions of the major ethnic and religious groups in your community regarding healthcare.
- The codependent individual is often involved in a relationship with someone with a drug or alcohol problem, mental illness, or chronic illness.
- The codependent person could hinder EMS intervention by covering up for the patient with an acute problem caused by addiction or illness.
- Economic burdens brought about by poverty affect all levels of society.
- Many poor people have chronic medical conditions caused by poor nutrition and poor living environments.
- Many of the poor have no medical coverage and, as such, must rely on local EDs even for minor illnesses or injuries.
- Paramedics must remember to treat all patients with the same level of respect and care regardless of the presence of social issues.
- An estimated 842,000 people are homeless on any given night in February, and 3.5 million experience homelessness during a year.
- Many homeless individuals also have mental illness and/or an addiction.
- Many homeless have untreated chronic medical conditions.

- Maintain a professional and nonjudgmental demeanor.
- Take additional body substance precautions.
- Do not let homelessness interfere with a patient's right to receive the best care possible.

SHORT ANSWER

1. What are the most common psychiatric disorders affecting homeless persons?

   _____
   _____
   _____
   _____

2. What effect does homelessness have on chronic disease processes such as diabetes and hypertension?

   _____
   _____
   _____
   _____

3. List four techniques for improving communications with homeless persons.

   _____
   _____
   _____
   _____

4. What is codependence?

   _____
   _____
   _____
   _____

5. Discuss the two principal challenges codependence creates for EMS personnel.

   _____
   _____

MULTIPLE CHOICE

1. Which of the following statements about homelessness is correct?
   A. Approximately 10% of the homeless population has a psychiatric disorder.
   B. Health problems found in the homeless population are similar to those seen in domiciled patients.
   C. Mortality among the homeless is four times that of the general population.
   D. Substance abuse is uncommon among the homeless because of their limited economic resources.

2. Which of the following statements about the incidence and effect of homelessness is correct?
   A. Homelessness is common in the United States and has a significant effect on EMS.
   B. Homelessness is common in the United States, but has a minimal effect on EMS.
   C. Homelessness is uncommon in the United States and has a minimal effect on EMS.
   D. Homelessness is uncommon in the United States, but has a significant effect on EMS in metropolitan areas.
3. The best place to stand when you are interacting with a homeless person is ________.
   A. 1 to 2 feet away, directly facing the patient
   B. 1 to 2 feet away, slightly turned
   C. 3 to 4 feet away, directly facing the patient
   D. 3 to 4 feet away, slightly turned
4. Which statement about codependence is least correct?
   A. Codependent individuals frequently deny the person in their care has a problem.
   B. Codependent persons are overly caring because they typically come from dysfunctional families.
   C. Codependent persons focus an excessive amount of attention and energy on the problems of another individual.
   D. Codependent persons often blame themselves for violent acts by the individual in their care.
5. The most appropriate response by EMS personnel to a suspected codependent relationship would be to:
   A. actively encourage the codependent individual to seek help and share your concerns about the relationship with personnel at the receiving hospital.
   B. focus on the relationship and actively encourage the codependent individual to seek help.
   C. ignore the codependency and treat the patients as in any other situation.
   D. share their impressions of the relationship with personnel at the receiving hospital.
6. Which statement about the impact of poverty is correct?
   A. Poverty does not significantly reduce life expectancy because of the availability of support programs.
   B. Poverty has little effect on persons in middle and upper income groups.
   C. The poor frequently use emergency departments and EMS as a source of primary healthcare.
   D. Use of EMS by the poor as a source of primary care should be actively discouraged because it is system abuse.
7. You are dispatched to the residence of a 45-year-old male who is complaining of chest pain. He says he does not want an ambulance and that his wife called. He says he cannot afford an ambulance and that he cannot afford to miss work. He asks you to leave. The patient's color is poor, his breathing is labored, and he is clutching his chest. His wife is crying, asking him to go with you. You best action would be to:
   A. call law enforcement to have the patient placed in protective custody so you can treat and transport him.
   B. explain the importance of early intervention in heart attack to the patient, contact the hospital by telephone, and have the patient talk to a physician.
   C. have the patient's wife drive him to the hospital while you follow in the ambulance in case something happens.
   D. tell the patient's wife there is nothing you can do and advise dispatch the patient refused care.

CASE STUDIES

Case one

You have responded to an area of your community where there is a large Vietnamese population. The patient is 3-year-old child who has a 3-day history of nausea, vomiting, and diarrhea. As you attempt to obtain a history, you notice that the child's mother will not talk to you and that the child's father refuses to look you in the eye as you question him.

1. What interpretation should you place on their behavior?

____

____

____

____

Copyright © 2010 by Mosby, Inc., an affiliate of Elsevier Inc. All rights reserved.

Case two

You respond to a call in an area of your community where a large number of recent immigrants from Mexico reside. When you arrive on the scene, you find that a curandera is present.

1. What is a curandera?

_____

_____

_____

_____

2. How should you interact with the curandera?

_____

_____

_____

_____

Case three

Your patient is a 56-year-old female who is complaining of weakness, dizziness, and shortness of breath. Her skin is pale, cool, and moist. Radial pulses are rapid and thready. Capillary refill time is 4 seconds. She has a history of chronic pain from osteoarthritis in both knees for which she frequently takes aspirin and ibuprofen. She has had repeated episodes of abdominal pain over the last 3 days and her bowel movements have become black in color and foul-smelling. Vital signs are: P—134 beats/min; R—24 breaths/min shallow, regular; BP—106/86 mm Hg.

1. What problem do you suspect?

_____

When you tell the patient what you suspect her problem is and ask permission to establish an IV with normal saline, she tells you, "I'm a Jehovah's Witness."

2. What religious objections do Jehovah's Witnesses have to modern healthcare?

_____

_____

_____

_____

3. How should you respond to this patient's concerns?

_____

_____

_____

_____

42 Care for the Patient with a Chronic Illness

READING ASSIGNMENT

Chapter 42, pages 230-262, in *Paramedic Practice Today: Above and Beyond*.

OBJECTIVES

After completing this chapter, you will be able to:
1. Compare the primary objectives of acute care, home care, and hospice care.
2. Summarize the types of home care and the services provided.
3. Compare the primary objectives of the advanced life support (ALS) professional and the home care professional.
4. Differentiate the role of EMS provider from the role of the home care provider.
5. Compare the cost, mortality rate, and quality of care for a given patient in the hospital versus the home care setting.
6. Discuss the aspects of home care that result in enhanced quality of care for a given patient.
7. Identify the importance of home healthcare medicine as related to the ALS level of care.
8. Discuss the aspects of home care that have the potential to become a detriment to the quality of care for a given patient.
9. Given a home care scenario, predict complications requiring ALS intervention and possible hospitalization.
10. Given a series of home care scenarios, determine which patients should receive follow-up home care and which should be transported to an emergency care facility.
11. List pathologic conditions and complications typical to home care patients.
12. Describe airway maintenance devices typically found in the home care environment.
13. List modes of artificial ventilation and prehospital situations where they each might be used.
14. Describe devices that provide or enhance alveolar ventilation in the home care setting.
15. Identify failure of ventilatory devices found in the home care setting.
16. List vascular access devices found in the home care setting.
17. Recognize standard central venous access devices used in the home care setting.
18. Describe the basic characteristics of central venous catheters and implantable drug administration ports, complications, and signs of malfunction associated with these devices.

19. List devices found in the home care setting that are used to empty, irrigate, or deliver nutrition or medication to the gastrointestinal or genitourinary tract.
20. Describe the indications, contraindications, and signs of equipment failure for urinary catheters in the prehospital setting.
21. Differentiate home care from acute care as a preferable situation for a given patient scenario.
22. Identify failure of drains.
23. Discuss the significance of palliative care programs related to a patient in a home care setting.
24. Define hospice care, comfort care, and resuscitation attempts as they relate to local practice, law, and policy.
25. List the stages of the grief process and relate them to an individual in hospice care.
26. Given a series of scenarios, demonstrate interaction and support with the family members and support persons for a patient who has died.
27. Discuss the relation between local home care treatment protocols and standard operating procedures and local EMS protocols and standard operating procedures.
28. Discuss differences in an individual's ability to accept and cope with his or her own impending death.
29. Discuss the rights of the terminally ill.

CHAPTER SUMMARY

- Acute care is short-term medical treatment usually provided in a hospital for patients who have an illness or injury or who are recovering from surgery. Home care is the provision of health services by formal and informal caregivers in the home to promote, restore, and maintain a person's maximal level of comfort, function, and health, including care toward a dignified death. Hospice is a care program that provides for the dying and their special needs.
- Examples of home care problems that usually require intervention by a home health professional or physician include chemotherapy, pain management, wound care, ostomy care, and hospice or palliative care. Examples of home care problems requiring acute intervention include altered mental status; airway complications; respiratory failure or acute respiratory events; cardiac decompensation or acute cardiac events; infection, acute sepsis, or septic complications; equipment malfunction; and gastrointestinal or genitourinary crisis. As a paramedic, you should be familiar with types of medical equipment found in the home, their uses, and how to troubleshoot potential problems.

59

SHORT ANSWER

1. If you are called to see a patient who is on a home ventilator system that is malfunctioning, what is your first step?

_____
_____
_____
_____

2. What is a PICC line?

_____
_____
_____
_____

3. If a patient's PICC line is broken, how should the bleeding from the damaged tube be stopped?

_____
_____
_____
_____

4. A patient who is receiving regular doses of morphine to control pain from terminal metastatic cancer has slow, shallow breathing and pinpoint pupils. Is the use of naloxone advisable in caring for this patient? Why or why not?

_____
_____
_____
_____

5. When patients with indwelling tubes in the gastrointestinal tract (NG tubes, G-tubes, J-tubes) are transported, in what position should they be placed? Why?

_____
_____
_____
_____

6. When a patient has an indwelling catheter in the urinary bladder, what is the most important point to remember about moving the patient and the urinary drainage system?

_____
_____
_____
_____

7. If a central venous catheter becomes uncapped or broken, what complication other than bleeding can occur?

_____
_____
_____
_____

8. How should a patient be managed if this central venous catheter complication is suspected?

_____
_____
_____
_____

9. Describe hazards you may encounter in a home care patient that you would not encounter in other patients.

_____
_____
_____
_____

10. What is a decubitus wound?

_____
_____
_____
_____

11. What are the stages of decubitus wounds?

_____
_____
_____
_____

MULTIPLE CHOICE

1. An infant or child with a gastrostomy tube should be transported _____.
   A. in a position of comfort or prone with the head lower than the trunk
   B. on his or her back or left side with the head lower than the trunk
   C. sitting or lying on the right side with the head elevated
   D. supine or prone with the head elevated

2. You respond to a report of a child with difficulty breathing. The patient is an 8-year-old male with a history of muscular dystrophy who is on a home mechanical ventilator system. An alarm on the ventilator is sounding. As you examine the patient, you notice he is becoming cyanotic and his chest is not rising as the ventilator cycles. What should you do?
   A. Contact on-line medical control for instructions on how to operate the ventilator.
   B. Disconnect the patient from the mechanical ventilator and assist his ventilations with a bag-mask and oxygen.
   C. Disconnect the patient from the ventilator and place him on a nonrebreather mask at 15 L/min.
   D. Refer to the instruction manual to determine how to operate the ventilator unit.

3. You respond to a report of a "child with bleeding." The patient is a 4-year-old female lying in bed. There is a large amount of blood on the sheets. The patient is quiet and very pale. Her father tells you she recently was diagnosed with leukemia. She had a PICC placed 3 days ago for administration of chemotherapy, and the external end of the catheter accidentally broke off about 5 minutes ago. Blood is still actively running from the broken end of the PICC. What would be the most appropriate response to this situation?
   A. Apply direct pressure at the point where the PICC enters the skin.
   B. Elevate the extremity above the level of the heart and transport immediately.
   C. Use a blood pressure cuff as a tourniquet to stop the flow of blood.
   D. Wrap the tips of a hemostat with gauze and use the hemostat to clamp the PICC.

4. A terminally ill patient in the home care environment who is experiencing respiratory distress should be _____.
   A. evaluated for a valid do not resuscitate order before any care is provided
   B. given a thorough initial assessment and provided with appropriate care
   C. given oxygen by nonrebreather mask and referred to the family physician
   D. taken to the emergency department for consultation and treatment

5. In the event of a life-threatening emergency, a patient with a signed, valid do not resuscitate order should receive _____.
   A. no care
   B. only comfort measures unless specifically outlined in the advance directives
   C. only the care directed by the home health provider
   D. only the care requested by the family

6. The anatomic location that would be least likely to be the site of a colostomy stoma would be the _____.
   A. LLQ; sigmoid colon
   B. LUQ; descending colon
   C. RUQ; ascending colon
   D. RUQ; transverse colon

7. You are treating a 48-year-old female who is having chest pain. She is diaphoretic, pale, and hypotensive. Chemotherapy has made the patient's veins extremely difficult to cannulate. You discover an implanted medication port in the right chest. You should _____.
   A. administer two more doses of nitroglycerin 0.4 mg by the sublingual route
   B. cannulate the medication port with the smallest over-the-needle catheter you have
   C. intubate to provide a route for giving resuscitation medications
   D. transport the patient to the nearest appropriate facility for further treatment

8. Which of the following statements regarding urinary catheterization is correct?
   A. Internal catheters, such as Foley catheters, are indicated in patients whose bladders cannot effectively collect urine.
   B. Suprapubic catheters, unlike urostomies, do not involve invasion into the abdominal wall.
   C. The most common complication of urinary catheters is infection.
   D. The Texas catheter is indicated for long-term use in a bed-bound patient.

9. If the family of a patient receiving hospice care calls EMS, the paramedics should _____.
   A. disregard the hospice principles and provide life-sustaining care
   B. encourage the family's hope for a cure of the family member's illness
   C. refuse to provide any adjunctive or supportive therapies
   D. respect the wishes of the patient and family and maintain patient dignity

10. You are dispatched to a report of a 7-year-old male who is having seizures. When you arrive, you find the patient in a postictal state, sitting in a wheelchair. He is in a brace with a halo traction device stabilizing his cervical spine. The patient's mother tells you he is recovering from a motor vehicle crash in which he sustained head and spinal injuries. He has been home for 1 week and was doing well until this seizure occurred. Your primary concern at this moment is _____.
   A. arranging padding for the halo device's posterior pins in the occipital area of the patient's skull
   B. ensuring the halo device and brace stay in position
   C. ensuring an adequate airway even though there is a spinal injury
   D. moving the patient from the chair to the ambulance stretcher so you can begin medication therapy

11. If a tracheostomy tube is dislodged from the stoma and cannot be replaced easily, you should _____.
   A. insert an appropriately sized endotracheal tube into the tracheostoma
   B. perform rapid sequence intubation
   C. place the patient on high-concentration oxygen using a nonrebreather mask
   D. rush the patient to the hospital immediately

12. A 46-year-old male with metastatic lung cancer has a decreased level of consciousness. His wife and children are present. The patient is cyanotic and appears to be in pain. There is vomitus in his airway. An appropriate question to ask would be:
    A. "Does the patient have a do not resuscitate order?"
    B. "Don't you have hospice care?"
    C. "What would you like us to do?"
    D. "Why did you call an ambulance?"

13. After you give 2 mg of morphine to the patient in the previous question, his respiratory rate drops to 4 breaths/min. What should you do?
    A. Ask the family what they would like you to do.
    B. Assist the patient's breathing with a bag-mask device and contact medical control for orders.
    C. Give naloxone to reverse respiratory depression.
    D. Intubate because it is your fault his breathing is depressed.

14. You are called to the home of a patient whose respirations are being supported by a mechanical ventilator. His wife says she dropped a book on the front panel of the machine. Some of the knobs were turned, and the alarms began sounding. The patient weighs approximately 70 kg. While contacting medical control for orders, what would be the most appropriate action?
    A. Disconnect the ventilator and ventilate with a bag-mask device and oxygen.
    B. Reset the ventilator to an FiO_2 of 0.4, a tidal volume of 500 mL, a rate of 12 breaths/min, and a PEEP of 5 cm.
    C. Reset the ventilator to an FiO_2 of 1.0, a tidal volume of 500 mL, a rate of 20 breaths/min, and a PEEP of 12 cm.
    D. Reset the ventilator to an FiO_2 of 1.0, a tidal volume of 700 to 1000 mL, a rate of 10 breaths/min, and a PEEP of 5 cm.

15. What is the primary difference between a PICC line and other central venous access devices?
    A. The PICC line enters a peripheral vein and extends into the central venous circulation.
    B. The PICC line enters directly into the central venous circulation.
    C. The PICC line has multiple lumens.
    D. The PICC line is shorter than the others.

16. During an interfacility transfer of a patient with a central venous line, the IV tubing becomes detached from the catheter. After reattaching the IV line, you notice the patient is having difficulty breathing and is becoming cyanotic. His pulse rate begins to rise, and his blood pressure falls. The best position in which to place this patient would be _____.
    A. on his left side, 30 degrees head down
    B. on his right side, 30 degrees head down
    C. semisitting
    D. supine

17. Your patient is a 73-year-old male who is suffering from end-stage Alzheimer's disease. He has aspirated the contents of his feeding tube and is in respiratory distress. His wife adamantly states she wants nothing done and produces her husband's advance directives, which correspond to those wishes. You should _____.
    A. comply with the wishes of the spouse and the advance directives and do nothing
    B. give 10 mg of morphine sulfate IV push
    C. intubate the patient, suction the trachea, and transport to the nearest hospital
    D. place the patient on a nonrebreather mask and call your supervisor

CASE STUDY

You are called to the home of a 5-year-old female who is severely developmentally delayed. The child's caregiver reports that the patient's gastrostomy tube was inadvertently dislodged 10 hours ago. The patient cannot swallow and is dependent on the gastrostomy tube for all intake of fluids and nutrients. The patient is unresponsive to verbal or painful stimuli. However, the caregiver reports this is her normal state. The patient's respirations are rapid, but unlabored. Her skin is cool and dry. Radial pulses are weak at 136 beats/min. Blood pressure is 82/56 mm Hg.

1. How would you manage this patient?
   _____
   _____
   _____
   _____

2. Is there an alternative to establishing an IV on this patient?

_____
_____
_____
_____

3. What problems may be associated with using this alternative?

_____
_____
_____
_____

43 Trauma Systems and Mechanism of Injury

READING ASSIGNMENT

Chapter 43, pages 264-303, in *Paramedic Practice Today: Above and Beyond.*

OBJECTIVES

After completing this chapter, you will be able to:
1. Describe the incidence and scope of traumatic injuries and death.
2. Identify the parts of a comprehensive trauma system and describe the roles of each part.
3. Describe the differences in the levels of trauma center.
4. Describe the considerations for ground versus air transport of a trauma patient.
5. Define the laws of motion and describe their relation to the effects of trauma.
6. Define and describe the roles of kinematics and index of suspicion as additional tools for assessing patients.
7. Describe each type of impact and its effect on the unrestrained victim (e.g., down and under, up and over, compression, deceleration).
8. Describe the role of restraints in injury prevention and injury patterns.
9. Identify and describe the injury patterns associated with motorcycle collisions.
10. Describe the injury patterns associated with vehicle collisions with pedestrians (adult and pediatric pedestrians).
11. Identify and describe the injury patterns associated with sports injuries, blast injuries, and vertical fall injuries.
12. Describe the damage caused by the different types of projectile velocities.

CHAPTER SUMMARY

- Maintain a high index of suspicion for multisystem trauma for pedestrians involved in motor vehicle crashes (MVCs). Differences exist between adult and pediatric victims and the body systems involved, even though the essential mechanism is similar.

- Penetrating trauma can affect multiple organ systems, causing damage to air-filled and solid organs, vascular injury, trauma to the vertebral column, and spinal cord injury. Assume a serious injury when managing victims of penetrating trauma.
- Trauma centers are specialty hospitals that have the necessary staff and expertise to deal with serious trauma. They are characterized as level I, II, III, or IV, with level I being the most comprehensive facility.
- Trauma is the leading cause of death in persons aged 1 to 45 years.
- The parts of a comprehensive trauma system include injury prevention, prehospital care, emergency department care, interfacility transport (if needed), definitive care, trauma critical care, rehabilitation, and data collection.
- The physical laws of motion have an effect on trauma:
  - The first law of motion (items in motion will stay in motion until acted on by an outside source) can be seen in unrestrained persons involved in an MVC.
  - Conservation of energy (energy cannot be destroyed but may change state) can be seen in trauma; energy such as electricity has thermal effects on tissue.
  - Kinetic energy (Mass/2 × V²) relates to trauma; the mass of an object and the velocity are directly related to the amount of damage sustained on the body.
  - Force (Mass × Acceleration = Mass × Deceleration) is the amount of energy applied to an object to set it in motion; an equal amount of energy is needed to stop the object. In penetrating injuries, for example, the same amount of force to propel a bullet must be met with the same amount of energy transfer within the body to stop the bullet.
- Base transport decisions regarding ground versus air on the patient's best interests of arriving at the appropriate facility as quickly as possible (approximately 60 minutes). Issues to consider include, but are not limited to, traffic conditions, time of day, weather, delay in transport, and whether the patient needs a higher critical level of care en route.

- Motorcycle collisions can include injury patterns such as those seen in car crashes as well as vertical falls.
- Vehicle collisions can result in multiple injury patterns (e.g., up and over, down and under) that produce highly predictable injuries to organs and organ systems.
- The use of restraint systems in motor vehicles has had a significant impact on decreasing injury and death in MVCs.

SHORT ANSWER

1. What is the purpose of the initial assessment (primary survey)?

_____

_____

_____

_____

2. What action should be taken if a trauma patient has a respiratory rate of less than 10 breaths/min or more than 30 breaths/min?

_____

_____

_____

_____

3. A patient has no palpable radial pulse, but does have a palpable carotid pulse. What do these findings indicate about the patient's perfusion?

_____

_____

_____

_____

4. In what three areas of the body do life-threatening injuries most commonly occur?

_____

_____

5. What is the "golden hour"? How much of the golden hour do EMS personnel have for on-scene patient assessment and management?

_____

_____

_____

_____

6. Which has a greater effect on an object's kinetic energy: mass or velocity?

_____

_____

_____

_____

7. During any motor vehicle crash, how many collisions actually occur? What are these collisions?

_____

_____

_____

_____

8. What is normal capillary refill time? How do cold environments affect capillary refill time?

_____

_____

_____

_____

9. If your rapid initial assessment (primary survey) of a trauma patient establishes that the patient is in shock, should IVs be established at the scene of the call or en route to the hospital? Why?

_____

_____

_____

_____

10. Can the probable locations of organs injured from a gunshot be determined by drawing a line between the entrance and exit wounds? Why?

_____

_____

_____

_____

11. When should the secondary survey (detailed history and physical examination) be performed on a critical trauma patient? Why?

_____

_____

_____

_____

12. What causes a "paper bag" pneumothorax?

_____

_____

_____

13. Your patient is a 30-year-old female who was thrown from a motorcycle she was riding. She is unconscious and unresponsive. Her skin is pale, cool, and moist. Her respirations are 28 breaths/min, shallow, and irregular. Radial pulses are absent. Her abdomen is rigid and distended. Breath sounds are absent on the left side of her chest. She has an open fracture of her right femur. What should be the focus of your initial efforts? Why?

_____

_____

_____

_____

14. What is the Don Juan syndrome?

_____
_____
_____
_____

15. What is Waddell's Triad?

_____
_____
_____
_____

16. At the scene of a explosion, you find a patient who is hemorrhaging from both ears and the nose. He is awake and alert and states that he was not struck by debris or thrown by the blast. What type of blast injury has he sustained?

_____
_____
_____
_____

17. Based on the mechanism of the injury the patient in the previous question has suffered, what other body organ systems are likely to have been damaged?

_____
_____
_____
_____

MULTIPLE CHOICE

1. You respond to a car-versus-tree crash. A 32-year-old male is sitting behind the steering wheel, which is cracked. He is conscious but confused and agitated. He is obviously dyspneic and complains he cannot breathe. His lips and nailbeds are cyanotic. His skin is cool, pale, and moist. His neck veins are distended. Examination of the chest reveals absent breath sounds on the right and subcutaneous emphysema. His radial pulses are weak and barely palpable. He is not pinned in the vehicle. The best course of action would be to _____.

   A. apply a cervical collar and KED, extricate him to a long board, apply oxygen and assist ventilation, apply PASG, and start IVs at the scene
   B. establish two IVs with Ringer's lactate with the patient still in the vehicle, apply a cervical collar, extricate the patient to a long board, apply oxygen and assist ventilation, apply PASG, and transport
   C. initiate oxygen therapy, apply a cervical collar, extricate the patient to a long board, assist ventilation, apply PASG, transport, and initiate IVs en route
   D. remove the patient from the vehicle, place him on the stretcher, give oxygen, and transport code 3

2. You respond to a motor vehicle crash where you find the following patients:
   Patient 1 is a 26-year-old male complaining of pain in the right arm. The injured area is swollen, tender, and discolored. A distal pulse is palpable. P—100 beats/min; BP—140/90 mm Hg; R—20 breaths/min.
   Patient 2 is a 22-year-old female with massive trauma to the face and neck. Cyanosis is present. P—140 beats/min; BP—96/50 mm Hg; R—40 breaths/min, stridorous.
   Patient 3 is a 23-year-old female complaining of severe lower abdominal pain. Her abdomen is rigid and tender. She was wearing a seat belt. P—130 beats/min; BP—80/50 mm Hg; R—26 breaths/min.
   Patient 4 is a 30-year-old male complaining of numbness in the upper and lower extremities. There is a deep laceration on his forehead. P—80 beats/min; BP—126/80 mm Hg; R—16 breaths/min.
   In what order would you treat these patients?
   A. 3, 2, 4, 1
   B. 2, 3, 4, 1
   C. 3, 2, 1, 4
   D. 2, 4, 3, 1

3. The purpose of triage is to ensure that _____.
   A. patients who are in the most pain are treated first
   B. patients with life-threatening conditions receive immediate treatment
   C. patients with potentially disabling injuries are treated first
   D. the "walking wounded" are treated first and evacuated from the scene to avoid crowd control problems

4. How much of the "golden hour" does the prehospital care provider have for on-scene patient assessment and management?
   A. 1 minute
   B. 10 minutes
   C. 15 minutes
   D. 30 minutes

5. In a motor vehicle crash, a patient's knees hit the dashboard, resulting in a fracture of the left hip. This is an example of _____.
   A. direct violence
   B. indirect violence
   C. pathologic fracture
   D. twisting injury (torsion)

6. A 23-year-old male suffered penetrating trauma to the chest from flying debris when a liquefied petroleum gas storage tank exploded. What type of blast injury is this?
   A. Primary
   B. Quaternary
   C. Secondary
   D. Tertiary

7. A medical care facility located in a remote area that stabilizes and prepares trauma patients with moderate or serious injuries for transport to a facility with capabilities for trauma surgery is a _____.
   A. level I trauma center
   B. level II trauma center
   C. level III trauma center
   D. level IV trauma center

8. A medical care facility, usually a university teaching center, that commits resources to address all types of specialty trauma 24 hours a day, 7 days a week is a _____.
   A. level I trauma center
   B. level II trauma center
   C. level III trauma center
   D. level IV trauma center

CASE STUDIES

Case one

A 25-year-old male was stabbed in the left anterior chest just below the nipple. No one knows anything about the situation or the length of the knife. The patient is extremely combative. His skin is cool and clammy. His neck veins are distended, but his trachea is midline. Heart sounds are distant and muffled. The knife still is embedded in the patient's chest. Vital signs are: BP—90/50 mm Hg; P—120 beats/min weak, regular; R—28 breaths/min shallow, regular. You notice that the pulse fades in and out as the patient inhales and exhales.

After 5 minutes, the patient's vital signs are: BP—70/56 mm Hg; P—138 beats/min weak, irregular; R—36 breaths/min gasping. At this point, you are 20 minutes away from a level I trauma center. A level IV trauma center is only 5 minutes away. Although the level IV facility is not equipped to manage multiple-systems trauma, it does have an emergency department with an advanced trauma life support–certified physician on-duty. It is foggy and the helicopter is on weather-hold.

1. What should you do? Defend your decision.

   _____
   _____
   _____
   _____

Case two

A 28-year-old male was driving a motor vehicle that struck a utility pole head-on. The patient was not restrained and the vehicle was not equipped with air bags.

1. What is the law of conservation of energy, and why is it relevant in this situation?

   _____
   _____
   _____
   _____

2. What is Newton's first law of motion, and why is it relevant in this situation?

   _____
   _____
   _____
   _____

3. Is mass or velocity the principal factor determining the amount of kinetic energy possessed by a moving body? Why?

   _____
   _____
   _____
   _____

4. During a collision involving a vehicle carrying unrestrained passengers, three collisions occur. What are these collisions?

_____

_____

_____

_____

5. Based on the mechanism of injury what thoracic injuries do you suspect?

_____

_____

_____

_____

As you prepare to rapidly extricate the patient, you notice that the dashboard is broken and pushed inward near the patient's right knee.

6. What mechanism of injury does this damage to the vehicle suggest?

_____

_____

_____

_____

7. What injuries do you suspect may be present?

_____

_____

_____

_____

Case three

A 6-year-old male ran into the street and was struck by a car. The patient is unresponsive. He is making snoring sounds as he breathes. Respirations are 38 breaths/min, shallow, and irregular. The lips and nailbeds are cyanotic. The patient's skin is pale, cool, and moist. Radial pulses are absent. A rapid, weak carotid pulse is present. Capillary refill is longer than 2 seconds. Obvious injuries include a bruise over the right frontal area of the head and a deep laceration of the right forearm from which dark red blood is flowing steadily. Pupils are equal and dilated and react sluggishly to light.

1. What is the typical pattern of injuries that characterizes children struck by automobiles?

_____

_____

_____

_____

2. What is the name of this injury pattern?

_____

3. Why does this injury pattern tend to occur in children?

_____

_____

_____

_____

Chapter **43** Trauma Systems and Mechanism of Injury

44 Bleeding

READING ASSIGNMENT

Chapter 44, pages 304-313, in *Paramedic Practice Today: Above and Beyond.*

OBJECTIVES

After completing this chapter, you will be able to:
1. Describe the etiology, history, and physical findings of external bleeding.
2. Predict hemorrhage on the basis of a patient's mechanism of injury.
3. Distinguish between controlled and uncontrolled hemorrhage.
4. Using the patient history and physical examination findings, develop a treatment plan for a patient with external bleeding.
5. Distinguish between the various techniques for hemorrhage control of open soft tissue injuries, including direct pressure and tourniquet application.
6. Distinguish between the administration rate and amount of intravenous fluid for a patient with controlled hemorrhage and the rate and amount for a patient with uncontrolled hemorrhage.
7. Describe the etiology, history, and physical findings of internal bleeding.
8. Using the patient history and physical examination findings, develop a treatment plan for a patient with internal bleeding.

CHAPTER SUMMARY

■ Internal and external hemorrhage can result from a variety of causes.
■ An adequate blood volume is critical to adequate perfusion.
■ Uncontrolled blood loss can quickly lead to hypovolemic shock and poor patient outcome.
■ The goal of treatment in the hemorrhaging patient is to stop the hemorrhage as quickly and efficiently as possible.
■ The patient should not be allowed to continue to bleed while ineffective methods of hemorrhage control are attempted.

MATCHING

1. Match the type of bleeding with its presentation.
   __ Bright red and spurting   A. Arterial
   __ Dark red and flowing   B. Capillary
   __ Dark red and oozing   C. Venous

SHORT ANSWER

1. What is the goal in controlling bleeding?

2. Define *hemorrhage*.

3. Define *perfusion*.

4. List at least four causes of major blood loss.

5. Define *exsanguination*.

6. What volume of sudden blood loss in the adult, child, and infant is considered serious?

7. List at least four signs and symptoms of blood loss.

8. Why should a tourniquet be considered if direct pressure and a pressure dressing are ineffective in controlling hemorrhage?

9. What is the typical target systolic blood pressure when administering IV fluids to a patient with severe hemorrhage?

_____

_____

_____

_____

10. What technique should be used first to control bleeding from an open wound?

_____

_____

_____

_____

11. If external extremity bleeding cannot be controlled with direct pressure, what is the next step in hemorrhage control?

_____

_____

_____

_____

12. What risks are associated with applying a tourniquet?

_____

_____

_____

_____

13. Why should tourniquets not be loosened or removed once they are in place?

_____

_____

_____

_____

14. What piece of equipment carried on the ambulance makes the most effective tourniquet?

_____

_____

_____

_____

MULTIPLE CHOICE

1. At the scene of a motor vehicle crash, a 23-year-old female has a scalp laceration that is spurting bright red blood. An avulsion on her left leg has dark red blood flowing from it steadily. Blood is oozing from abrasions on her elbows. Your first action should be to _____.
   A. check for spinal injuries by assessing movement and sensation in all four extremities
   B. control the hemorrhage from her leg
   C. control the hemorrhage from her scalp
   D. dress and bandage the abrasions

2. If a dressing and bandage become soaked with blood, you should _____.
   A. apply a tourniquet
   B. do nothing
   C. reinforce the bandage with more gauze and pressure
   D. remove the blood-soaked dressing and replace it with a dry one

3. A patient has a 5-inch laceration on his right upper arm. Dark red blood is flowing from the wound. Your first action to control the hemorrhage should be to _____.
   A. apply a tourniquet
   B. apply direct pressure
   C. apply pressure to the brachial artery
   D. elevate the extremity

4. Which statement best describes arterial bleeding?
   A. Bright red, spurting
   B. Bright red, steadily flowing
   C. Dark red, spurting
   D. Dark red, steadily flowing

5. What is the average blood volume?
   A. 50 mL/kg
   B. 60 mL/kg
   C. 70 mL/kg
   D. 80 mL/kg

6. What amount of blood loss is usually well tolerated in patients?
   A. 10% to 15%
   B. 15% to 20%
   C. 20% to 25%
   D. 25% to 30%

7. Which of the following medications can reduce a patient's ability to form blood clots?
   A. Carbamazepine
   B. Furosemide
   C. Propranolol
   D. Warfarin

8. Your patient has internal bleeding. Which of the following will be of the most benefit?
   A. Elevating the patient's legs
   B. Administering high-flow oxygen
   C. Applying a PASG
   D. Rapidly administering IV fluids

9. Which of the following are signs of internal hemorrhage?
   A. Tachycardia, hypertension, narrowed pulse pressure
   B. Tachycardia, hypertension, widened pulse pressure
   C. Tachycardia, hypotension, narrowed pulse pressure
   D. Tachycardia, hypotension, widened pulse pressure

10. A 25-year-old man with a history of schizo-phrenia amputated his penis with a knife. You should control the bleeding by _____.
    A. applying cold packs
    B. applying direct pressure
    C. applying moist sterile dressings
    D. using a tourniquet

45 Soft Tissue Trauma

READING ASSIGNMENT

Chapter 45, pages 314-347, in *Paramedic Practice Today: Above and Beyond.*

OBJECTIVES

After completing this chapter, you will be able to:

1. Describe the incidence, morbidity, and mortality rates of soft tissue injuries.
2. Describe the layers of the skin, specifically the epidermis and dermis (cutaneous), superficial fascia (subcutaneous), and deep fascia.
3. Identify the major functions of the integumentary system.
4. Describe the anatomy and physiology of joints.
5. Discuss the pathophysiology of wound healing, including hemostasis, inflammation, epithelialization, neovascularization, and collagen synthesis.
6. Describe common interruptions in the wound healing process.
7. Identify wounds that have a high risk for infection or complications.
8. Discuss the pathophysiology of soft tissue injuries.
9. Distinguish between open and closed soft tissue injuries.
10. Distinguish between the types of closed soft tissue injuries.
11. Describe the etiology, history, and physical findings of a closed soft tissue injury.
12. Using the mechanism of injury, patient history, and physical examination findings, develop a treatment plan for a patient with a closed soft tissue injury.
13. Distinguish between the types of open soft tissue injuries.
14. Describe the etiology, history, and physical findings of an open soft tissue injury.
15. Using the mechanism of injury, patient history, and physical examination findings, develop a treatment plan for a patient with an open soft tissue injury.
16. Describe the etiology, history, and physical findings of crush injuries.
17. Using the mechanism of injury, patient history, and physical examination findings, develop a treatment plan for a patient with a crush injury.
18. Discuss the effects of reperfusion and rhabdomyolysis on the body.
19. Define the following conditions: crush injury, crush syndrome, and compartment syndrome.
20. Distinguish between the types of injuries that require the use of an occlusive dressing versus those that require a nonocclusive dressing.
21. Define and discuss the following:
    - Dressings
        - Sterile and nonsterile
        - Occlusive and nonocclusive
        - Adherent and nonadherent
        - Absorbent and nonabsorbent
        - Wet and dry
    - Bandages
        - Absorbent and nonabsorbent
        - Adherent and nonadherent
    - Tourniquets
22. Predict the possible complications of an improperly applied dressing, bandage, or tourniquet.

CHAPTER SUMMARY

- The skin and its structures serve key roles in maintaining body temperature and moisture and protecting the body from disease. Any disruption of the skin caused by trauma can result in significant threats to the patient's life.
- Soft tissue injuries encompass all types of injuries, from superfical to life threatening.
- You must carefully assess a patient's injuries and apply the appropriate knowledge to distinguish superficial from life-threateninig soft tissue injuries and provide the proper care.
- Soft tissue injuries can be classified as either open or closed. The critical difference is whether the skin remains intact. Both injuries present the potential for complications when they are not identified and properly managed
- You will mainly control hemorrhage by applying direct pressure. Check your local protocols regarding approved methods of bleeding control in your EMS system
- Wound healing can be complicated by age, unrelated medical conditions, wound contamination, location of the injury, and severity of the injury.
- Wound management of open soft tissue injuries is focussed on the control of hemorrhage and the protection of the wound from contamination.
- Ultimately you must prioritize the care of injuries to ensure the most life-threatening ones receive the most attention instead of spending excessive amounts of time on insignificant but graphic soft tissue trauma.
- You must take special care when treating amputations, avulsions, chest injuries, abdominal injuries, and crush injuries.

MATCHING

1. Match the type of soft tissue injury with its description.

_____ Abrasion
_____ Amputation
_____ Avulsion
_____ Contusion
_____ Laceration
_____ Puncture

A. Closed injury with local swelling and bruising
B. Open injury caused by top layer of skin being scraped
C. Open injury consisting of a cut that is longer than it is deep
D. Open injury in which the skin/body part is completely separated from the rest of the body
E. Open injury in which the wound is deeper than it is long
F. Open injury where skin is partially pulled away as a flap

2. Match the stage of wound healing with its description.

_____ Collagen synthesis
_____ Epithelialization
_____ Hemostasis
_____ Inflammation
_____ Neovascularization

A. Body's control of bleeding through natural clotting
B. Body's nonspecific response to tissue damage
C. Growth of new capillaries within wound
D. Migration of body covering cells over wound surface
E. Production of new structural protein within wound

3. Match the type of dressing with its properties.

_____ Absorbent
_____ Adherent
_____ Nonabsorbent
_____ Nonadherent
_____ Nonocclusive
_____ Occlusive
_____ Sterile

A. Clean, but not free of bacteria and other organisms
B. Does not prevent movement of air though itself
C. Does not stick to drying blood and fluid
D. Free of bacteria and other microorganisms
E. Prevents movement of air or fluid through itself
F. Sticks to drying blood and fluid
G. Unable to soak up blood or other fluids

SHORT ANSWER

1. List the layers of the skin.

_____
_____
_____
_____

2. Which layer contains specialized structures such as hair follicles, sweat glands, oil glands, and nerve endings?

_____
_____
_____
_____

3. Describe how amputated body parts should be managed in the prehospital setting.

_____
_____
_____
_____

4. When you are managing an avulsion, what should be done with the skin flap before bandaging the injury?

_____
_____
_____
_____

5. How should an impaled object be managed in the prehospital setting?

_____
_____
_____
_____

6. Once a wound has been dressed and bandaged, should the dressing and bandage ever be removed in the field? Why or why not? If the patient bleeds through the dressing or bandage, what should you do?

_____
_____
_____
_____

7. What is crush syndrome?

_____
_____
_____
_____

8. What is rhabdomyolysis?

_____
_____
_____
_____

9. Why are patients with crush syndrome at risk for renal failure?

_____

_____

_____

_____

10. How can the risk of renal failure from crush syndrome be minimized?

_____

_____

_____

_____

11. What is compartment syndrome?

_____

_____

_____

_____

12. Describe prehospital management of suspected compartment syndrome.

_____

_____

_____

_____

MULTIPLE CHOICE

1. At the scene of a motorcycle crash, a 22-year-old male has a 7-inch scalp laceration from just over his right eye to the top of his head. He is conscious and alert. Bright red blood is spurting from the laceration. There are multiple avulsions on the arms and legs from which dark red blood is flowing steadily. There are also several abrasions on the knees and elbows with slow oozing bleeding. Your first action should be to have your partner control the head and neck while you _____.
   A. control the bleeding from the avulsions
   B. control the spurting bleeding from the scalp
   C. dress and bandage the abrasions
   D. evaluate for spinal injury by assessing extremity motor/sensory function

2. Avulsed or amputated parts present at a motor vehicle crash should be _____.
   A. left at the scene since they now may be part of the evidence at a crime scene
   B. transported only if less than 10 minutes have elapsed
   C. transported only if they are parts of extremities
   D. transported with the patient

3. A 32-year-old female's ring became caught in moving machinery. The skin has been partially stripped from her finger and is hanging as a flap. What type of soft tissue injury is present?
   A. A contusion
   B. A laceration
   C. An abrasion
   D. An avulsion

4. A dressing and bandage applied over a wound have become soaked with blood. What should you do?
   A. Remove the bandage and apply a tourniquet.
   B. Do nothing.
   C. Reinforce the bandage with more gauze and pressure.
   D. Remove the blood-soaked dressing and replace it with a dry one.

5. A patient recently was released from the hospital after undergoing abdominal surgery. The patient had a coughing spell that caused the stitches to rupture. You find part of the man's intestines protruding from the open incision. Management would include _____.
   A. applying direct pressure to prevent internal bleeding
   B. covering the exposed organs with a dry, clean sheet
   C. covering the organs with a moist, sterile dressing
   D. replacing the organs in the abdominal cavity

6. How should avulsed or amputated body parts be managed?
   A. They should be packed in ice to increase the amount of time available for reattachment.
   B. They should be transported if fewer than 20 minutes have passed, because this is the time limit for reattachment.
   C. They should be transported with the patient since it may be possible to reattach them.
   D. They should be transported only if they are parts of extremities since other tissue cannot be reattached.

7. Which of the following is an acceptable technique for bandaging open extremity wounds?
   A. Bandage tightly to control bleeding by reducing blood flow to the injured extremity.
   B. Leave the ends of the bandage unsecured so the physician can inspect the wound more easily.
   C. Leave the tips of fingers and toes exposed to permit monitoring of circulation.
   D. Lift the bandage occasionally to check the wound for clotting.

8. The soft tissue injury that produces edema and ecchymosis from crushing of skin and subcutaneous tissues is _____.
   A. an abrasion
   B. an avulsion
   C. a contusion
   D. a laceration

9. A localized collection of blood forming a lump in the tissues is _____.
   A. an ecchymosis
   B. an erythrocyte
   C. a hematoma
   D. a hemothorax

10. When you are managing a patient with a partial avulsion or amputation, you should _____.
    A. apply direct pressure to the skin flap to control bleeding
    B. complete the amputation with sterile scissors
    C. gently straighten and align any skin bridges
    D. leave the part in the position found

11. What is the most important indicator that compartment syndrome may be present?
    A. Altered distal motor and sensory function
    B. Pain out of proportion to physical findings
    C. Presence of paresthesia and pulselessness
    D. Rapid onset of signs and symptoms following extremity trauma

12. Which of the following is an advantage of an adherent over a nonadherent dressing?
    A. Adherent dressings act as a more effective barrier against bacterial contamination.
    B. Adherent dressings are less likely to disturb clots when they are removed from wounds.
    C. Adherent dressings prevent air and fluid movement through the dressing.
    D. Adherent dressings promote clot formation more effectively than nonadherent dressings.

CASE STUDY

You respond to a report of a person injured in a fight at a high school. The patient is a 16-year-old female who is lying on the floor in the cafeteria. A knife wound on the anterolateral surface of her right forearm is spurting bright red blood. The wound is longer than it is deep and has smooth edges. The patient is awake, alert, and very anxious.

1. What type of wound is present?

2. What action should you take to control bleeding from the wound?

3. The wound continues to bleed. What should you do next?

4. Bleeding has been controlled. The patient's skin is pale, cool, and moist. Her respirations are rapid and shallow. The distal pulses in all extremities are weak, and rapid. What should you do now?

5. When you obtain a history from the patient, she tells you she has diabetes mellitus. Why will this be significant during the long-term management of her wound?

46 Burn Injury

READING ASSIGNMENT

Chapter 46, pages 348-382, in *Paramedic Practice Today: Above and Beyond.*

OBJECTIVES

After completing this chapter, you will be able to:
1. Describe the epidemiology, including incidence, mortality and morbidity rates, risk factors, and prevention strategies for the patient with a burn injury.
2. Describe the anatomy and physiology pertinent to burn injuries.
3. Describe the pathophysiologic complications and systemic complications of a burn injury.
4. Identify and describe types of burn injuries, including thermal, inhalational, chemical, and electrical, as well as radiation exposure.
5. Describe the epidemiology of a chemical burn injury and a chemical burn injury to the eye.
6. Describe the specific anatomy and physiology pertinent to a chemical burn injury and a chemical burn injury to the eye.
7. Describe the pathophysiology of a chemical burn injury, including types of chemicals and their burning processes and a chemical burn injury to the eye.
8. Identify and describe the depth classifications of a chemical burn injury.
9. Identify and describe the severity of a chemical burn injury.
10. Describe considerations that affect management and prognosis of the patient with a chemical burn injury and a chemical burn injury to the eye.
11. Discuss mechanisms of burn injury and conditions associated with a chemical burn injury.
12. Describe the management of a chemical burn injury and a chemical burn injury to the eye, including airway and ventilation, circulation, pharmacologic and nonpharmacologic treatment, transport considerations, and psychological support and communication strategies.
13. Describe the epidemiology of an electrical burn injury.
14. Describe the specific anatomy and physiology pertinent to an electrical burn injury.
15. Describe the pathophysiology of an electrical burn injury.
16. Identify and describe the depth classifications of an electrical burn injury.
17. Identify and describe the severity of an electrical burn injury.
18. Describe considerations that affect management and prognosis of the patient with an electrical burn injury.
19. Discuss mechanisms of burn injury and conditions associated with an electrical burn injury.
20. Describe the management of an electrical burn injury, including airway and ventilation, circulation, pharmacologic and nonpharmacologic treatment, transport considerations, and psychological support and communication strategies.
21. Describe special considerations for a pediatric patient with a burn injury.
22. Identify and describe the depth classifications of a radiation exposure.
23. Identify and describe the severity of a radiation exposure.
24. Describe considerations that affect management and prognosis of the patient with a radiation exposure.
25. Discuss mechanisms of burn injury associated with a radiation exposure.
26. Discuss conditions associated with a radiation exposure.
27. Describe the management of a radiation exposure, including airway and ventilation, circulation, pharmacologic and nonpharmacologic treatment, transport considerations, and psychological support and communication strategies.

CHAPTER SUMMARY

- Approximately 1 million people are burned each year in the United States.
- The majority of burn patients are male.
- Persons at high risk for sustaining burn injuries include infants (10% of all patients), the elderly (14%), and those in high-risk occupations.
- Burns are categorized by their cause, size (BSA involved), and depth.
- The major categories of burns are thermal, chemical, radiation, and electrical.
- BSA, although difficult to estimate in the field, is approximated by using the rule of nines or the Lund-Browder chart. Approximating the size of the burn is critical.
- Burn depth is categorized as superficial thickness (first degree), partial thickness (second degree), or full thickness (third degree).
- The skin is the largest organ in the body and is quite complex. It exists in layers and, as such, these layers correlate with the depth of burn injury. The skin is responsible for, among other functions, controlling

- body temperature, preventing the invasion of infectious organisms, and maintaining water balance.
- Burns that are partial or full thickness have three zones of injury: (1) zone of coagulation and necrosis (innermost), (2) zone of ischemia (middle, outer zone), and (3) zone of hyperemia (outermost zone). These zones correlate with the potential for spontaneous healing (zone of hyperemia), the potential for spontaneous healing but at risk for complete loss of integrity (zone of ischemia), and loss requiring surgical treatment if larger than 1% or 2% TBSA (zone of coagulation and necrosis).
- Superficial burns are painful, nonblistered, and best represented by the common sunburn.
- Partial-thickness burns are pink, moist appearing, quite painful, and blistered and have an intact blood supply.
- Full-thickness burns have a grayish-white appearance, are insensate, and have lost blood supply.
- Inhalation injury (commonly called *smoke inhalation*) is a serious injury pattern in which the upper and lower airways are compromised by the inhalation of byproducts of combustion. Alone, significant inhalation injury results in a 30% mortality rate.
- The signs of inhalation injury include cough (productive and nonproductive), tachypnea, and hypoxemia.
- The symptoms of inhalation injury include dyspnea, air hunger, and fatigue.
- The treatment of inhalation injury includes high-flow oxygen and intubation if necessary.
- Early intubation is the key to preventing early, devastating loss of airway.
- The treatment of the cutaneous component of burn injury is basic. It involves dry, clean, and sterile dressings; IV fluid resuscitation for burns larger than 15% TBSA; and pain control.
- With the exception of tar and asphalt or chemical burns, lavage or irrigation of burns should not be done. This will result in hypothermia, which substantially increases morbidity in burn patients.
- Cutaneous exposure to chemicals causes varying burn depth, primarily from two factors: pH of the chemical and length of exposure time.
- Chemicals are broadly categorized as either acidic (pH less than 7) or alkaline (pH greater than 7).
- A basic understanding of chemistry is essential for treating chemical burns.
- Chemical and tar burns are the rare exceptions to the "no irrigation" rule in burn care. Chemicals should be diluted to prevent ongoing burn injury. Tar and asphalt burns are cooled with water to prevent ongoing, deep burn injury when trapped heat is contained beneath a blanket of molten material.
- The inhalation of chemicals can cause serious lung injury. Whether trapped within a building containing chemicals in gaseous form or in the outdoors with a widespread chemical cloud, inhalation remains a significant threat to those involved in the initial incident and those responding to the incident.
- Other manners of exposure to chemicals include absorption, ingestion, and injection.
- Electrical injuries may occur in the home, as part of occupational hazards, and in recreation.
- The most common cause of immediate death with electrical injury is ventricular fibrillation.
- Electrical injuries are categorized as either high or low voltage. Energy of less than 1000 V is low voltage, and energy greater than 1000 V is high voltage.
- An example of low voltage is household current; an example of high voltage is lightning.
- Low-voltage injuries cause flash burns and minor muscle or cutaneous injury from direct contact. High-voltage injuries cause devastating muscle, bone, and nerve injury. Long-term effects include kidney damage, paralysis, blindness, and hearing loss.
- High-voltage injuries are treated with spinal and long bone immobilization and aggressive fluid resuscitation.
- Pediatric burn injuries are common. Infants alone account for 10% of all burn injuries (100,000) annually.
- Among the most common burn injuries to children are those caused by scalding hot liquids.
- The dermal portion of the skin of children is much thinner than that of adults. This puts children at increased risk for deep burn injury.
- Fluid resuscitation in children must be undertaken with caution. Children are at significant risk for fluid overload compared with healthy adults because of limited cardiovascular reserve.
- Burn shock is a unique form of shock best characterized as a distributive shock. Its hallmark is capillary leak. Intravascular loss of fluid is in the form of plasma, leaked through capillaries, into the third space.
- Burn shock is treated with fluid resuscitation in a staged manner. That is, fluids are replaced at a rate roughly equal to the rate of loss into the surrounding tissues. Administration is then slowed as fluid moves back into the intravascular space.
- Fluid resuscitation for burn injury is undertaken with a balanced salt solution. The most commonly used fluid is Ringer's lactate.
- More fluid in burns is not necessarily better. During resuscitation of the burn patient, fluids should be given in a controlled manner, never as a wide-open therapy.
- The formula used for adult burn resuscitation is known as the *consensus formula*.
- The consensus formula for burn resuscitation calls for 2 to 4 mL/kg/TBSAB of IV fluid given over the first 24 hours after the burn injury.
- Rarely will a significant amount of fluid be given in the prehospital setting.
- Paramedics should understand that an IV rate of more than 250 mL/hour is rarely needed.
- Radiation-associated burn injuries are rare but pose an exceptional danger to both the patient and provider.
- The three types of radioactive particles are alpha, beta, and gamma.
- Of the three types of radioactive particles, gamma radiation is the most dangerous.
- All types of radioactive particles exist in the communities paramedics serve.

- The treatment of radiation exposure focuses on the principles of decreased exposure time, removal from the source, and decontamination. For all types of radiation, aggregate quantity should be limited.
- Pain is a significant problem with all types of burn injury. Controlling pain is an important step in the care of the burn patient.
- The preferred route of administration in the acutely injured burn patient is IV. Subcutaneous and intramuscular routes can be used but are less effective because of the poor perfusion of these tissues.
- The following types of burns should be referred to a qualified burn center for care:
  - Partial-thickness burns of more than 10% TBSA
  - Burns involving the hands, feet, genitalia, face, perineum, or major joints
  - Third-degree burns in any age group
  - Electrical burns, including lightning injury
  - Chemical burns
  - Inhalation injury (with or without burns)
  - Burns with associated trauma of any type
  - Burns in patients with special social, emotional, or long-term rehabilitative needs
  - Burns in children if the current institution lacks qualified personnel or equipment necessary to care for children
- Care at the burn center is a continuation of the care begun in the prehospital setting.
- In addition to ongoing fluid resuscitation, specific wound care (including surgery if needed), nutritional support, occupational and physical therapy, and psychological care are provided by burn centers.
- The goal in the treatment of the burn patient is to restore function, at all levels, to as close to the preburn injury state as possible.
- The surgical care of burn wounds includes simple wound care with debridement; surgical excision of wounds with skin grafting; and reconstructive surgery to restore the normal contour of the body, function of motion, and improve cosmesis.
- One of the key goals of the ABA and the burn centers of the world is prevention. The overwhelming majority of burn injuries are preventable.

MATCHING

1. Match the description of the burn with its depth.

   _____ Burned areas are red and painful. They blanch under pressure. No blisters are present.

   _____ Burn is gray, white, or charred. Looks thickened and leathery. Pain is absent.

   _____ Burn is salmon-pink and moist. Severe pain is present. Blisters may be present.

   A. Superficial
   B. Partial thickness
   C. Full thickness

2. Classify these burns as minor, moderate, or critical.

   _____ 3% third degree caused by an electrical shock

   _____ 9% third degree, excluding face, feet, hands, and genitalia

   _____ 15% first degree caused by exposure to the sun

   _____ 20% second degree in a patient with a femur fracture

   _____ 35% second degree, including face and hands

   A. Critical
   B. Minor
   C. Moderate

SHORT ANSWER

1. What are the layers of the skin?

   _____
   _____
   _____
   _____

2. Which skin layer contains the nerve endings, blood vessels, sweat glands, sebaceous glands, and hair follicles?

   _____
   _____
   _____
   _____

3. List three problems that can result from loss of a large amount of skin surface because of a burn.

   _____
   _____
   _____
   _____

4. Using the rule of nines, indicate the percentage of the total body surface area that each of the following parts comprises in an adult.

   _____ Head
   _____ Anterior trunk
   _____ Posterior trunk
   _____ Each upper extremity
   _____ Each lower extremity
   _____ Perineum

5. Using the rule of nines, indicate the percentage of the total body surface area comprised by the following in a 1-year-old child.

   _____ Head
   _____ Anterior trunk
   _____ Posterior trunk
   _____ Each upper extremity
   _____ Each lower extremity
   _____ Perineum

6. A patient's palm represents approximately what percentage of his or her total body surface area?

_____

_____

_____

7. A 34-year-old male has burns on the front and back of both arms from the shoulder to the fingertips. Approximately what percentage of his body surface area is burned?

_____

_____

_____

_____

8. A 6-month-old infant is rescued from a house fire. Physical examination reveals burns to the anterior aspect of the chest and abdomen. Approximately what percentage of the child's body is burned?

_____

_____

_____

_____

9. A 3-year-old patient has burns covering his back, buttocks, and the posterior aspect of both legs. Approximately what percentage of the child's body is burned?

_____

_____

_____

_____

10. An 80-kg patient has been burned over 70% of his body surface. State the IV fluid you would use to resuscitate him and use the Parkland formula to determine how much fluid this patient should be given during the first 24 hours after he was burned.

_____

_____

_____

11. A 50-kg patient has been burned over 50% of her body surface. How much fluid should be given during the first 8 hours after she was burned?

_____

_____

_____

_____

12. Why is Ringer's lactate preferred to normal saline for management of fluid loss produced by a burn?

_____

_____

_____

_____

13. If a burn patient shows rapid onset of signs of hypovolemic shock after being burned, what should you suspect?

_____

_____

_____

14. A patient has burns on the hands and forearms of both upper extremities. Where should you obtain vascular access? Why?

_____

_____

_____

_____

15. Should the IV or Sub-Q route be used for medication administration to a patient with a large burn? Why or why not?

_____

_____

_____

_____

16. If you suspect that a patient has been injured by contact with an electrical current, what should your first action be?

_____

_____

_____

_____

17. A 33-year-old dockworker had a large amount of dry chemical spilled on him from a ruptured 55-gallon drum. He is complaining of burning pain in his armpits and groin. What should you do?

_____

_____

_____

18. A 16-year-old female was burned on her face, neck, and chest by a gas stove explosion. Her nasal hair is singed, the mucosa of her mouth and pharynx are red and dry, and she is hoarse. What is the most immediate danger facing this patient?

_____

_____

_____

19. A 26-year-old man was injured when a television antenna he was installing came into contact with a power line. His only complaint is slight stiffness of his right arm and leg. Small burns are present on the palm of his right hand and the sole of his right foot. How would you manage this patient?

_____
_____
_____

20. What is the difference between the paths followed through the body by low-voltage and high-voltage current?

_____
_____
_____
_____

21. You respond to a report of an injured person at a house fire. Your patient is a 60-year-old male who was found unconscious in a burning building by the fire department. Why is the patient's loss of consciousness significant?

_____
_____
_____
_____

22. List three questions you should ask if you suspect that a patient may have inhaled smoke or another toxic gas.

_____
_____
_____

23. Why is carbon monoxide toxic?

_____
_____
_____
_____

24. What are the color and odor of carbon monoxide?

_____
_____
_____
_____

25. If a child and an adult are both burned over the same amount of their body surface areas, why does the child not tolerate the burn as well as the adult?

_____
_____
_____
_____

26. If a pediatric patient has burns on the extremities in a "stocking" or "glove" pattern, what problem should you suspect?

_____
_____
_____
_____

27. What is burn shock?

_____
_____
_____
_____

28. What are the three types of radioactive particles.

_____
_____
_____

MULTIPLE CHOICE

1. A 16-year-old female had carbolic acid (phenol) splashed in her eyes during chemistry class. You should immediately _____.
   A. bandage her eyes with moist dressings and transport, because phenol can only be removed at the hospital
   B. flush her eyes with alcohol because phenol is not soluble in water
   C. flush her eyes with sodium bicarbonate solution to neutralize the acid
   D. flush her eyes with water or saline solution

2. A 70-kg patient has suffered burns over 60% of his body surface area. During the first 8 hours after being burned, he should receive _____.
   A. 8400 mL of Ringer's lactate
   B. 8400 mL of normal saline
   C. 16,800 mL of Ringer's lactate
   D. 16,800 mL of normal saline

3. A 22-year-old male has burns on the front and back of both of his legs and arms. Approximately what percentage of his body has been burned?
   A. 18%
   B. 27%
   C. 36%
   D. 54%

4. You are dispatched to "assist the fire department" at the scene of a house fire. When you arrive, you are met by a fire captain, who leads you to the patient. The patient, a 62-year-old male who was exposed to smoke, is sitting on the tailboard of a fire engine receiving oxygen, by simple facemask. The history should include_____.
   A. the duration of the exposure; whether the fire was located in an enclosed space; whether the patient lost consciousness
   B. the material that was burning; the duration of the exposure; whether the fire was located in an enclosed space; whether the patient lost consciousness
   C. the material that was burning; the duration of the exposure; whether the patient lost consciousness
   D. the material that was burning; whether the fire was located in an enclosed space

5. A 4-year-old child was rescued from a house fire. Physical examination reveals burns of the entire head, anterior thorax, and anterior abdomen. What percentage of the child's body is burned?
   A. 27%
   B. 33%
   C. 36%
   D. 45%

6. A patient sustained second-degree burns to her entire right leg in an auto fire. She also has an open fracture of the right femur. The severity of her burn is:
   A. critical
   B. either critical or moderate depending on her age
   C. minor
   D. moderate

7. A patient has sustained a 30% to 40% second-degree burn in a house fire. In the prehospital setting the most appropriate management for the burn wound would be to _____
   A. apply an antibiotic ointment to lessen pain and reduce the risk of infection
   B. cover the injury with a dry, clean sheet to reduce pain and limit contamination
   C. rupture all blisters immediately to speed healing of the wound
   D. wash the burn immediately with cool water to stop the burning process

8. An area equal in size to the area of a patient's palm is approximately _____.
   A. 1% of the patient's body surface area
   B. 2% of the patient's body surface area
   C. 3% of the patient's body surface area
   D. 4% of the patient's body surface area

9. Children and infants who are burned are more likely to suffer significant fluid loss than adults because _____.
   A. a higher proportion of their body weight consists of water
   B. a lower proportion of their body weight consists of water
   C. their body surface area is larger in proportion to their body volume, compared to adults
   D. their body surface area is smaller in proportion to their body volume, compared to adults

10. Which of the following would be a moderate burn?
    A. 5% first-degree burn of the face associated with hoarseness and drooling
    B. 5% third-degree burn excluding the face, feet, hands, and genitalia
    C. 5% third-degree burn including the face and hands
    D. 20% second-degree burn in a patient with a history of diabetes mellitus

11. A 28-year-old employee of an agricultural chemical firm had a large amount of an unknown dry chemical spilled over her from a broken bag. She complains of difficulty breathing. A safety shower is available. You are 30 minutes from a hospital. You should _____.
    A. brush away as much of the chemical as possible, and then transport to the hospital
    B. brush away as much of the chemical as possible, and then wash with water
    C. immediately wash off the chemical with alcohol
    D. immediately wash off the chemical with water

12. A patient has skin burns caused by dry lime. Your first step should be to _____.
    A. brush away as much of the lime as possible before washing
    B. remove the lime by washing with a dilute solution of vinegar or another acid
    C. remove the lime by washing with alcohol
    D. wash the area with large amounts of water

13. A 6-month-old infant is rescued from a house fire. Physical examination reveals burns to the child's entire head and the anterior aspect of the chest and abdomen. Approximately what percent of his total body surface area has been burned?
    A. 18%
    B. 27%
    C. 36%
    D. 54%

14. An 8-year-old male was found in a burned house. He is not burned, but is unconscious and unresponsive. His nasal hairs and eyebrows are not singed. There is no apparent injury to the oral mucosa. Breath sounds are present and equal bilaterally without crackles, rhonchi, or wheezing. Radial pulses are present, strong, and regular. Capillary refill is less than 2 seconds. Vital signs are: P—130 beats/min weak, regular; R—6 breaths/min shallow, gasping, irregular; BP—128/30 mm Hg. What is his problem?
    A. Carbon monoxide poisoning
    B. Hypovolemic shock
    C. Pulmonary burns
    D. Upper airway burn

15. The patient in the previous question should be managed by giving _____.
    A. 60% oxygen via simple facemask
    B. 90% oxygen via bag-mask device
    C. 90% oxygen via nasal cannula
    D. 90% oxygen via nonrebreather mask

16. A 26-year-old male received an electrical shock while trying to remove his son's kite from a power line. He is awake and alert. His only injuries appear to be small burns on his right hand and right foot. You should _____.
    A. advise the patient to go to the hospital immediately by private vehicle because he could develop an infection
    B. advise the patient to make an appointment to see his physician for a follow-up visit within the next few days
    C. immediately transport the patient to the hospital
    D. tell the patient he has no need for medical attention if he keeps the burns clean and well-bandaged

17. A power company lineman came in contact with a high-voltage source while working on a transformer bank. He apparently was thrown several feet. He has obvious electrical burns on his hands. Other injuries that should be anticipated could include _____.
    A. cardiopulmonary arrest or cardiac dysrhythmias and spinal fractures
    B. cardiopulmonary arrest, dysrhythmia, extremity orthopedic injuries, and spinal fractures
    C. extremity fractures and dislocations and cardiac dysrhythmias
    D. spinal and extremity fractures

18. A burn that is painful, salmon-pink, moist, and blistered would be classified as _____.
    A. first degree (superficial)
    B. second degree (partial thickness)
    C. third degree (full thickness)
    D. fourth degree (full thickness)

19. According to the rule of nines _____.
    A. an adult's head is 9% of the body surface area and an infant's head is 18%
    B. an adult's head is 18% of the body surface area and an infant's head is 9%
    C. both an adult's head and an infant's head are 9% of the body surface area
    D. both an adult's head and an infant's head are 18% of the body surface area

20. What is the first step to take when dealing with an accident in which high-voltage power lines have fallen onto a car?
    A. Get help from trained power company personnel.
    B. Ground the power lines with another wire.
    C. Use a nonconductive rope to remove the power lines from the car.
    D. Use the ambulance public address system to tell the patients to jump from the vehicle.

21. What is the prehospital treatment for a chemical burn of the eyes?
    A. Cover the eyes with moistened sterile dressings and transport.
    B. Flush out the eyes with an appropriate chemical antidote, such as vinegar or baking soda solution.
    C. Flush out the eyes with large amounts of water or saline solution.
    D. Transport immediately since nothing else should be placed in the eyes until the chemical is identified.

22. What problems may a patient who has extensive burns develop?
    A. Excessive loss of fluid, leading to hypovolemic shock; peripheral vasoconstriction, leading to decreased body temperature; infection by bacteria
    B. Inability to regulate body temperature, leading to hypothermia; peripheral vasodilation from pain, leading to neurogenic shock; infection by bacteria
    C. Infection by bacteria; extensive fluid loss, leading to hypovolemic shock; inability to regulate body temperature, leading to hypothermia
    D. Infection by bacteria; peripheral vasoconstriction from pain, leading to neurogenic shock; inability to regulate body temperature and hypothermia secondary to peripheral vasoconstriction

23. Commercial gel (and wet dressings) may be applied to burned areas covering _____.
    A. 33% or less of the body surface area
    B. 9% or less of the body surface area
    C. no more than 5% of the body surface area
    D. up to 21% of the body surface area

24. Which type of radiation causes the most damage to human tissues?
    A. Alpha
    B. Beta
    C. Gamma
    D. Ionizing

You have been dispatched to a report of an explosion and fire with injuries in a residential area. When you arrive, you are met by a fire department officer who tells you the patient is a male in his late 30s who apparently was attempting to work on the furnace in the basement of his home when an explosion occurred followed by a fire.

The patient is unresponsive to verbal or painful stimuli. However, a gag reflex is present. His respirations are rapid and labored. Inspiratory stridor is present. Burns of the face and neck are present with singeing of the eyebrows. Chest auscultation reveals wheezing and crackles throughout the lung fields. A weak, rapid carotid pulse is present. Burns also are present on the anterior chest and abdomen, circumferentially on the left upper extremity from the shoulder to the fingertips, circumferentially on the right forearm, and on the anterior aspects of both thighs.

1. What is your highest priority in managing this patient?

   _____
   _____
   _____
   _____

2. What other problem should you assume is present while you deal with your highest priority for management?

   _____
   _____
   _____
   _____

3. Because the patient has crackles and wheezes in the lung fields, would you administer a diuretic? Why or why not?

   _____
   _____
   _____
   _____

4. An oximeter placed on the patient indicates an SpO_2 of 100%. What is the significance of this finding?

   _____
   _____
   _____
   _____

5. The patient's pulse rate continues to rise steadily. His blood pressure is 76/52 mm Hg. What is the significance of this finding?

   _____
   _____
   _____
   _____

47 Head and Face Trauma

READING ASSIGNMENT

Chapter 47, pages 383-423, in *Paramedic Practice Today: Above and Beyond*.

OBJECTIVES

After completing this chapter, you will be able to:
1. Describe the etiology, history, and physical findings of facial injuries.
2. Using the mechanism of injury, patient history, and physical examination findings, develop a treatment plan for a patient with facial injuries.
3. Describe the etiology, history, and physical findings of eye injuries.
4. Using the mechanism of injury, patient history, and physical examination findings, develop a treatment plan for a patient with an eye injury.
5. Describe the etiology, history, and physical findings of ear injuries.
6. Using the mechanism of injury, patient history, and physical examination findings, develop a treatment plan for a patient with an ear injury.
7. Describe the etiology, history, and physical findings of neck injuries.
8. Using the mechanism of injury, patient history, and physical examination findings, develop a treatment plan for a patient with a neck injury.
9. Explain anatomy and relate physiology of the central nervous system to head injuries.
10. Distinguish between head injury and brain injury.
11. Describe the etiology, history, and physical findings of a skull fracture.
12. Using the patient history and physical examination findings, develop a treatment plan for a patient with a skull fracture.
13. Explain the pathophysiology of head and brain injuries.
14. Predict head injuries on the basis of mechanism of injury.
15. Explain the pathophysiology of increasing intracranial pressure and the process involved with each of the levels of increase.
16. Describe the etiology, history, and physical findings of each of the following:
    - Concussion
    - Diffuse axonal injury
    - Cerebral contusion
    - Epidural hematoma
    - Subdural hematoma
    - Intracerebral hemorrhage
    - Subarachnoid hemorrhage

17. Using the patient history and physical examination findings, develop a treatment plan for a patient with any of the following:
    - Concussion
    - Diffuse axonal injury
    - Cerebral contusion
    - Epidural hematoma
    - Subdural hematoma
    - Intracerebral hemorrhage
    - Subarachnoid hemorrhage
18. Develop a management plan for the removal of a helmet for a head-injured patient.

CHAPTER SUMMARY

- Facial injuries may be the result of blunt or penetrating trauma. Airbag deployment can cause abrasions to the face, neck, and upper chest.
- An orbital fracture is any fracture that involves the bony cavity containing the eyeball. Orbital fractures may occur as an isolated injury or in conjunction with another injury, such as a zygomatic fracture or fractures of the midface.
- The nose is the most commonly fractured bone of the face. Most nasal fractures are the result of blunt trauma.
- Zygomatic fractures are common and are usually the result of an assault or MVC. Maxillary or midface fractures are usually a combination of fractures involving several structures of the face. Significant force is required to fracture this area of the face.
- Mandibular fractures are common. They are caused by blunt trauma to the face, most commonly domestic violence and contact sports. A mandibular fracture also can be caused by penetrating trauma, such as gunshot wounds, blast injuries, or industrial injuries (e.g., chain saw).
- Two million brain injuries occur every year. Most brain injuries are mild, with a ratio of 8:1:1 (mild/moderate/severe). Assessment is the key to proper care and evaluation of the injury. Correctly identifying and prioritizing injuries can greatly improve patient outcome. Appropriately treat injuries, always assessing airway, breathing, circulation, and deficits. Never occlude the nose or ear, especially if CSF fluid leaks are present.
- In loss of consciousness with facial or head injuries, protect the spinal cord.
- If in doubt, treat the patient for a traumatic brain injury.

SHORT ANSWER

1. State the primary function of each of the following structures:

   Cerebrum:_____

   Cerebellum:_____

   Brainstem:_____

2. Cerebral perfusion pressure =

   _____ minus _____

3. What is Cushing's triad? What problem does Cushing's triad indicate?

   _____
   _____
   _____
   _____

4. Why does controlled hyperventilation lower increased intracranial pressure?

   _____
   _____
   _____
   _____

5. What are the risks associated with overly aggressive hyperventilation of a patient with a head injury?

   _____
   _____
   _____
   _____

6. What is the significance of a rising pulse rate and a decreased blood pressure in an adult patient with a closed head injury?

   _____
   _____
   _____
   _____

7. Why should levels of consciousness be described in terms of the patient's responses to the environment rather than with terms such as *stuporous, lethargic,* or *obtunded*?

   _____
   _____
   _____
   _____

8. What is the IV fluid and the infusion rate that should be used in the management of a patient with an isolated head injury? Why?

   _____
   _____
   _____
   _____

9. Complete the following chart by indicating whether the pulse rate and blood pressure will increase or decrease.

	Pulse Rate	Blood Pressure
Head injury		
Neurogenic shock		
Hypovolemia		

10. List four signs of a basilar skull fracture.

    _____
    _____
    _____
    _____

11. Why should nasogastric tube placement or nasotracheal intubation not be attempted on a patient who has signs of a basilar skull fracture or mid-face trauma?

    _____
    _____
    _____

12. What is decorticate posturing?

    _____
    _____
    _____
    _____

13. What is decerebrate posturing?

    _____
    _____
    _____
    _____

14. What beneficial effect does mannitol have in the management of a patient with cerebral edema?

    _____
    _____
    _____
    _____

15. Why is mannitol always administered through an IV set that contains an in-line filter?

    _____
    _____
    _____

16. Why should pressure never be applied to a lacerated eyeball?

    _____
    _____
    _____
    _____

17. Why should both eyes be covered when an eye injury is bandaged?

_____
_____
_____
_____

18. A 22-year-old male was struck in the left eye with a fist during a fight. He is experiencing heavy discharge from the left nostril and is complaining of numbness over the left side of the upper lip. He also states that he has double vision. When you ask him to look up, the upward gaze of his left eye is paralyzed. What is wrong with this patient?

_____
_____
_____
_____

19. While examining a patient who was struck in the right eye with a tennis ball, you notice blood behind the cornea in the anterior chamber of the eye. What is this problem called?

_____
_____
_____
_____

20. Why is the problem described in the previous question significant?

_____
_____
_____
_____

21. A 26-year-old male had chemicals splashed in his eyes. You have a number of chemical antidotes available, including alcohol, sodium bicarbonate, and acetic acid. What should you do? Why?

_____
_____
_____
_____

22. What are your principal concerns when you are managing a patient with maxillofacial trauma?

_____
_____
_____
_____

23. At the scene of a motor vehicle crash, a police officer presents you with several of the patient's teeth and a dental bridge that he found in the floorboard of the vehicle. What should you do with these? Why?

_____
_____
_____
_____

24. A patient has suffered a laceration that involves a jugular vein. What special concern is associated with this injury? How do you manage it?

_____
_____
_____
_____

25. Describe each of the three types of Le Fort fractures.

_____
_____
_____
_____

26. Identify the structures that a light ray passes through on its way from the outside of the eye to the retina.

_____
_____
_____
_____

27. A patient who was working in a machine shop without proper protective eyewear felt a sharp pain in his right eye followed by an onset of blurred vision. You cannot see any obvious trauma when you examine the eye. What problem do you suspect?

_____
_____
_____
_____

28. Your initial assessment of a trauma patient reveals a slow, bounding pulse; rapid, deep respirations; unresponsiveness to painful stimuli; and unequal pupils. What problem do you suspect?

_____
_____
_____
_____

MULTIPLE CHOICE

1. A 15-year-old male has a pellet gun wound to his right eye. There is an obvious injury to the sclera through which a jelly-like material is escaping. You should apply a _____.
   A. loose dressing to both eyes
   B. loose dressing to the right eye
   C. pressure dressing to both eyes
   D. pressure dressing to the right eye

2. At a construction site, a patient has been struck on the head by a piece of falling pipe. He is unconscious and unresponsive. The left pupil is dilated and unreactive. The right pupil is mid-position and reacts sluggishly. Peripheral pulses are slow and weak. Respirations are shallow and irregular. You should _____.
   A. open the airway with cervical spine control, administer high-concentration oxygen via nonrebreather mask, stabilize the spine, and transport
   B. open the airway with cervical spine control, insert an oral airway, administer high-concentration oxygen via nonrebreather mask, and transport
   C. open the airway with cervical spine control, insert an oral airway, hyperventilate with oxygen using a bag-mask device at 24 to 30 breaths/min, stabilize the spine, and transport
   D. open the airway with cervical spine control, intubate the trachea, ventilate with oxygen using a bag-mask device at 20 to 24 breaths/min, stabilize the spine, and transport.

3. A patient involved in an automobile accident was initially unconscious. As you were evaluating him, he regained consciousness and was awake, alert, and oriented. En route to the hospital, however, his level of consciousness began to decrease. What injury would most likely be responsible for his condition?
   A. Cerebral contusion
   B. Concussion
   C. Epidural hematoma
   D. Subdural hematoma

4. You respond to a report of an injured person at the university's recreation center. A 19-year-old female was struck in the eye by the ball during a racquetball game. There is blood in the anterior chamber between the cornea and the iris. This injury is called a _____.
   A. blow-out fracture
   B. detached retina
   C. hyphema
   D. subconjunctival hemorrhage

5. Which of the following is usually the earliest sign of an expanding intracranial mass lesion?
   A. A unilateral fixed, dilated pupil
   B. Alterations in consciousness
   C. Decorticate or decerebrate posturing
   D. Rapid, deep respirations

6. The brainstem functions primarily as the _____.
   A. coordination center for posture, balance, and equilibrium
   B. regulator of involuntary activity such as respiration and heart rate
   C. speech center
   D. vision center

7. When you are managing a patient with maxillofacial trauma, your first consideration should be that the patient may have _____.
   A. a mandibular fracture
   B. broken or avulsed teeth
   C. cervical spine injuries
   D. lacerations of the tongue and lips

8. Appropriate treatment for a patient who has clear fluid flowing from his ears following a hard blow to the head would be to _____.
   A. cover the ears with a loose, sterile dressing
   B. irrigate the ears with Ringer's solution
   C. pack the ears to stop the flow
   D. suction as much fluid as possible out of the ears

9. The most reliable indication of a head-injured patient's condition is the patient's _____.
   A. blood pressure
   B. level of consciousness
   C. pulse rate
   D. respiratory rate and pattern

10. Which of the following statements best describes *decerebrate* posturing?
    A. Extension of the lower extremities; extension and external rotation of the upper extremities
    B. Extension of the lower extremities; flexion of the upper extremities
    C. Flexion of the lower extremities; extension and external rotation of the upper extremities
    D. Flexion of the lower extremities; flexion of the upper extremities

11. Which of the following statements best describes *decorticate* posturing?
    A. Extension of the lower extremities; extension and external rotation of the upper extremities
    B. Extension of the lower extremities; flexion of the upper extremities
    C. Flexion of the lower extremities; extension and external rotation of the upper extremities
    D. Flexion of the lower extremities; flexion of the upper extremities

12. The elements of the Glasgow Coma Scale include _____.
    A. eye opening; motor response; verbal response
    B. motor response; blood pressure; pulse rate
    C. respiratory pattern; pulse rate; blood pressure
    D. verbal response; respiratory pattern; blood pressure

13. A 16-year-old female had carbolic acid (phenol) splashed in her eyes during chemistry laboratory. You should immediately _____.
    A. cover her eyes with moist dressings and transport, because phenol can only be removed at the hospital
    B. flush her eyes with alcohol, because phenol is more soluble in alcohol than in water
    C. flush her eyes with baking soda solution to neutralize the carbolic acid
    D. flush her eyes with water or saline solution

14. A 23-year-old oil field worker was struck on the head by a falling piece of pipe. The impact split his hardhat. Brain tissue is protruding through an open fracture of the right parietal area. You would manage this patient by _____.
    A. applying a sterile dressing and a pressure bandage and giving high-concentration oxygen
    B. applying a sterile dressing without pressure and restricting motion of the patient's spine
    C. irrigating the wound with saline solution and then applying direct pressure to control bleeding
    D. not treating the wound, opening the airway, giving high-concentration oxygen, and transporting immediately

15. Your patient received a blow to his head. He now is conscious, but his friends say he was unconscious for approximately 2 minutes. He cannot remember the events surrounding the accident. The patient probably has suffered _____.
    A. a cerebral contusion
    B. a concussion
    C. an epidural hematoma
    D. a subdural hematoma

16. A patient has a fishhook protruding from his right eye. The object should be _____.
    A. covered with a pressure dressing
    B. left unbandaged and unstabilized
    C. protected with a cup
    D. removed immediately

17. Your patient has a foreign body on the surface of his eye. How should you attempt to manage this object initially?
    A. Ask the patient to rub his eye vigorously.
    B. Attempt to blow the object out of the eye.
    C. Close both of the patient's eyes and patch them.
    D. Gently wash the eye with water or saline solution.

18. You are called to see a patient with a closed head injury. The patient is pale, cool, and sweaty. Radial pulses are absent. The carotid pulse is weak, and rapid. You should recall that _____.
    A. a patient cannot lose enough blood inside his skull to cause shock; the patient is bleeding elsewhere
    B. head injuries often produce shock from blood loss within the skull
    C. shock associated with closed head injury seldom causes complications
    D. the signs and symptoms of hypovolemic and neurogenic shock are similar and easily confused

19. A patient's jugular vein has been lacerated in a knife fight. What should you do?
    A. Apply a tight pressure bandage completely encircling the neck to ensure adequate control of the heavy bleeding.
    B. Apply an occlusive dressing to the laceration to prevent possible air embolism.
    C. Compress the carotid artery on the injured side to reduce blood return through the jugular vein and slow bleeding.
    D. Locate and clamp the ends of the bleeding jugular vein since a pressure dressing is unlikely to control the bleeding.

20. A patient suffered a facial injury that resulted in his right eye being partly extruded from its orbit. The eye should be _____.
    A. covered with a moist dressing and bandaged tightly to prevent excessive movement
    B. covered with a moist dressing and protected with a loose bandage or cup
    C. replaced into the socket and then dressed and bandaged
    D. washed continuously with saline solution while the patient is transported to the hospital

21. You are called to the scene of a motor vehicle crash in which a car rear-ended a tractor-trailer. The driver of the car is unconscious and slumped over the steering wheel. Her face is covered with blood and is grossly swollen. Which problem should you consider first as you begin to assess and evaluate this patient?
    A. Cervical spine injury
    B. Head injury
    C. Mandibular fracture with loss of teeth
    D. Skull fracture

22. A 30-year-old male fell from a second-story window and landed on his head. He is unconscious and unresponsive. His pupils are unequal. Vital signs are: BP—260/140 mm Hg; P—42 beats/min strong, regular; R—10 breaths/min shallow, irregular. The most appropriate treatment would be to _____.
    A. open and maintain the airway and transport
    B. open and maintain the airway, immobilize the spine, and transport
    C. open and maintain the airway, immobilize the spine, give high-concentration oxygen, and transport
    D. open and maintain the airway, immobilize the spine, give oxygen by controlled hyperventilation, and transport

23. What is the best indicator of a head-injured patient's condition?
    A. Blood pressure
    B. Level of consciousness
    C. Pulse
    D. Pupils

Chapter **47** **Head and Face Trauma**

24. Which set of vital signs leads you to suspect increased intracranial pressure?
    A. P—40 beats/min; BP—210/110 mm Hg; R—36 breaths/min deep, irregular
    B. P—100 beats/min; BP—140/70 mm Hg; R—20 breaths/min shallow, regular
    C. P—120 beats/min; BP—100/60 mm Hg; R—16 breaths/min normal, regular
    D. P—140 beats/min; BP—84/60 mm Hg; R—26 breaths/min shallow, regular

25. A patient with periorbital ecchymosis ("raccoon eyes") would be suspected of having _____.
    A. a basilar skull fracture
    B. an epidural hematoma
    C. an intracerebral hematoma
    D. a subdural hematoma

26. What structure regulates the amount of light entering the eye?
    A. Cornea
    B. Iris
    C. Optic nerve
    D. Retina

27. The covering of the brain located directly against the brain's surface is the _____.
    A. arachnoid
    B. dura mater
    C. pia mater
    D. subarachnoid

28. Which structure coordinates posture and balance?
    A. Cerebellum
    B. Cerebrum
    C. Medulla
    D. Spinal cord

29. A patient who is bleeding into his cranial cavity but who has no other injuries would be expected to have _____.
    A. decreased blood pressure, rapid pulse rate
    B. decreased blood pressure, slow pulse rate
    C. increased blood pressure, rapid pulse rate
    D. increased blood pressure, slow pulse rate

30. Controlled hyperventilation is effective in managing severe cases of increased intracranial pressure (ICP) because it _____.
    A. decreases the $PaCO_2$, which will cause cerebral vasoconstriction and decreased ICP
    B. increases the $PaCO_2$, which will cause cerebral vasodilation and improved blood flow
    C. increases the $PaCO_2$, which will sedate the patient and decrease the probability of seizures
    D. increases the PaO_2, which will prevent cerebral edema

CASE STUDIES

Case one

A patient who was struck on the head lost consciousness immediately. By the time EMS arrived on the scene, he had regained consciousness and seemed to be fine except for a scalp laceration in the left temporal region. En route to the hospital, he began to become drowsy. He vomited, experienced about a minute of seizure activity, and became unconscious. His left pupil dilated and became unreactive to light.

1. What problem is this patient most likely to have?
   _____

2. Does this problem usually result from an injury to an artery or a vein?
   _____
   _____
   _____
   _____

3. Why is this problem commonly associated with injuries to the temporal area of the head?
   _____
   _____
   _____
   _____

4. What is the significance of the patient's losing consciousness initially, regaining consciousness, and then once again becoming unconscious?

_____
_____
_____
_____

5. Why is the patient's left pupil dilated and unreactive?

_____
_____
_____
_____

6. What changes would you anticipate seeing in the pulse and blood pressure?

_____
_____
_____
_____

Case two

A nursing home patient fell and struck his head approximately 1 week ago. He did not experience loss of consciousness and at the time seemed to have no significant injuries. Earlier today he complained of a headache. Over a period of several minutes he developed slurred speech and weakness on the right side of his body.

1. What problem do you suspect?

_____

2. Does this problem result from an injury to an artery or a vein?

_____
_____
_____
_____

3. Why do signs and symptoms of this problem tend to develop more slowly than with the disease process presented in Case One?

_____
_____
_____
_____

4. Why are the elderly particularly prone to a slow onset of signs and symptoms with the disease process presented in this case?

_____
_____
_____
_____

5. Which side of the patient's brain is being affected by his injury?

_____
_____
_____
_____

48 Spinal Trauma

READING ASSIGNMENT

Chapter 48, pages 424-467, in *Paramedic Practice Today: Above and Beyond*.

OBJECTIVES

After completing this chapter, you will be able to:

1. Describe the incidence, morbidity, and mortality rates of spinal injuries in the trauma patient.
2. Describe the anatomy and physiology of the following structures related to spinal injuries:
   - Cervical
   - Thoracic
   - Lumbar
   - Sacrum
   - Coccyx
   - Spinal cord
   - Nerve tract
   - Dermatome
3. Predict spinal injuries on the basis of mechanism of injury.
4. Describe the pathophysiology of spinal injuries.
5. Explain traumatic and nontraumatic spinal injuries.
6. Describe the assessment findings associated with spinal injuries.
7. Integrate pathophysiologic principles to the assessment of a patient with a spinal injury.
8. Differentiate spinal injuries on the basis of assessment and history.
9. Formulate a field impression on the basis of assessment findings.
10. Develop a patient management plan on the basis of field impression.
11. Describe the assessment findings associated with traumatic spinal injuries.
12. Describe the management of spinal injuries.
13. Integrate pathophysiologic principles to the assessment of a patient with a traumatic spinal injury.
14. Describe the pathophysiology of traumatic spinal injury related to the following:
    - Spinal shock
    - Neurogenic shock
    - Tetraplegia and paraplegia
    - Incomplete cord injury and cord syndromes
      - Central cord syndrome
      - Anterior cord syndrome
      - Brown-Séquard syndrome
      - Cauda equina syndrome
      - Conus medullaris syndrome
      - Spinal cord injury without radiologic abnormality
15. Differentiate traumatic and nontraumatic spinal injuries on the basis of assessment and history.
16. Describe the pathophysiology of nontraumatic spinal injury, including the following:
    - Low back pain
    - Herniated intervertebral disk
    - Spinal cord tumors
    - Degenerative disk disease
    - Spondylosis
17. Describe the assessment findings associated with nontraumatic spinal injuries.
18. Describe the management of nontraumatic spinal injuries.
19. Integrate pathophysiologic principles to the assessment of a patient with nontraumatic spinal injury.
20. Formulate a field impression for nontraumatic spinal injury on the basis of assessment findings.
21. Develop a patient management plan for nontraumatic spinal injury on the basis of field impression.

CHAPTER SUMMARY

- The spinal column is composed of 33 vertebrae: 7 cervical, 12 thoracic, 5 lumbar, 5 sacral, and 4 coccygeal.
- The spinal cord runs through the spinal foramen, beginning at the base of the skull and terminating between vertebrae L2 and L3 in adults at the conus medullaris.
- Many mechanisms can potentially injure a spinal column and cord; the EMS professional is responsible for determining when a mechanism is significant enough to cause injury and when it is not.
- Any patient who has a mechanism of injury for a spine injury must undergo a thorough spine assessment. If a spine assessment cannot be performed, fully immobilize the patient.
- A complete spine assessment includes determining patient reliability; evaluating the history for spine pain, numbness, tingling, or electrical shooting sensations; and performing a specific examination, evaluating for spine tenderness and specific motor and sensory skills.
- If a patient fails the spine assessment, immobilize the patient and document the findings; spine pain and tenderness indicate a column injury, whereas numbness, tingling, electrical shooting sensations, and impaired motor or sensory skills all indicate a cord injury.
- PMS (*p*ulses, *m*ovement, and *s*ensation) best evaluates musculoskeletal injuries, not spine injuries.

- When immobilizing a pediatric patient, remember to pad beneath the shoulders, not the head.
- Do not hesitate to place a patient in a lateral recumbent position while on the long board. You can safely immobilize a patient in that position; it simply takes additional padding.
- Provide ample padding to eliminate all terrible triangles.
- Secure the patient to a long board with X's across the shoulders and chest, hips, and head and straps across the legs.
- Not all spine injuries are trauma related. If no trauma has occurred, immobilization is not indicated; look for and identify another cause.

SHORT ANSWER

1. What is the most important indication that a patient may have a spinal injury?

_____
_____
_____
_____

2. What technique should be used to open the airway of a patient who has a possible cervical spine injury?

_____
_____
_____
_____

3. If the airway of a patient with a possible cervical spine injury cannot be opened using the technique identified in the previous question, what should you do?

_____
_____
_____
_____

4. What is the most important action in the management of a patient with possible spinal trauma?

_____
_____
_____
_____

5. A 67-year-old male fell in the bathroom, hitting his chin on the edge of the bathtub. He is awake and alert. He has no pain or deformity of the cervical spine. He complains of weakness and tingling in both of his upper extremities. However, he has normal sensation and movement in both lower extremities. What problem do you suspect?

_____
_____
_____
_____

6. Why does the problem present in the previous question cause weakness that is more pronounced in the upper extremities than in the lower extremities?

_____
_____
_____
_____

7. What is Brown-Séquard syndrome?

_____
_____
_____
_____

8. Describe the pattern of motor and sensory deficits that characterizes Brown-Séquard syndrome.

_____
_____
_____
_____

9. What is cauda equina syndrome?

_____
_____
_____

10. Describe the changes you would anticipate in the pulse and blood pressure readings of a patient who is in neurogenic shock secondary to trauma to the spinal cord, and explain why these changes occur.

_____
_____
_____
_____

11. How should the hypotension associated with neurogenic shock be managed?

_____
_____
_____

12. Explain why patients with spinal cord injuries are at risk for becoming hypothermic. (HINT: Think of the effect on the vasculature, specifically in neurogenic shock.)

_____
_____
_____

13. What beneficial effect do steroids have in the management of head-injured or spinal cord–injured patients?

_____
_____
_____
_____

14. A patient thrown from a horse presents with bradycardia; hypotension; pale, cool, moist skin on the face and upper extremities; dry, flushed skin on the abdomen and lower extremities; and absence of sensation and motion in the lower extremities. What problem do you suspect?

_____

_____

_____

_____

MULTIPLE CHOICE

1. A patient who was thrown from a horse has sensation at the nipple line but no sensation below the umbilicus. You should suspect damage to the spinal cord between _____.
   A. C4 and C7
   B. L1 and L3
   C. T5 and T10
   D. T1 and T4

2. A 32-year-old female fell down a flight of stairs at an apartment complex. She is unconscious with a deep forehead laceration and is lying with her forearms flexed across her chest. When you extend one of her arms and then release it, the arm returns to the flexed position. Her intercostal muscles appear to be paralyzed, but she is breathing with her diaphragm. You suspect spinal cord damage at _____.
   A. C1
   B. C3
   C. C6
   D. T4

3. A patient fell from a scaffold at a construction site. His skin is cool and dry. Respirations are present and equal bilaterally. Vital signs are: BP—82/60 mm Hg; P—54 beats/min; R—28 breaths/min shallow, regular. The problem that would best account for all of the changes in the patient's physical findings and vital signs is _____.
   A. aortic tear with intrathoracic hemorrhage
   B. closed head injury with increased intracranial pressure
   C. ruptured spleen with intra abdominal hemorrhage
   D. spinal cord injury with neurogenic shock

4. A patient with a possible spinal cord injury should be covered with blankets because _____.
   A. damage to the parasympathetic nervous system may cause vasoconstriction and result in increased heat loss
   B. damage to the parasympathetic nervous system may cause vasodilation and result in increased heat loss
   C. spinal cord trauma may damage the sympathetic nervous system, cause vasodilation, and result in increased heat loss
   D. spinal cord trauma may damage the sympathetic nervous system, cause vasoconstriction, and result in increased heat loss

5. Damage to the sympathetic nervous system as a result of a spinal fracture can produce _____.
   A. hypothermia because of increased heat loss through constricted peripheral vessels
   B. peripheral vasodilation, leading to pooling of blood in the vascular system and a fall in blood pressure
   C. peripheral vasodilation, leading to flushed, dry skin and a rise in systemic blood pressure
   D. severe tachycardia, leading to decreased preload and cardiac output

6. Which of the following best describes the proper procedure for opening the airway of a patient with a possible cervical spine injury?
   A. Hyperextend the neck and insert an oropharyngeal airway.
   B. Maintain the neck in a neutral position; open the airway with a jaw thrust or chin lift.
   C. Open the airway with a jaw thrust or chin lift and neck hyperextension.
   D. Place the neck in hyperflexion.

7. The shock that follows spinal cord injury is due to _____.
   A. hypovolemia
   B. increased sympathetic tone
   C. loss of peripheral vascular resistance
   D. pump failure

8. A 34-year-old male with a history of diabetes mellitus fell from the roof of a house and landed on his feet. His only complaint is of pain in both heels. The most important aspect of your management of this patient would be to _____.
   A. give oxygen by nonrebreather mask and check his blood sugar level
   B. immobilize his lumbar spine
   C. immobilize the entire spine
   D. remove his shoes and apply pillow splints to his feet

9. Which set of vital signs leads you to suspect neurogenic shock?
   A. P—60 beats/min; BP—180/110 mm Hg; R—42 breaths/min deep, regular
   B. P—62 beats/min; BP—70/50 mm Hg; R—26 breaths/min shallow, regular
   C. P—72 beats/min; BP—120/80 mm Hg; R—16 breaths/min normal, regular
   D. P—140 beats/min; BP—60/40 mm Hg; R—24 breaths/min shallow, irregular

10. As you perform your initial assessment of a trauma patient, when do you stabilize the cervical spine?
    A. As soon as you are sure the patient has an open airway
    B. As soon as you finish evaluating the patient's ABCs
    C. At the same time you open and evaluate the airway
    D. Only if you are sure there has been an injury to the head or neck

97

11. What is the most important indication that a patient may have a spinal injury?
    A. Mechanism of injury
    B. Numbness and tingling in the extremities
    C. Pain in the neck or back
    D. Paralysis or weakness in the extremities

12. With any spinal injury, what is the primary treatment?
    A. Keep the entire spine immobilized.
    B. Keep the patient from losing body heat.
    C. Transport as soon as possible.
    D. Treat for neurogenic shock.

13. The two most common complications to anticipate in a patient who has a spinal cord injury are _____.
    A. hypovolemic shock, decreased body temperature
    B. hypovolemic shock, respiratory paralysis or failure
    C. neurogenic shock, elevated body temperature
    D. neurogenic shock, respiratory paralysis or failure

14. A patient has sensation and movement in the upper extremities, but none in the lower extremities. This is a sign of _____.
    A. injury to the cervical spinal cord
    B. injury to the cervical vertebrae
    C. injury to the lumbar or thoracic spinal cord
    D. injury to the lumbar or thoracic vertebrae

15. Which part of the spinal column forms the lower back?
    A. Cervical spine
    B. Lumbar spine
    C. Sacral spine
    D. Thoracic spine

16. The patient is a 23-year-old male who was driving a motor vehicle that struck a fixed object. He is awake and alert. His skin is warm and dry. Radial pulses are present. He complains only of neck and lower back pain. As you prepare to extricate him, the first step would be to _____.
    A. check pulses, movement, and sensation in all four extremities; then place the Kendrick extrication device (KED) on the seat behind the patient
    B. manually stabilize the head and neck and apply a rigid cervical collar
    C. place a long spine board on the front seat of the vehicle next to the patient
    D. secure the patient's head to the KED with sufficient padding to maintain the head in a neutral position

17. Shock may be produced by spinal cord injury because _____.
    A. spinal cord injury always involves internal bleeding, which rapidly produces hypovolemic shock
    B. the blood vessels below the injury become dilated and there is no longer enough blood to fill them
    C. the heart no longer receives electrical impulses to pump blood, resulting in a slow heart rate and low blood pressure
    D. the patient's skeletal muscles become paralyzed, which slows the return of the blood to the heart

18. If an injury to the head or spinal cord is suspected, you should _____.
    A. ask the patient whether it hurts to move his or her head
    B. check for pulses, sensation, and movement in all four extremities
    C. check reflexes and capillary refill in all four extremities
    D. have the patient sit up and ask if he or she feels dizzy

19. When applying a cervical collar, you should remember _____.
    A. that all cervical collars are sized the same way
    B. that most of the population requires a "no-neck" collar
    C. to continue manual stabilization until the patient's head can be secured to a back board
    D. to use whatever size collar is most comfortable for the patient

20. At the scene of a single-car crash, bystanders have already removed the patient from the vehicle. He is standing and complains of neck and back pain. There is a "spiderweb" pattern on the windshield. Your partners have already placed a cervical collar on the patient. The best way to place him on the stretcher is to _____.
    A. perform a standing takedown using a long spineboard
    B. perform an emergency move to place him on the spine board as quickly as possible
    C. place a back board on the cot and have the patient sit down on the board
    D. place a KED on the patient and then have him lie down on the stretcher

21. When managing infants and small children with spinal injuries, you should _____.
    A. not immobilize the patient if it causes excessive restlessness and agitation
    B. not secure the patient's head to the back board because this may interfere with airway management
    C. not use a long back board for immobilization since it is too large to adequately immobilize a child
    D. place padding from the shoulders to the heels to provide proper immobilization

22. A helmet worn by an athlete wearing shoulder pads should be left in place unless _____.
    A. the helmet is loose and allows for excessive movement
    B. you are unable to adequately assess and manage the patient's airway and breathing
    C. you cannot perform proper spinal immobilization because of the helmet
    D. any of the situations described in A, B, or C is present

A 17-year-old female fell down a flight of stairs at her school, striking her head on a concrete floor. She is unconscious and unresponsive. A laceration is present on her forehead. Movement of her chest wall is diminished, and she appears to be breathing primarily with her diaphragm. She does not respond to painful stimuli applied to any of her extremities. Vital signs are: P—62 beats/min weak, regular; BP—76/50 mm Hg; R—28 breaths/min shallow, regular.

1. In what section of her spine has she sustained injury?

2. What problem is suggested by her vital signs?

3. Explain why this patient is breathing with her diaphragm, but not with her chest wall.

4. Why does this patient not have a tachycardia?

5. Why is this patient not diaphoretic?

6. Why is the patient's blood pressure decreased?

7. What IV solution should be used to treat her? Why?

49 Thoracic Trauma

READING ASSIGNMENT

Chapter 49, pages 468-488, in *Paramedic Practice Today: Above and Beyond.*

OBJECTIVES

After completing this chapter, you will be able to:
1. Explain the relevance of thoracic injuries as a part of overall mortality rate from major trauma.
2. List the thoracic injuries that may result in early death if left untreated in the prehospital setting.
3. Describe the incidence, morbidity, and mortality rates of thoracic injuries in the trauma patient.
4. Discuss the types of thoracic injuries.
5. Discuss the anatomy and physiology of the organs and structures related to thoracic injuries.
6. Discuss the pathophysiology of thoracic injuries.
7. Discuss the assessment findings associated with thoracic injuries.
8. Discuss the management of thoracic injuries.
9. Identify the need for rapid intervention and transport of the patient with thoracic injuries.
10. Discuss the management of chest wall injuries.
11. Describe the impact of rib fractures on oxygenation and ventilation.
12. Predict thoracic injuries on the basis of mechanism of injury.
13. Discuss the pathophysiology of specific chest wall injuries, including the following:
    - Rib fracture
    - Flail segment
    - Sternal fracture
    - Third-degree burns in any age group
14. Discuss the management of lung injuries.
15. Explain the physiologic consequences of flail chest.
16. Discuss the assessment findings associated with chest wall injuries.
17. Identify the need for rapid intervention and transport of the patient with lung injuries.
18. Discuss the pathophysiology of traumatic asphyxia.
19. Discuss the assessment findings associated with traumatic asphyxia.
20. Discuss the management of traumatic asphyxia.
21. Identify the need for rapid intervention and transport of the patient with traumatic asphyxia.
22. Discuss the assessment findings associated with lung injuries.
23. Discuss the pathophysiology of injury to the lung, including the following:
    - Simple pneumothorax
    - Open pneumothorax
    - Tension pneumothorax
    - Hemothorax
    - Hemopneumothorax
    - Pulmonary contusion
24. Define *pneumothorax* and *hemothorax*.
25. List the signs and symptoms of a tension pneumothorax.
26. Identify the need for rapid intervention and transport of the patient with chest wall injuries.
27. Discuss the pathophysiology of tracheobronchial injuries.
28. Discuss the assessment findings associated with tracheobronchial injuries.
29. Discuss the management of tracheobronchial injuries.
30. Identify the need for rapid intervention and transport of the patient with tracheobronchial injuries.
31. Discuss the pathophysiology of myocardial injuries, including the following:
    - Pericardial tamponade
    - Myocardial contusion
    - Myocardial rupture
32. Discuss the assessment findings associated with myocardial injuries.
33. Discuss the management of myocardial injuries.
34. Define *Beck's triad.*
35. Identify the need for rapid intervention and transport of the patient with myocardial injuries.
36. Describe the pathophysiology of aortic rupture.
37. Discuss the pathophysiology of vascular injuries, including injuries to the following:
    - Aorta
    - Venae cavae
    - Pulmonary arteries and veins
38. Discuss the assessment findings associated with vascular injuries.
39. Discuss the management of vascular injuries.
40. Identify the need for rapid intervention and transport of the patient with vascular injuries.
41. Discuss the pathophysiology of diaphragmatic injuries.
42. Discuss the assessment findings associated with diaphragmatic injuries.
43. Discuss the management of diaphragmatic injuries.
44. Identify the need for rapid intervention and transport of the patient with diaphragmatic injuries.
45. Discuss the pathophysiology of esophageal injuries.
46. Discuss the assessment findings associated with esophageal injuries.
47. Discuss the management of esophageal injuries.
48. Identify the need for rapid intervention and transport of the patient with esophageal injuries.

CHAPTER SUMMARY

- Thoracic trauma includes a wide range of injuries, many of which may result in death if not recognized early. You must take into account the mechanism of injury to suspect potential injury to the heart, lungs, or great vessels.
- You must suspect and treat certain injuries, such as tension pneumothorax, in the field.
- You must be able to identify and treat these injuries rapidly to provide potentially lifesaving care.

SHORT ANSWER

1. Why are fractures of ribs 1 through 3 typically associated with high mortality rates?

2. What problem usually is associated with fractures of ribs 8 to 12 on the right side of the chest?

3. What problem usually is associated with fractures of ribs 9 to 11 on the left side of the chest?

4. A patient with penetrating trauma to the chest below the nipple line would be suspected of having injuries to organs in which body cavity, or cavities, until proven otherwise? Why?

5. What is paradoxical motion of the chest wall?

6. If paradoxical motion is observed, what chest injury is present?

7. Why is flail chest associated with inadequate ventilation?

8. What are the two most important treatments for flail chest?

9. What is a pulmonary contusion?

10. What mechanism of injury should suggest the presence of pulmonary contusion?

11. A patient with a mechanism of injury suggesting pulmonary contusion presents with shortness of breath and restlessness. Oxygen saturation is 91%. Chest expansion is symmetric. Radial pulses are present, strong, and regular. Blood pressure is 134/96 mm Hg. Should this patient receive rapid infusion of an isotonic crystalloid? Why or why not?

12. What is a myocardial contusion?

13. What is the most common complication of a myocardial contusion?

14. How should a sucking chest wound be managed?

15. For what complication should a patient with a sealed sucking chest wound be monitored? If this complication develops, what should be done?

16. What is subcutaneous emphysema?

_____
_____
_____
_____

17. What other chest injury is suggested by the presence of subcutaneous emphysema on the chest wall?

_____
_____
_____
_____

18. What changes would you anticipate in the capillary refill time, pulse rate, and blood pressure measurement of a patient who has an expanding tension pneumothorax? Why do these changes occur?

_____
_____
_____
_____

19. When a pleural decompression is performed, should the needle be inserted into the intercostal space just below the upper rib or just above the lower rib? Why?

_____
_____
_____
_____

20. Why do the neck veins become distended in a patient with a tension pneumothorax?

_____
_____
_____
_____

21. What is Beck's triad? With what problem is Beck's triad associated?

_____
_____
_____
_____

22. Why do the neck veins become distended in a patient who has cardiac tamponade?

_____
_____
_____
_____

23. What is pulsus paradoxus? Why does pulsus paradoxus occur in cardiac tamponade?

_____
_____
_____
_____

24. Where is the aorta most likely to tear during a sudden deceleration? Why?

_____
_____
_____
_____

25. A patient with chest trauma presents with tachycardia, hypotension, distended neck veins, muffled heart sounds, and a narrow pulse pressure. What problem do you suspect?

_____
_____
_____
_____

26. A patient with chest trauma presents with tachycardia, hypotension, distended neck veins, tracheal deviation to the left, and absent breath sounds on the right. What problem do you suspect?

_____

MULTIPLE CHOICE

1. A 26-year-old male was struck in the right lateral chest with a baseball bat during a barroom brawl. He complains of severe shortness of breath. He is anxious and agitated. Cyanosis of the lips and nailbeds is present. The neck veins are not distended with the patient in a semisitting position. Examination of the chest reveals decreased lung sounds on the right with a localized area of ecchymosis and tenderness over the sixth and seventh ribs in the right midaxillary line. The chest is hyperresonant to percussion on the right. Radial pulses are present, strong, and regular. This patient is probably suffering from _____.
   A. hemothorax
   B. pulmonary contusion
   C. simple pneumothorax
   D. tension pneumothorax

2. At the scene of a motor vehice crash, a patient complains of dyspnea and chest pain. A segment of the chest wall displays paradoxical motion. Vital signs are: BP—136/98 mm Hg; P—120 beats/min strong, regular; R—32 breaths/min shallow, regular. You should _____.
   A. administer high-concentration oxygen via nonrebreather mask, establish an IV with Ringer's lactate and run it wide open, and stabilize the segment to reduce patient discomfort.
   B. administer high-concentration oxygen via nonrebreather mask and establish an IV with Ringer's lactate to keep open.
   C. assist the patient's ventilations with a bag-mask and oxygen, and establish an IV with Ringer's lactate to keep open.
   D. assist the patient's ventilations with a bag-mask, establish an IV with Ringer's lactate, and run it wide open.

3. You are dispatched to a car-versus-utility pole crash. A 27-year-old male is unconscious behind the steering wheel. His head, neck, and shoulders are dark blue. His eyes are bloodshot and bulging. His lips are swollen and cyanotic. The trachea is midline. His neck veins are distended. Breath sounds are present and equal bilaterally. Examination of the chest reveals subcutaneous emphysema and multiple areas of ecchymosis and instability. Vital signs are: P—130 beats/min weak, regular; BP—70 mm Hg palpable; R—38 breaths/min shallow, regular. The patient is suffering from:
   A. cardiac tamponade
   B. hemothorax
   C. tension pneumothorax
   D. traumatic asphyxia

4. A 23-year-old male, who was involved in a motor vehicle crash, complains of chest pain and shortness of breath. A steering wheel bruise is present over the anterior chest. Breath sounds are present and equal bilaterally. Radial pulses are present, weak, and irregular. When an ECG monitor is applied to the patient, it shows a sinus tachycardia with frequent premature ventricular contractions. Based on these signs and symptoms you suspect this patient is suffering from _____.
   A. a myocardial contusion
   B. a pneumothorax
   C. a traumatic acute myocardial infarction
   D. fractured ribs

5. At the scene of a motor vehicle crash, a 32-year-old male is unconscious and unresponsive. His skin is pale, cool, and moist. Peripheral cyanosis is present. The trachea is midline, and the neck veins are flat with the patient supine. There is an area of ecchymosis and abrasions on the left lateral chest at the level of the fifth and sixth ribs in the anterior axillary line. Lung sounds are absent over the left lower lung field, which is dull to percussion. This patient is probably suffering from _____.
   A. cardiac tamponade
   B. hemothorax
   C. simple pneumothorax
   D. tension pneumothorax

6. A 30-year-old male has been stabbed in the left anterior chest in the mid-clavicular line at the level of the fourth intercostal space. He is unconscious and unresponsive. Vital signs are: BP—90/50 mm Hg; P—120 beats/min weak, regular; R—30 breaths/min shallow, regular. The patient's skin is cool and moist. The trachea is midline. The neck veins are markedly distended with the patient supine. Breath sounds are present and equal bilaterally. Heart sounds are distant and muffled. After 5 minutes vital signs are: BP—70/50 mm Hg; P—136 beats/min weak, regular; R—36 breaths/min shallow, regular. You suspect _____.
   A. cardiac tamponade
   B. hemothorax
   C. simple pneumothorax
   D. tension pneumothorax

7. Leakage of air into the pleural space through a wound that acts as a one-way valve may produce _____.
   A. simple pneumothorax
   B. a sucking chest wound
   C. tension pneumothorax
   D. traumatic asphyxia

8. Which of the following signs and symptoms would you expect to see in a patient with a cardiac tamponade?
   A. Jugular vein distention; tracheal deviation; hyper-resonance to percussion
   B. Narrowing pulse pressure; jugular vein distention; tracheal deviation
   C. Rapid, weak pulse; jugular vein distention; tracheal deviation
   D. Rapid, weak pulse; narrowing pulse pressure; jugular vein distention

9. A 27-year-old female has been shot in the right upper chest with a large-caliber handgun. When the patient breathes, air can be heard moving in and out of the wound. Her respirations are rapid, shallow, and gasping. You should _____.
   A. elevate the patient's head and shoulders and assist her ventilations with a bag-mask
   B. give oxygen by nonrebreather mask and position the patient with her injured side up
   C. give oxygen via nasal cannula at 4 L/min and then seal the wound with an occlusive dressing
   D. immediately seal the wound with an occlusive dressing and then assist her ventilations as needed

10. A 22-year-old male has a sucking chest wound caused by a gunshot. You have sealed the wound with an occlusive dressing and are giving oxygen at 12 L/min by nonrebreather mask. The patient is experiencing severe shortness of breath. He is cyanotic. His neck veins are distended, and his trachea is deviating away from the injured side of his chest. You should _____.
    A. decrease the flow rate of the patient's oxygen to 10 L/min
    B. increase the flow rate of the patient's oxygen to 15 L/min
    C. temporarily remove the occlusive dressing
    D. ventilate the patient with a bag-mask and oxygen

11. A 19-year-old male has a knife impaled in the left anterior chest. When he breathes, air bubbles from around the knife. You should _____.
    A. give oxygen, apply an occlusive dressing at the base of the knife, stabilize the knife with a bulky bandage, and transport
    B. open the airway, give high-concentration oxygen by nonrebreather mask, and transport immediately
    C. open the airway, stabilize the knife, and transport immediately with no further treatment
    D. remove the knife, apply an occlusive dressing, give oxygen by nonrebreather mask, and transport

12. At the scene of a motor vehicle crash, a patient whose chest struck the steering wheel complains of dyspnea and chest pain. A segment of the chest wall displays paradoxical motion. What should you do?
    A. Assist the patient's ventilations with a bag-mask and oxygen at 12 to 15 L/min.
    B. Place gentle pressure over the segment to stop the paradoxical motion and reduce pain.
    C. Transport the patient in a semisitting position and give oxygen at 15 L/min by nonrebreather mask.
    D. Transport the patient with his injured side up and assist his ventilations with a bag-mask and oxygen.

13. A motor vehicle crash victim who struck the steering wheel has a crackling sensation in the soft tissues of the chest wall. This crackling sensation is called _____.
    A. pleural effusion
    B. pulmonary emphysema
    C. subcutaneous emphysema
    D. tension pneumothorax

14. The finding in the previous question suggests the patient may have a _____.
    A. cardiac tamponade
    B. hemothorax
    C. myocardial contusion
    D. pneumothorax

15. A condition in which two or more ribs are broken in two or more places and the chest wall lying between the fractures becomes a free-floating segment is _____.
    A. flail chest
    B. pneumothorax
    C. tension pneumothorax
    D. traumatic asphyxia

16. A patient has penetrating trauma to the right lateral chest below the nipple line. Which of the following injuries might be suspected?
    A. A lacerated liver
    B. A lacerated liver or a pneumothorax
    C. A perforated lung with a pneumothorax
    D. A perforated stomach

17. Paradoxical movement means that a segment of the chest wall _____.
    A. moves in and out with the rib cage as the patient breathes
    B. moves in the opposite direction from the rest of the chest cage as the patient breathes
    C. moves outward an excessive distance in relation to the rest of the rib cage during breathing
    D. remains perfectly still while the chest cage moves in and out

18. What is air in the pleural space called?
    A. Hemothorax
    B. Pneumothorax
    C. Pulmonary embolism
    D. Subcutaneous emphysema

19. A 24-year-old female was the driver of a motor vehicle that struck a utility pole. She is awake, alert, and complaining of chest pain. Breath sounds are present and equal bilaterally. Heart sounds can be heard clearly. The neck veins are not distended. Radial pulses are present, rapid, weak, and irregular. You suspect this patient is suffering from _____.
    A. cardiac tamponade
    B. hemothorax
    C. myocardial contusion
    D. pneumothorax

CASE STUDIES

Case one

A 56-year-old farmer fell approximately 20 feet from a hayloft to the floor of a barn. He has bruising over the mid-sternal area and complains of deep, aching chest pain. His right radial pulse is significantly stronger than the left. When you take his blood pressure bilaterally, it is elevated in the right upper extremity, but is diminished in the left. The patient tells you he is beginning to experience difficulty breathing and swallowing. His voice is becoming hoarse. Chest auscultation reveals equal breath sounds bilaterally.

1. What problem do you suspect?

   _____
   _____
   _____
   _____

2. At what location is this problem most likely to occur? Why?

   _____
   _____
   _____
   _____

3. What accounts for the patient's difficulty breathing? (HINT: Think about the anatomic relationships of structures in the mediastinum.)

_____
_____
_____
_____

4. What accounts for the difficulty swallowing?

_____
_____
_____
_____

5. Why is the patient developing hoarseness?

_____
_____
_____
_____

Case two

A 25-year-old male was found lying in a ditch beside his overturned vehicle. He is unconscious and unresponsive. Respirations are rapid, shallow, and gasping. His skin is pale and cool. His trachea is deviated to the right. His neck veins are flat when he is in the supine position. Breath sounds are absent on the left side. The left lung field is hyperresonant to percussion. The abdomen is rigid and distended. There is an open fracture of the right tibia at mid-shaft.

1. Where does the tibia fracture rank on your list of priorities? Why?

_____
_____
_____
_____

2. What type of chest injury probably is present?

_____

3. Are the patient's flat neck veins consistent with the type of chest injury you suspect? If not, how do you explain this?

_____
_____
_____
_____

Case three

A 28-year-old male was driving a motor vehicle that struck a utility pole head-on. The patient was not restrained and the vehicle was not equipped with air bags. The patient is unresponsive. Cyanosis of the face, neck, and shoulders is present. The patient's eyes have a bloodshot appearance. The neck veins are distended. The trachea is midline. Respirations are shallow and gasping. Radial pulses are weak and irregular.

1. What term is used to describe a patient who presents with this appearance?

_____

2. What mechanism accounts for the persistent cyanosis of the face, neck, and shoulders?

_____
_____
_____
_____

3. Based on the mechanism of injury and the patient's appearance, what thoracic injuries do you suspect?

_____
_____
_____
_____

As you observe the patient's respirations, you notice that the sternum and adjacent portions of the rib cage are moving asymmetrically as the patient attempts to breathe.

4. What term is used to describe the asymmetric movement of the chest wall?

_____

5. What problem is present?

_____
_____
_____
_____

6. What is the principal reason this problem interferes with adequate oxygenation and ventilation?

_____
_____
_____
_____

7. How is this problem managed?

_____
_____
_____
_____

At the hospital, the patient continued to experience respiratory distress and tachypnea. Mechanical ventilation was required to maintain the patient's PaO_2 above 60 torr and the hemoglobin saturation above 90%. A chest radiograph revealed localized, nonsegmental pulmonary infiltrates in the right and left lung fields.

8. What injury do you suspect is present?

_____
_____
_____
_____

9. Why does this injury interfere with adequate gas exchange?

_____
_____
_____
_____

10. When this injury is present, what precaution must be taken during fluid administration?

_____
_____
_____
_____

The ECG monitor showed frequent premature ventricular contractions. A 12-lead ECG recorded nonspecific ST segment and T-wave abnormalities in multiple leads. The patient's cardiac enzymes became elevated.

11. What problem probably is present?

_____

_____

_____

_____

12. What complications can result from this problem?

_____

_____

_____

_____

50 Abdominal Trauma

READING ASSIGNMENT

Chapter 50, pages 489-504, in *Paramedic Practice Today: Above and Beyond*.

OBJECTIVES

After completing this chapter, you will be able to:

1. Describe the epidemiology, including the morbidity and mortality rates and prevention strategies, for a patient with abdominal trauma.
2. Describe the anatomy and physiology of the organs and structures related to abdominal injuries.
3. Predict abdominal injuries on the basis of blunt and penetrating mechanisms of injury.
4. Describe open and closed abdominal injuries.
5. Explain the pathophysiology of abdominal injuries.
6. Describe the assessment findings associated with abdominal injuries.
7. Identify the need for rapid intervention and transport of the patient with abdominal injuries based on the assessment findings.
8. Integrate pathophysiologic principles into the assessment of a patient who has abdominal injury.
9. Differentiate abdominal injuries on the basis of assessment of the patient and his or her history.
10. Formulate a field impression for patients with abdominal trauma on the basis of assessment findings.
11. Apply the epidemiologic principles to develop prevention strategies for abdominal injuries.
12. Integrate pathophysiologic principles into the assessment of a patient with abdominal injuries.
13. Describe the management of abdominal injuries.
14. Develop a management plan for patients with abdominal trauma on the basis of field impression.
15. Describe the epidemiology, including the morbidity and mortality rates and prevention strategies, for hollow organ injuries.
16. Explain the pathophysiology of hollow organ injuries.
17. Describe the assessment findings associated with hollow organ injuries.
18. Describe the treatment plan and management of patients with hollow organ injuries.
19. Describe the epidemiology, including the morbidity and mortality rates and prevention strategies, for solid organ injuries.
20. Explain the pathophysiology of solid organ injuries.
21. Describe the assessment findings associated with solid organ injuries.
22. Describe the treatment plan and management of patients with solid organ injuries.
23. Describe the epidemiology, including the morbidity and mortality rates and prevention strategies, for abdominal vascular injuries.
24. Explain the pathophysiology of abdominal vascular injuries.
25. Describe the assessment findings associated with abdominal vascular injuries.
26. Describe the treatment plan and management of patients with abdominal vascular injuries.
27. Describe the epidemiology, including the morbidity and mortality rates and prevention strategies, for pelvic fractures.
28. Explain the pathophysiology of pelvic fractures.
29. Describe the assessment findings associated with pelvic fractures.
30. Describe the treatment plan and management of patients with pelvic fractures.
31. Describe the epidemiology, including the morbidity and mortality rates and prevention strategies, for other related abdominal injuries.
32. Explain the pathophysiology of other related abdominal injuries.
33. Describe the assessment findings associated with other related abdominal injuries.
34. Describe the treatment plan and management of patients with other related abdominal injuries.
35. Describe the epidemiology, including the morbidity and mortality rates and prevention strategies, for diaphragmatic injuries.
36. Explain the pathophysiology of diaphragmatic injuries.
37. Describe the assessment findings associated with diaphragmatic injuries.
38. Describe the treatment plan and management of patients with diaphragmatic injuries.
39. Describe the epidemiology, including the morbidity and mortality rates and prevention strategies, for retroperitoneal injuries.
40. Explain the pathophysiology of retroperitoneal injuries.
41. Describe the assessment findings associated with retroperitoneal injuries.
42. Describe the treatment plan and management of patients with retroperitoneal injuries.
43. Describe the epidemiology, including the morbidity and mortality rates and prevention strategies, for penetrating abdominal injuries.
44. Explain the pathophysiology of penetrating abdominal injuries.
45. Describe the assessment findings associated with penetrating abdominal injuries.

46. Describe the treatment plan and management of patients with penetrating abdominal injuries.
47. Describe the epidemiology, including the morbidity and mortality rates and prevention strategies, for trauma in pregnancy.
48. Explain the pathophysiology of trauma in pregnancy.
49. Describe the assessment findings associated with trauma in pregnancy.
50. Describe the treatment plan and management of a pregnant patient with trauma.
51. Describe the epidemiology, including the morbidity and mortality rates and prevention strategies, for genitourinary trauma.
52. Explain the pathophysiology of genitourinary trauma.
53. Describe the assessment findings associated with genitourinary trauma.
54. Describe the treatment plan and management of a patient with genitourinary trauma.

CHAPTER SUMMARY

- Morbidity and mortality from abdominal trauma are primarily related to hemorrhage.
- The goal of prehospital care for abdominal trauma is to prevent or control hemorrhage when possible and rapidly transport the patient to a facility capable of surgical intervention when necessary.
- Abdominal trauma may involve solid organs, hollow organs, and vascular structures in any combination.
- The spillage of abdominal contents from the rupture of hollow organs leads to peritonitis, the second leading cause of morbidity and mortality.
- You should maintain a high index of suspicion in the assessment of patients with potential abdominal injuries.
- Your assessment of a patient with abdominal trauma should proceed in a staged fashion, beginning with a search for critical findings.
- You should rapidly transport patients with critical findings on a primary survey to an appropriate receiving facility.
- For victims of significant abdominal trauma, conduct further assessment and initial treatment for shock while en route to the hospital.

SHORT ANSWER

1. Indicate whether the following organs are hollow or solid.
_____ Appendix
_____ Gallbladder
_____ Liver
_____ Pancreas
_____ Right kidney
_____ Sigmoid colon
_____ Spleen
_____ Stomach

2. Indicate the quadrant in which each organ is found.
_____ Appendix
_____ Gallbladder
_____ Liver
_____ Pancreas
_____ Right kidney
_____ Sigmoid colon
_____ Spleen
_____ Stomach

3. What is the usual effect of trauma to an abdominal hollow organ?
_____
_____
_____
_____

4. What is the usual effect of trauma to an abdominal solid organ?
_____
_____
_____
_____

5. What is Cullen's sign?
_____
_____
_____
_____

6. What is Grey Turner's sign?
_____
_____
_____
_____

7. What is Kehr's sign?
_____
_____
_____
_____

8. Kehr's sign suggests injury to which abdominal organ?
_____
_____
_____
_____

9. Why is a PASG useful in the management of patients who have intraabdominal hemorrhage?
_____
_____
_____
_____

10. What is a diaphragmatic hernia?
_____
_____
_____
_____

11. Should the PASG be used to manage a patient with a suspected diaphragmatic hernia? Why or why not?

_____
_____
_____
_____

12. Why should patients with abdominal trauma or abdominal pain generally *not* be given anything by mouth?

_____
_____
_____
_____

13. A male patient slipped and "straddled" the top of a fence over which he was attempting to climb. He has a swollen, blue-red scrotum and bruising that extends to the medial aspects of both thighs. You should suspect injury to what structure?

_____
_____
_____
_____

14. In what position should a trauma patient who is in late-term pregnancy be transported? Why?

_____
_____
_____
_____

15. If a patient in late-term pregnancy needs application of the PASG, what restrictions apply? Why?

_____
_____
_____
_____

16. When you are administering fluid to a patient who is in late-term pregnancy, have you reached a state of adequate resuscitation when the mother shows signs of reversal of hypovolemic shock? Why?

_____
_____
_____
_____

17. In the management of a pregnant patient with multiple systems' trauma, where do your priorities lie, with the mother or the fetus? Why?

_____
_____
_____
_____

MULTIPLE CHOICE

1. An automobile struck a 10-year-old boy. He has fractures of the eighth through tenth ribs on the right side. He is pale, confused and sweating heavily. Radial pulses are absent. Carotid pulses are weak and rapid. Breath sounds are present bilaterally, but the right upper quadrant of the abdomen is tender. You should suspect an injury of the _____.
   A. gallbladder
   B. liver
   C. pancreas
   D. spleen

2. A car struck a 16-year-old male. Palpation of the pelvis reveals pain and instability. While you are preparing to transport, the patient passes a large amount of bloody urine. He probably has suffered an injury of the _____.
   A. gallbladder
   B. liver
   C. spleen
   D. urinary bladder

3. Which of the following groups of signs and symptoms would be most suggestive of a ruptured spleen?
   A. Rapid, shallow breathing; rapid pulse rate; left upper quadrant pain radiating to the left shoulder
   B. Rapid, shallow breathing; slow pulse rate; vomiting of blood; left upper quadrant bruising
   C. Rapid, shallow breathing; rapid pulse rate; right lower quadrant pain
   D. Slow, shallow breathing; restlessness; discoloration of the right upper quadrant

4. A patient has penetrating trauma to the right lateral chest below the nipple line. Which of the following injuries would most likely be present?
   A. A lacerated liver or a pneumothorax
   B. A lacerated liver or spleen
   C. A perforated lung with a pneumothorax
   D. A perforated stomach or a pneumothorax

5. A patient with a stab wound in the anterior abdomen 3 to 4 inches inferior to the umbilicus probably would have an injury of the _____.
   A. gallbladder or urinary bladder
   B. small intestine or urinary bladder
   C. spleen or small intestine
   D. stomach or liver

6. At the scene of a knife fight, a 16-year-old male has a large laceration of the left anterior abdominal wall. Several loops of small bowel are protruding through the wound. Which of the following actions would be least appropriate while caring for this patient?
   A. Covering the exposed bowel with a moist, sterile dressing
   B. Monitoring the vital signs for shock
   C. Replacing the bowel into the abdominal cavity
   D. Securing an airway and starting high-concentration oxygen

7. The preferred choice of coverings for an abdominal evisceration would be a sterile dressing saturated with _____.

A. D$_{50}$W
B. distilled water
C. normal saline
D. sodium bicarbonate

8. An automobile struck a 12-year-old boy when he rode his bicycle into traffic from between two parked cars. He has fractures of the ninth through eleventh ribs on the left side. He is pale and confused, and sweating heavily. Breath sounds are present bilaterally. The left upper quadrant of the abdomen is tender. He also complains of pain in his left shoulder, which appears to be uninjured. You suspect an injury of the _____.

A. gallbladder
B. liver
C. pancreas
D. spleen

9. A patient involved in a motor vehicle crash is unconscious and unresponsive. Breath sounds are present and equal bilaterally. His right leg is shortened and abducted. His right forearm is swollen and deformed. The patient's skin is pale, cool, and moist. Vital signs are: BP—76/50 mm Hg; P—126 beats/min weak, regular; R—30 breaths/min shallow, regular. The injury which would most likely account for the changes in the patients vital signs is _____.
A. closed head injury
B. hemothorax
C. pelvic fracture
D. radius/ulna fracture

CASE STUDY

A 22-year-old female who is 22-weeks' pregnant has been involved in a motor vehicle crash. She is unconscious and unresponsive. Her skin is pale, cool, and diaphoretic. Radial pulses are absent. Capillary refill is prolonged. Respirations are rapid, shallow, and labored.

1. In the management of an injured pregnant patient, where does your highest priority lie, with the mother or with the fetus? Why?

_____
_____
_____
_____

2. What restrictions apply to the use of PASG with this patient? Why?

_____
_____
_____
_____

3. In what position should this patient be placed for transport? Why?

_____
_____
_____
_____

After application of a PASG and rapid infusion of 2000 mL of Ringer's lactate, the patient's radial pulses return and she begins to respond to verbal stimuli.

4. Is this an indication that the patient has been adequately resuscitated? Why or why not?

_____
_____
_____
_____

51 Musculoskeletal Trauma

READING ASSIGNMENT

Chapter 51, pages 505-534, in *Paramedic Practice Today: Above and Beyond*.

OBJECTIVES

After completing this chapter, you will be able to:
1. Describe the incidence, morbidity, and mortality rates of musculoskeletal injuries.
2. Predict injuries on the basis of mechanism of injury, including the following:
   - Direct
   - Indirect
   - Pathologic
3. Discuss the anatomy and physiology of the musculoskeletal system.
4. Describe changes in bones associated with age.
5. Discuss the following types of musculoskeletal injuries:
   - Fracture (open and closed)
   - Dislocation and fracture
   - Sprain
   - Strain
   - Compartment syndrome
6. Discuss the pathophysiology of musculoskeletal injuries, including the following:
   - Fracture (open and closed)
   - Dislocation and fracture
   - Sprain
   - Strain
   - Compartment syndrome
7. Discuss the usefulness of the pneumatic antishock garment in managing fractures.
8. Discuss the relation between the volume of hemorrhage and open or closed fractures.
9. Discuss the assessment findings associated with the following musculoskeletal injuries:
   - Fracture (open and closed)
   - Dislocation and fracture
   - Sprain
   - Strain
   - Compartment syndrome
10. List the "six *P*'s" of assessing a musculoskeletal injury.
11. Identify the need for rapid intervention and transport when dealing with musculoskeletal injuries.
12. Discuss how to manage the following musculoskeletal injuries:
    - Fracture (open and closed)
    - Dislocation and fracture
    - Sprain
    - Strain
    - Compartment syndrome
13. Discuss why you need to assess pulses, movement, and sensation before and after splinting.
14. Discuss the general guidelines for splinting.
15. Explain the benefits of cold application for musculoskeletal injury.
16. Explain the benefits of heat application for musculoskeletal injury.
17. Discuss the prehospital management of dislocation/fractures, including splinting and realignment.
18. Describe the special considerations involved in managing femur fracture.
19. Describe the procedure for the reduction of a shoulder, finger, or ankle dislocation and fracture.
20. Explain the importance of manipulating a knee dislocation and fracture with an absent distal pulse.

CHAPTER SUMMARY

- Musculoskeletal injuries are seldom life threatening; however, they do need prompt medical attention to prevent permanent damage.
- Blood loss is probable with fractured bones and injured muscles.
- The care you provide in the field will depend on the patient's overall condition and other presenting injuries, and it may determine if the patient incurs a long-term disability or regains full use of the injured area.
- Musculoskeletal injuries can be distracting. You must focus on life threats before treating injuries to bones and muscles.
- You must also provide for the psychological support of the patient and give reassurance as you treat and transport the patient to a care facility.
- You must be complete and thorough in your assessment to avoid missing hidden injuries or underlying illnesses.
- The reassessment of injuries is crucial.
- Aggressive pain control benefits the patient and helps facilitate procedures.
- When in doubt, splint it.

MATCHING

1. ____ Bone ends are crushed or broken into more than two pieces

    ____ Bone ends are driven together at fracture site

    ____ Bone is only partially broken on one side

    ____ Fracture line crosses shaft at an angle other than right angle

    ____ Fracture line coils through bone like a spring

    ____ Fracture line is at a right angle to the bone's shaft

A. Comminuted
B. Greenstick
C. Impacted
D. Oblique
E. Spiral
F. Transverse

SHORT ANSWER

1. What type of joint connects the femur to the pelvis?

2. What type of joint connects the humerus to the ulna at the elbow?

3. What type of joint connects the mandible to the skull?

4. Name the anatomic structure that connects bone to bone.

5. Name the anatomic structure that connects muscles to bone.

6. What is the name of the fibrous outer covering of the bone?

7. What is the origin of a muscle?

8. What is the insertion of a muscle?

9. What is a fracture?

10. What is a dislocation?

11. What structures should be immobilized when splinting a fracture?

12. What structures should be immobilized when splinting a dislocation?

13. What is the principal problem associated with any orthopedic injury?

14. What is the principal danger associated with a fractured pelvis?

15. What is the potential blood loss from a closed femur fracture?

16. What are the only orthopedic injuries that are likely to become life threatening?

17. What is the splint of choice for an isolated femur fracture? Why?

18. What is the splint of choice for a fracture of the ankle or foot?

_____
_____
_____
_____

19. If a trauma patient has multiple extremity fractures and also is in respiratory distress and shock, how would you immobilize the extremity injuries?

_____
_____
_____
_____

20. What structures should be immobilized when a fracture of the tibia and fibula is properly splinted?

_____
_____
_____
_____

21. How is circulation checked when an injury involves the hand or foot?

_____
_____
_____
_____

22. What is the difference between a strain and a sprain?

_____
_____
_____
_____

23. What is crepitation? Should crepitation actively be sought as a sign of a fracture during patient assessment? Why?

_____
_____
_____
_____

24. What structure is injured in a patient who has a Colles' fracture?

_____

25. What is the preferred device for stabilizing a possible pelvic fracture?

_____

26. What two orthopedic injuries are unique to children? Why?

_____
_____

MULTIPLE CHOICE

1. A 23-year-old female has a possible dislocation of her right knee. Her leg and foot are cool and pale. Pulses are absent. When you attempt to straighten her leg, she complains of intense pain. You should _____.
   A. apply cold packs to the knee, elevate the leg to reduce edema, and transport
   B. document her pain and straighten her leg anyway
   C. give high-concentration oxygen and transport immediately without splinting the leg
   D. immobilize the leg as you found it and transport

2. A 69-year-old man fell at home. His left leg is shortened and externally rotated. His left hip is bruised and tender. You should _____.
   A. apply a traction splint to the left leg
   B. transport the patient with the leg immobilized as it was found
   C. transport the patient with the leg straightened and secured to the other leg
   D. transport without attempting to immobilize his leg

3. A patient with a midshaft right tibia fracture complains of pain in the distal extremity as well as at the fracture site. The extremity is cold and pale. Pedal and posterior tibial pulses are absent. The most probable cause of these signs and symptoms is _____.
   A. compression of nerves at the site of the fracture
   B. occlusion of the arterial supply to the extremity
   C. occlusion of the venous supply to the extremity
   D. vasoconstriction in response to pain from the fracture

4. In what position should an injured hand usually be splinted?
   A. With the fingers slightly flexed as if holding a baseball
   B. With the fingers straight and spread apart
   C. With the fingers straight and the fingertips exposed
   D. With the hand curled in a tight fist

5. A 67-year-old female "twisted" her ankle when she stepped off of a curb. The ankle is painful, swollen, discolored, and deformed. Distal pulses are present. Skin color and temperature are normal. What would be the best splint to apply?
   A. Elastic bandage
   B. Pillow splint
   C. Short board splint
   D. Traction splint

6. A 19-year-old male working on a construction site was struck in the leg by a steel beam. His midthigh is painful, swollen, and deformed. Coworkers say the patient immediately fell to the ground after being struck. He tells you he did not hit his head and denies any neck or back pain. A major concern with this type of extremity injury is _____.
   A. a high incidence of infection
   B. amputation below the injury often is indicated
   C. blood loss leading to hypovolemia
   D. conversion into an open fracture

115

7. A 12-year-old male injured his leg while playing soccer. The lower leg is painful, swollen, and deformed. After applying a splint and moving the patient to the cot _____.
   A. elevate the leg and apply a cold pack to the injury site
   B. elevate the leg and apply a heat pack to the injury site
   C. lower the leg and apply a cold pack to the injury site
   D. lower the leg and apply a heat pack to the injury site

8. Which statement about orthopedic injuries is correct?
   A. All orthopedic injuries are immediately life threatening and have a high treatment priority in multiple systems' trauma.
   B. In a critical patient, orthopedic injuries can be splinted by securing the patient to a long spine board.
   C. In the multiple systems' trauma patient, all orthopedic injuries must be splinted individually before the patient is moved.
   D. The principal concern in orthopedic injury is the trauma to the bone rather than to the surrounding soft tissues.

9. A properly applied splint immobilizes the _____.
   A. fracture site and the joint above the fracture
   B. fracture site and the joint below the fracture
   C. fracture site and the joints above and below the fracture
   D. fracture site only

10. What is the *most common* complication of fractures and dislocations?
    A. Amputation
    B. Hypovolemic shock
    C. Infection
    D. Injury to peripheral nerves and blood vessels

11. What is your goal when you apply manual traction to a fractured femur?
    A. Force all of the bone fragments back into alignment.
    B. Reduce the fracture.
    C. Separate the fractured bone ends.
    D. Stabilize the bone fragments and improve alignment of the limb.

12. A fracture of which of the following bones would be most likely to produce hypovolemic shock?
    A. Humerus
    B. Pelvis
    C. Radius/ulna
    D. Tibia

13. A partial dislocation where ligaments are stretched or torn, but the bone ends realign when the stress is removed is a _____.
    A. first-degree dislocation
    B. second-degree subluxation
    C. sprain
    D. strain

14. When applied to an injured extremity, a splint should _____.
    A. be at least one and one-half times the length of the bone
    B. be the same length as the bone
    C. immobilize at least 6 inches above and below the injury
    D. immobilize one joint above and one joint below the injury

15. What are the three types of muscle tissue?
    A. Involuntary, smooth, cardiac
    B. Skeletal, involuntary, striated
    C. Skeletal, smooth, cardiac
    D. Striated, skeletal, smooth

16. Which of the following statements is correct?
    A. A fracture is the same as a broken bone.
    B. In fractures the bone is cracked, but in broken bones the bone is broken through completely.
    C. In fractures the bone ends are displaced, but in broken bones they are not.
    D. In fractures the bone ends protrude through the skin, but in broken bones they do not.

17. What are the flat, cordlike bands of connective tissue that connect bone to bone?
    A. Cartilages
    B. Ligaments
    C. Smooth muscles
    D. Tendons

18. In a motor vehicle crash, a patient's knees hit the dashboard, resulting in a fracture of the left patella. This is an example of _____.
    A. direct violence
    B. indirect violence
    C. pathologic fracture
    D. twisting injury (torsion)

19. What bone is involved in a Colles' fracture?
    A. Distal radius
    B. Distal ulna
    C. Proximal radius
    D. Proximal ulna

20. What type of joint attaches the femur to the pelvis at the hip?
    A. Ball and socket
    B. Condylar
    C. Hinge
    D. Pivot

21. The traction splint is indicated if the patient has _____.
    A. a hip injury
    B. a mid-shaft femur fracture
    C. a partial midthigh amputation or mid-thigh avulsion where the distal limb is connected only by tissue
    D. a pelvic injury

Case one

You patient is a 13-year-old female who fell from a jungle gym. She is complaining of pain and tenderness in her right knee. When you examine the affected area, you note a deformity of the knee joint. The leg distal to the affected joint is pale and cool. Dorsal pedal and posterior tibial pulses are absent.

1. What problem do you suspect?

   _____

2. Should you attempt to realign the knee? Why or why not?

   _____
   _____
   _____
   _____

3. When you attempt to straighten the affected extremity, the patient complains of severe pain and the joint will not move easily. What should you do at this point?

   _____
   _____
   _____
   _____

Case two

A 17-year old female fractured her femur during a fall from a horse. On open reduction with internal fixation using an intramedullary rod was performed. Approximately 48 hours post injury, the patient began to develop restlessness and anxiety. She complained of shortness of breath and chest pain on inspiration. Rales and wheezing were audible throughout the lung fields. A petechial rash formed on the patient's upper chest and shoulders. The hemoglobin saturation fell to 87% and ABGs showed pH 7.48, PaO_2 78, $PaCO_2$ 30. A chest radiograph showed a "snowstorm" pattern of diffuse alveolar infiltrates throughout the lung fields.

1. What problem probably is present?

   _____

2. What is the relationship between this problem and the patient's initial injury?

   _____
   _____
   _____
   _____

3. What intervention by EMS personnel can reduce the probability of this problem occurring?

   _____
   _____
   _____
   _____

Case three

You are standing by at a high school football game. A running back is attempting to turn up field when he is tackled from the front at the level of his kness. When he has difficulty getting up, you and the team trainer go onto the field to assess him. The player tells you he felt his right knee "bend backwards" at the moment of impact. The knee is tender and swollen, but seems to be stable. Distal circulation, motion, and sensation are intact. The trainer says, "It's probably just a sprain. We'll ice it for the rest of the game, then wrap it with an elastic bandage. I'll take another look at it on Monday at practice".

1. What problem should you suspect based on the mechanism of injury?
    _____

2. Do you agree with the trainer's recommendation?
    _____
    _____
    _____
    _____

3. If not, what would you suggest?
    _____
    _____
    _____
    _____

52 Environmental Conditions

READING ASSIGNMENT

Chapter 52, pages 535-571, in *Paramedic Practice Today: Above and Beyond*.

OBJECTIVES

After completing this chapter, you will be able to:
1. Define *environmental emergency*.
2. Describe the incidence, morbidity, and mortality rates associated with environmental emergencies.
3. Identify risk factors most predisposing to environmental emergencies.
4. Identify environmental factors that may cause illness or exacerbate a preexisting illness.
5. Identify environmental factors that may complicate treatment or transport decisions.
6. List the principal types of environmental illnesses.
7. Define *homeostasis* and relate the concept to environmental influences.
8. Identify normal, critically high, and critically low body temperatures.
9. Describe several methods of temperature monitoring.
10. Identify the components of the body's thermoregulatory mechanism.
11. Describe the general process of thermal regulation, including substances used and wastes generated.
12. Describe the body's compensatory process for overheating.
13. Describe the body's compensatory process for excess heat loss.
14. List the common forms of heat and cold disorders.
15. List the common predisposing factors associated with heat and cold disorders.
16. List the common preventative measures associated with heat and cold disorders.
17. Integrate the pathophysiologic principles and complicating factors common to environmental emergencies and discuss differentiating features between emergent and urgent presentations.
18. Define *heat illness*.
19. Describe the pathophysiology of heat illness.
20. Identify signs and symptoms of heat illness.
21. List the predisposing factors for heat illness.
22. List measures to prevent heat illness.
23. Discuss the symptomatic variations presented in progressive heat disorders.
24. Relate symptomatic findings to the commonly used terms of *heat cramps, heat exhaustion*, and *heat stroke*.

25. Correlate the abnormal findings in assessment with their clinical significance in the patient with heat illness.
26. Describe the contribution of dehydration to the development of heat disorders.
27. Describe the differences between classic and exertional heat stroke.
28. Define *fever* and discuss its pathophysiologic mechanism.
29. Identify the fundamental thermoregulatory difference between fever and heat stroke.
30. Discuss how to differentiate fever and heat stroke.
31. Discuss the role of fluid therapy in the treatment of heat disorders.
32. Differentiate the various treatments and interventions in the management of heat disorders.
33. Integrate the pathophysiologic principles and the assessment findings to formulate a field impression and implement a treatment plan for the patient who has dehydration, heat exhaustion, or heat stroke.
34. Define *hypothermia*.
35. Describe the pathophysiology of hypothermia.
36. List predisposing factors for hypothermia.
37. List measures to prevent hypothermia.
38. Identify differences between mild and severe hypothermia.
39. Describe differences between chronic and acute hypothermia.
40. List signs and symptoms of hypothermia.
41. Correlate abnormal findings in assessment with their clinical significance in the patient with hypothermia.
42. Discuss the impact of severe hypothermia on standard basic and advanced life support algorithms and transport considerations.
43. Integrate pathophysiologic principles and the assessment findings to formulate a field impression and implement a treatment plan for the patient who has either mild or severe hypothermia.
44. Define *frostbite*.
45. Define *superficial frostbite* (frostnip).
46. Differentiate superficial frostbite and deep frostbite.
47. List predisposing factors for frostbite.
48. List measures to prevent frostbite.
49. Correlate abnormal findings in assessment with their clinical significance in the patient with frostbite.
50. Differentiate the various treatments and interventions in the management of frostbite.
51. Integrate pathophysiologic principles and the assessment findings to formulate a field impression and implement a treatment plan for the patient with superficial or deep frostbite.

119

52. Define *drowning*.
53. Describe the pathophysiology of drowning.
54. List signs and symptoms of drowning.
55. Describe the lack of significance of fresh versus saltwater immersion in relation to drowning.
56. Discuss the incidence of wet versus dry drownings and the differences in their management.
57. Discuss the complications and protective role of hypothermia in the context of drowning.
58. Correlate the abnormal findings in assessment with the clinical significance in the patient with drowning.
59. Differentiate the various treatments and interventions in the management of drowning.
60. Integrate pathophysiologic principles and assessment findings to formulate a field impression and implement a treatment plan for the drowning patient.
61. Define *self-contained underwater breathing apparatus*.
62. Describe the laws of gasses and relate them to diving emergencies.
63. Describe the pathophysiology of diving emergencies.
64. Define *decompression illness*.
65. Identify the various forms of decompression illness.
66. Identify the various conditions that may result from pulmonary overpressure accidents.
67. Differentiate the various diving emergencies.
68. List signs and symptoms of diving emergencies.
69. Correlate abnormal findings in assessment with their clinical significance in the patient with a diving-related illness.
70. Describe the function of the Divers Alert Network and how its members may aid in the management of diving-related illnesses.
71. Differentiate the various treatments and interventions for the management of diving accidents.
72. Describe the specific function and benefit of hyperbaric oxygen therapy for the management of diving accidents.
73. Integrate pathophysiologic principles and assessment findings to formulate a field impression and implement a management plan for the patient who has had a diving accident.
74. Define *altitude illness*.
75. Describe the application of gas laws to altitude illness.
76. Describe the etiology and epidemiology of altitude illness.
77. List predisposing factors for altitude illness.
78. List measures to prevent altitude illness.
79. Define *acute mountain sickness*.
80. Define *high-altitude pulmonary edema*.
81. Define *high-altitude cerebral edema*.
82. Discuss the symptomatic variations presented in progressive altitude illnesses.
83. List signs and symptoms of altitude illnesses.
84. Correlate abnormal findings in assessment with their clinical significance in the patient with altitude illness.
85. Discuss the pharmacology appropriate for the treatment of altitude illnesses.
86. Differentiate the various treatments and interventions for the management of altitude illness.
87. Integrate pathophysiologic principles and assessment findings to formulate a field impression and implement a treatment plan for the patient who has altitude illness.
88. Integrate the pathophysiologic principles of the patient affected by an environmental emergency.
89. Differentiate environmental emergencies on the basis of assessment findings.
90. Correlate abnormal findings in the assessment with their clinical significance in the patient affected by an environmental emergency.
91. Develop a patient management plan based on the field impression of the patient affected by an environmental emergency.
92. Describe the etiology, signs and symptoms, and management of a patient struck by lightning.
93. Describe the etiology, signs and symptoms, and management of patients with envenomations.

CHAPTER SUMMARY

■ Management of environmental emergencies requires integration of pathophysiologic principles. Key to this is an understanding of anatomy, physiology, and metabolic mechanisms the body uses to maintain homeostasis. When these mechanisms are overwhelmed, a careful history and physical examination should allow the paramedic to differentiate environmental emergencies based on assessment findings and develop a patient management plan. Abnormal findings in the assessment should be correlated with their clinical significance as detailed in the individual sections of this chapter.

■ The differentiation between urgent and emergent conditions may be different in remote or austere areas than in "street" paramedicine. In remote or rugged environments, conditions that may only be urgent in urban medicine may need to be managed emergently because of difficulties in adequately treating and transporting patients in a timely fashion. On the other hand, truly emergent conditions may need to be managed for longer periods than would be typically allowed in traditional EMS systems, making them take on more features of urgent medical management rather than emergent medical management.

■ As with most injuries and illnesses, many preventive measures can be taken in advance of a trip. Unfortunately many victims of environmental injuries do not prepare properly and subsequently suffer dire consequences.

■ Basic knowledge of how the environment can affect the human body is helpful to the paramedic attempting to reverse the events that have occurred within the patient. Paramedics may not encounter primary injuries and illnesses from the environment on a regular basis. This should not preclude the paramedic from suspecting environmental disorders in patients.

■ Paramedics encounter a wide variety of calls in their careers—all carry with them the risk of personal injury. The paramedic must remember to not act hastily when handling environmental incidents. This will keep the paramedic from becoming another victim or part of the problem. Scene safety is always important to the paramedic, and never more so in the environment. Consider, for example, the paramedic who approaches the home of an elderly patient on a cold winter day for a report of a fall victim. Consideration must be given to the overt reason for the call (a fall) but consideration must also be given to the location of the incident and the fact that the environment plays a role in the condition of the patient. Will you be able to look beyond the obvious and search for circumstances that exacerbate patient conditions? A good paramedic will.

SHORT ANSWER

1. What is an environmental emergency?

2. What are the principal risk factors that predispose patients to environmental emergencies?

3. Define *homeostasis*.

4. What are the mechanisms by which heat normally is lost from the body?

5. Temperature regulation is centered in what area of the brain?

6. What mechanism(s) does the body use to compensate for increased heat production or high environmental temperatures?

7. What mechanism(s) does the body use to compensate for decreased heat production or low environmental temperatures?

8. Why are the elderly predisposed to heat-related illness?

9. What medications predispose patients to heat-related illness?

10. Why are patients with diabetes predisposed to heat-related illness?

11. Your patient is a 40-year-old male found unconscious in a non–air-conditioned apartment by a neighbor. The temperature has been in excess of 100° F for 2 weeks. The patient is unresponsive to verbal and painful stimuli. His skin is flushed, dry, and warm. He has a history of alcoholism and is morbidly obese.
    A. What problem do you suspect?

    B. What is your primary objective in managing this patient?

12. How does the appearance of a patient with exertional heat stroke differ from that of a patient with classic heat stroke?

13. Why should active cooling of a heat stroke victim be stopped when the victim's temperature falls to 102° F?

121

14. Your patient is a 56-year-old male with a history of hypertension who had a syncopal episode while mowing his lawn on a hot, humid July afternoon. He is mildly confused. His skin is pale, cool, and moist. Vital signs are: P—98 beats/min weak, regular; BP—100/70 mm Hg; R—22 breaths/min shallow, regular. He takes atenolol and hydrochlorothiazide to manage his hypertension.
    A. What problem do you suspect?

    _____

    B. How would you manage this patient?

    _____
    _____
    _____
    _____

15. The patient is a 25-year-old male complaining of severe cramping in his legs for approximately 15 minutes. He states that before the onset of the pain, he had been jogging for approximately 30 minutes. It is a hot day and the humidity is high. The patient is perspiring profusely. He is awake and alert.
    A. What problem do you suspect?

    _____

    B. Describe your management of this patient.

    _____
    _____
    _____
    _____

16. Why should a patient with heat cramps not be given water without supplemental salt?

    _____
    _____
    _____

17. Why are pediatric patients at increased risk of developing hypothermia?

    _____
    _____
    _____
    _____

18. Why are the elderly at increased risk of developing hypothermia?

    _____
    _____
    _____
    _____

19. Why does alcohol consumption increase the risk of developing hypothermia?

    _____
    _____
    _____
    _____

20. Your patient is a homeless man who has been found by the police unconscious in an alley following an ice storm. He responds only to painful stimuli and is very cold to the touch. Vital signs are: P—50 beats/min weak, regular; BP—80/40 mm Hg; R—6 breaths/min shallow, regular.
    A. What problem do you suspect?

    _____

    B. How would you manage this patient?

    _____
    _____
    _____
    _____

    C. Should this patient be actively rewarmed? Why or why not?

    _____
    _____
    _____
    _____

21. How does the presence of hypothermia affect the management of cardiac arrest?

    _____
    _____
    _____
    _____

22. Should frostbitten body parts be rubbed to help rewarm them? Why or why not?

    _____
    _____
    _____
    _____

23. If a frostbitten part is to be rewarmed outside a hospital, what should be the temperature of the water used in the rewarming?

    _____
    _____
    _____

24. You respond to a report of a drowning in an apartment complex swimming pool. Your patient is a 6-year-old female who was pulled from the water before your arrival. She reportedly was submerged for about 3 minutes but has been successfully resuscitated and is crying vigorously. What action should you recommend? Why?

    _____
    _____
    _____
    _____

25. In early April, you respond to a report of a drowning at a spot on a river that is popular with local teenagers. The patient is a 15-year-old male who was seen to have jumped from a rock outcropping into the water. When he did not surface immediately, his friends began to search for him. He finally was discovered about 30 yards downstream 10 minutes later. He is unconscious and unresponsive, but is breathing at a rate of 10 breaths/min and has a pulse rate of 60 beats/min. What problems might be associated with this drowning?

_____
_____
_____
_____

26. You respond to a report of a drowning at an area lake. When you arrive, you find that your patient is a 24-year-old female who was trying out her boyfriend's SCUBA equipment. She reportedly panicked when her mask filled with water and she was unable to clear it. She surfaced rapidly and lost consciousness almost immediately. What problem do you suspect?

_____
_____
_____
_____

27. What is the pathophysiology of decompression sickness?

_____
_____
_____
_____

28. What is nitrogen narcosis ("rapture of the deep")?

_____
_____
_____
_____

29. What are the signs and symptoms of high-altitude cerebral edema?

_____
_____
_____
_____

30. What are the signs and symptoms of high-altitude pulmonary edema?

_____
_____
_____
_____

MULTIPLE CHOICE

1. Heat loss by the movement of air over the surface of the body is called _____.
   A. conduction
   B. convection
   C. evaporation
   D. radiation

2. Which statement about prehospital management of frostbite is correct?
   A. Cover the affected area with loosely applied, moist, sterile dressings.
   B. Do not thaw the affected area if there is a risk of refreezing.
   C. Slowly rewarm the affected area with warm packs, blankets or other warm objects.
   D. Vigorously massage the frozen area or rub with snow.

3. Heat is generated within the body by _____.
   A. cellular metabolism and physical activity
   B. evaporation and cellular metabolism
   C. radiation and physical activity
   D. shivering and convection

4. The most effective means of cooling a heat exhaustion patient is to _____.
   A. cover the patient with wet sheets and fan the patient
   B. have the patient drink cold liquids
   C. infuse cool IV fluids
   D. place the patient in an air-conditioned environment

5. The temperature control center of the body is located in the _____.
   A. cerebellum
   B. cerebrum
   C. hypothalamus
   D. pons

6. When administering medications to hypothermic patients they should be _____.
   A. given at longer intervals
   B. given at shorter intervals
   C. given at twice the normal dose since circulation and absorption are delayed
   D. withheld unless the patient is severely hypothermic ($< 86° F$)

7. Which of the following persons is at greatest risk for classic heat stroke assuming the environment's temperature and humidity are high?
   A. A 40-year-old man out on his daily morning jog
   B. A 65-year-old man with a history of type 1 diabetes taking a walk outside
   C. A 70-year-old woman with a history of congestive heart failure who is inside her air-conditioned apartment
   D. A healthy 14-year-old boy out playing baseball

8. Mild alterations of mental status are most likely to occur in a patient who has _____.
   A. frost bite
   B. heat cramps
   C. heat exhaustion
   D. heat stroke

9. A 73-year-old female with a history of heart disease and type 2 diabetes mellitus was found unconscious in her backyard on a July afternoon. The temperature has been 103 F or higher for 5 days. The patient's skin is hot and dry, and her respirations are rapid and labored. A neighbor tells you the patient complained of a headache earlier in the day and has been "acting funny" all afternoon. The patient probably is suffering from _____.
   A. classic heat stroke
   B. exertional heat stroke
   C. heat cramps
   D. heat exhaustion

10. The most important action in treating the patient in the previous question would be to _____.
    A. assist her ventilations with a bag-mask and oxygen
    B. begin cooling her immediately
    C. give high-concentration oxygen by nonrebreather mask
    D. take frequent body temperatures

11. An 18-year-old male's car went off a bridge through the ice into a frozen lake. When the fire department finally extricated him 40 minutes later, he was unconscious with no pulse and no blood pressure. His pupils were fixed and dilated. His skin was cold to the touch. The fire department tells you the vehicle was completely filled with water. You should _____.
    A. assist the patient's ventilations and transport to the hospital without doing CPR
    B. call for the police and the medical examiner
    C. start CPR immediately and attempt to rewarm the patient rapidly
    D. start CPR immediately and transport

12. At the scene of a traffic accident, a state trooper tells you that his hands "feel funny." His fingers are white and feel "doughy." He tells you he has been outside for 45 minutes without gloves. The wind chill factor is −5° F. You are approximately 60 minutes from the closest hospital. You should _____.
    A. have him keep his hands below the level of his heart to promote blood flow
    B. rapidly rewarm his hands
    C. rapidly rewarm his hands while rubbing his fingers to stimulate circulation
    D. rub his fingers vigorously to stimulate circulation

13. *Active* external rewarming techniques are indicated for hypothermia patients who are _____.
    A. either not responding appropriately or unconscious
    B. not responding appropriately
    C. responding appropriately
    D. unconscious

14. *Passive* external rewarming techniques are indicated for hypothermia patients who are _____.
    A. either not responding appropriately or unconscious
    B. not responding appropriately
    C. responding appropriately
    D. unconscious

15. Which statement about assessing the pulse in a victim of extreme generalized hypothermia is correct?
    A. Carotid pulse assessment should be performed for as long as 30 to 45 seconds. If a pulse is felt during that time, chest compressions should not be performed.
    B. Carotid pulse assessment should take no longer than 30 seconds. If the pulse rate is less than 60 beats/min, start CPR.
    C. If a radial pulse is not present, begin CPR.
    D. If a radial pulse is present but is less than 60 beats/min, begin CPR.

16. Which statement about emergency care of deep cold injury (frostbite) is correct?
    A. Apply hot packs to all deeply cold-injured (frost-bitten) parts as soon as possible, especially if reexposure to cold will occur before or during transport.
    B. Do not massage the injured area; cover it with dry dressings. If any jewelry is present, remove it.
    C. Remove jewelry, apply hot packs as soon as possible, and then cover the injured area with dry dressings.
    D. Since the patient is unlikely to be able to massage the part, gently massage the part for him or her to stimulate circulation of warm blood to the injured areas.

124

Case one

A 56-year-old female had a syncopal episode while returning from a walk to the grocery store on a warm August afternoon. She is not oriented to place or time. Respirations are rapid and shallow. Breath sounds are present and equal bilaterally. Radial pulses are rapid and weak. The patient has a history of mild chronic essential hypertension for which she takes hydrochlorothiazide (HydroDIURIL). Vital signs are: BP—100/70 mm Hg; P—116 beats/min weak, regular; R—22 breaths/min shallow, regular.

1. From what problem is the patient suffering?

2. Why is the patient's skin cool and pale?

3. Why is the patient tachycardic?

4. Is the patient's blood pressure what you would anticipate? Why or why not?

5. What problems account for the changes in the patient's blood pressure and pulse rate?

6. What would you anticipate finding if you took this patient's temperature?

7. What is significant about the patient's history of hypertension and her medication history?

8. How would you manage this patient?

125

Case two

A 25-year-old male complains of severe muscle spasms in his legs and abdomen that began after he played tennis in 90-degree heat for 4 hours. The patient is awake and alert. His respirations are rapid and shallow. His radial pulses are rapid and strong, and his skin is pale, cool, and moist. The patient has no significant past medical history and takes no medications. Vital signs are: BP—132/82 mm Hg; P—98 beats/min strong, regular; R—20 breaths/min shallow, regular.

1. From what problem is the patient suffering?

2. What is the principal difference in signs and symptoms that distinguishes this problem from the problem in Case One?

3. What is the difference in the pathophysiology of the problem in this case from the problem in Case One?

4. What is causing the muscle spasms?

5. How would you manage this patient?

6. If you gave this patient large amounts of pure water to drink, what effect would you anticipate? Why?

Case three

At the scene of a traffic accident a highway patrolman tells you his hands "feel funny." When you examine his fingers you discover they are white and feel "doughy" to the touch. The patient tells you his fingers were "burning" earlier, but that they now are numb. He has been outside for 45 minutes without any gloves. The air temperature is 20° F, and the wind chill is −5° F. You are 90 minutes from the closest hospital.

1. From what problem is the patient suffering?

2. What is the pathophysiology of this problem?

3. How should this patient be managed?

_____
_____
_____
_____

4. If you were only 15 minutes from a hospital, how would your management of this patient change?

_____
_____
_____
_____

5. Should you allow the patient to rub or slap his hands together to warm them? Why?

_____
_____
_____
_____

Case four

You respond to a report of a drowning at a large apartment complex. The patient is a 22-year-old female who is unconscious and unresponsive. Her pupils are dilated and sluggishly responsive to light. You are told she was trying out her boyfriend's SCUBA equipment in the swimming pool just before she collapsed. Auscultation of the chest reveals breath sounds bilaterally. Vital signs are: P—58 beats/min weak, regular; R—24 breaths/min shallow, regular; BP—168/100 mm Hg.

1. From what problem is the patient probably suffering?

_____

2. What is the pathophysiology of this problem?

_____
_____
_____
_____

3. Describe the management of this patient.

_____
_____
_____
_____

Case five

Your patient is a 23-year-old male who has just arrived at the local airport. He is complaining of aching pain in his shoulder, elbows, and knees, and of blank spots in his visual fields. He is awake and alert. Respirations are rapid and shallow. His skin is pale and cool. Radial pulses are rapid and bounding. The patient tells you he had been diving in Mexico over the weekend and got on the plane just after his last dive. Vital signs are: BP—146/98 mm Hg; R—22 breaths/min shallow, regular; P—110 beats/min strong, regular.

1. From what problem is the patient suffering?

_____

2. What is the pathophysiology of this problem?

_____
_____
_____
_____

127

3. How does the pathophysiology of this problem differ from that of the patient in Case Four?

_____
_____
_____
_____

4. Why is the patient's recent air travel significant?

_____
_____
_____
_____

5. How would you manage this patient?

_____
_____
_____
_____

Case six

While on a skiing trip, you are asked to "check out" a 32-year-old male who has suddenly become ill. The patient is complaining of headache, nausea, and fatigue. Although he denies alcohol and drug abuse, he has a staggering gait. He tells you he left Houston, Texas, by plane yesterday and arrived in a nearby city that is located at an altitude of 5000 feet. He then rented a car and immediately drove to the mountains. By 0900 this morning, he was at the 13,000-foot level.

1. From what problem is this patient suffering?

_____

2. What is the pathophysiology of this problem?

_____
_____
_____
_____

3. How would you manage him?

_____
_____
_____
_____

Case seven

Later in the day, you encounter a 42-year-old female who is experiencing difficulty breathing. She says she has been developing worsening dyspnea on exertion for the last 8 hours and that she cannot breathe when she lies down. She has a dry cough, and rales are present in her lung bases.

1. What problem do you suspect?

_____

2. How should this patient be managed?

_____
_____
_____
_____

3. Are morphine and furosemide (Lasix) indicated in the management of this patient?

   _____

   _____

   _____

   _____

4. Why or why not?

   _____

   _____

   _____

   _____

53 Farm Response

READING ASSIGNMENT

Chapter 53, pages 572-596, in *Paramedic Practice Today: Above and Beyond*.

OBJECTIVES

After completing this chapter, you will be able to:
1. Discuss common mechanisms of injury in the farm setting.
2. Explain the differences in approach to a patient with crush injury compared with a laceration injury.
3. Discuss the causes and management of compartment syndrome.
4. Explain the urgency of caring for a patient who has received a hydraulic injection injury.
5. Describe how to recognize organophosphate poisoning.
6. Identify the hazards associated with farm confined spaces and risks posed to potential rescuers.

CHAPTER SUMMARY

- Managing emergencies on a farm often requires modified procedures and protocols.
- Most farms use at least one tractor daily, and tractor overturns result in half of all farm deaths.
- Crush injury syndrome is a condition that can be seen in farm trauma situations because of the length of time a person often is entrapped.
- Numerous hazard points on farm machines can cause a severe entanglement that can challenge even seasoned rescue technicians.
- Power take-off entanglements can result in severe crushing injuries as well as acute amputations.
- Hydraulic oil pressure is normally 2000 psi but can exceed 7000 psi through a pinhole leak. Under this pressure, the fluid can easily penetrate the skin and cause serious complications.
- A host of hazardous materials are present on farms to which farmers, their families, and employees can be exposed. Some of the materials are derivatives of nerve agents.
- Many areas on farms are considered confined spaces by OSHA definition. Although the majority of farmers are exempt from OSHA inspections, emergency responders must recognize confined spaces and follow OSHA confined space standards when managing these emergencies.
- Emergency responders must recognize the potential for deadly gases generated inside silos and manure storage because they may respond to calls involving these aspects of farming.

SHORT ANSWER

1. Why should EMS personnel always anticipate a serious situation when they respond to an incident at a farm?

2. What is the cause of most deaths and serious injuries on farms?

3. What is the pathophysiology of crush syndrome?

4. What is the preferred IV solution for a patient with suspected crush syndrome? Why?

5. State three reasons why sodium bicarbonate is used in the management of crush syndrome.

6. What changes on a patient's ECG might suggest crush syndrome is present? What abnormality produces these changes?

7. What is the pathophysiology of compartment syndrome?

8. Describe the prehospital management of compartment syndrome.

_____
_____
_____
_____

9. Describe the three factors that contribute to tissue damage in hydraulic injection injury.

_____
_____
_____
_____

10. By what route do most pesticide exposures occur?

_____
_____
_____
_____

11. Discuss the pathophysiology of organophosphate toxicity.

_____
_____
_____
_____

12. Why is atropine used as an initial antidote for organophosphate toxicity?

_____
_____
_____
_____

13. What is the definitive antidote for organophosphate toxicity?

_____
_____
_____
_____

14. How does management of carbamate toxicity differ from the management of an organophosphate poisoning?

_____
_____
_____
_____

15. Should oxygen be given to a patient who has been poisoned with Paraquat? Why or why not?

_____
_____
_____
_____

16. What is silo gas?

_____
_____
_____

17. Describe the situations in which silo gas is most likely to be present.

_____
_____
_____
_____

18. Describe the pathophysiology of silo filler's disease.

_____
_____
_____
_____

19. Describe the pathophysiology of anhydrous ammonia exposure.

_____
_____
_____
_____

20. Discuss the management of a patient who has been exposed to anhydrous ammonia.

_____
_____
_____
_____

21. Describe the situations on a farm in which hydrogen sulfide is most likely to be present. What is another name used for hydrogen sulfide found in these situations?

_____
_____
_____
_____

MULTIPLE CHOICE

1. Most serious injuries and deaths on farms are caused by _____.
   A. attacks by farm animals
   B. confined space incidents
   C. pesticide exposure
   D. tractors and other machinery

2. Crush syndrome should be suspected if a patient has had a large muscle mass compressed for longer than _____.
   A. 15 minutes
   B. 30 minutes
   C. 45 minutes
   D. 60 minutes

3. Which of these statements about management of crush syndrome is correct?
   A. Because crush syndrome can produce critical injuries, IVs should be started during transport.
   B. Once rescue equipment has arrived, the patient should be freed from entrapment as quickly as possible.
   C. Ringer's lactate is preferred over normal saline because it contains potassium.
   D. Sodium bicarbonate should be given to correct acidosis and to decrease the risk of renal failure.

4. Which of the following statements about hydraulic injection injury is correct?
   A. For injection to occur, the patient must have come into direct contact with the leak.
   B. Severe pain will be present immediately after the injection occurs.
   C. Swelling typically begins 1 to 3 hours after the patient is injected.
   D. The problem typically resolves quickly with elevation, application of cold packs, and administration of anti-inflammatory drugs.

Questions 5 through 8 relate to the following scenario:
A farmer was riding a tractor when a crop duster accidentally sprayed him. The patient responds only to painful stimuli. He is salivating heavily, his pupils are pinpoint, and he is incontinent of bladder and bowel. Auscultation of his chest reveals crackles and rhonchi. Vital signs are: BP—96/50 mm Hg; P—40 beats/min weak, regular; R—6 breaths/min shallow, labored.

5. To what type of toxin has the patient probably been exposed?
   A. A bipyridial
   B. A polychlorinated biphenyl
   C. An organochlorine
   D. An organophosphate

6. What is causing his excess salivation, incontinence, and pupillary constriction?
   A. Decreased parasympathetic tone
   B. Decreased sympathetic tone
   C. Increased parasympathetic tone
   D. Increased sympathetic tone

7. What drug should be given to this patient initially?
   A. Atropine
   B. Flumazenil
   C. Furosemide
   D. Narcan

8. What drug is the definitive antidote for this toxin?
   A. 2-PAM
   B. Amyl nitrite
   C. Methylene blue
   D. Sodium bicarbonate

9. Which of the following statements about Paraquat poisoning is correct?
   A. Death usually results from respiratory failure.
   B. IV fluids should be withheld to avoid worsening pulmonary edema.
   C. Patients should be treated with high-concentration oxygen and assisted ventilations as quickly as possible.
   D. The most likely route for poisoning is through skin absorption.

10. Which of the following statements about confined spaces on farms is correct?
    A. Although confined spaces are common on farms, most of them do not meet the OSHA definition of a "permitted" confined space.
    B. Because most farms are exempt from OSHA inspection, farmers often do not follow OSHA-mandated confined space entry procedures.
    C. Because most farms are exempt from OSHA inspection, rescuers do not have to follow OSHA regulations during responses to farm incidents.
    D. Confined spaces are uncommon on farms.

11. What are the effects of breathing moderate concentrations of silo gas?
    A. Burning of the eyes and throat, rapid onset of pharyngeal edema, and loss of the airway
    B. Few immediate symptoms followed by inflammation of the lower airway and pulmonary edema 6 to 12 hours later
    C. Few immediate symptoms followed by severe pharyngeal edema and loss of the airway 6 to 12 hours later
    D. Laryngospasm, immediate collapse, and respiratory arrest

12. A patient who complains of eye irritation after smelling an odor "like rotten eggs" most likely was exposed to _____.
    A. anhydrous ammonia
    B. hydrogen sulfide
    C. Paraquat
    D. silo gas

On a Tuesday afternoon at 1330 hours you are dispatched to a report of a "man pinned under a tractor." The temperature is 93° F and the relative humidity is 80%. The weather is clear; however, there has been heavy rain from thunderstorms during the afternoons of each of the past 3 days. Your response takes 30 minutes. When you arrive, a young man meets you. He tells you that the patient, his father, left the house at about 0630 hours. When he did not return for the noon meal, a search was started immediately. The patient was discovered pinned under a tractor approximately 30 minutes ago. The patient is about 75 yards from a roadway in a very muddy field. The tractor is resting on the patient's pelvis and thighs. His skin is pale and dry. Transport time to the closest hospital is 40 minutes. A level II trauma center is 90 minutes away. The local volunteer fire department is responding.

1. Are there any additional resources that should be requested?

   _____
   _____
   _____
   _____

2. Discuss any special considerations in gaining access to this patient.

   _____
   _____
   _____
   _____

3. What hazards might need to be identified and managed before patient care and disentanglement can begin?

   _____
   _____
   _____
   _____

4. Identify any special problems that should be taken into consideration when managing this patient. Describe how these problems should be addressed.

   _____
   _____
   _____
   _____

5. Describe any other issues that may effect the health and safety of the rescuers as the call progresses.

   _____
   _____
   _____
   _____

6. Are there any special considerations for patient transport?

   _____
   _____
   _____
   _____

54 Wilderness EMS

READING ASSIGNMENT

Chapter 54, pages 597-614, in *Paramedic Practice Today: Above and Beyond.*

OBJECTIVES

After completing this chapter, you will be able to:
1. Define and describe wilderness medicine and wilderness EMS.
2. Define and describe a wilderness EMS system.
3. Describe the differences in practice environments between traditional EMS and wilderness EMS.
4. Describe the differences in protocols between traditional EMS and wilderness EMS.
5. Describe the differences in certification and training between traditional EMS and wilderness EMS.
6. Demonstrate techniques used to clear a cervical spine clinically in a wilderness setting.
7. Describe the differences in equipment between traditional EMS and wilderness EMS.
8. Describe the differences in resources between traditional EMS and wilderness EMS.
9. Describe the differences in team interfaces between traditional EMS and wilderness EMS.
10. Identify current wilderness EMS systems in the United States.
11. Identify challenges facing wilderness EMS systems.

CHAPTER SUMMARY

- *Wilderness medicine* is a term that must be understood contextually. In this chapter it is defined as medical management in situations where care and prevention are limited by environmental considerations, prolonged extrication, or resource availability.
- Wilderness EMS systems plan and help implement the provision of wilderness medical care to a discrete region or type of activity and help integrate wilderness medical principles into the greater EMS system. Wilderness EMS systems differ from traditional (street) systems in important ways. Some of these include differences in environment in which the provider delivers care, protocols and online and offline medical direction, certification and training, equipment, resources, and organizations with which the providers are expected to interact. Wilderness EMS systems currently are in place that provide standards and resources for medical care and rescue in certain environments (e.g., MRA and the NCRC). Others provide wilderness medical care for certain regions (e.g., the Parkmedic program or local EMS or nonprofit rescue services) or temporary care in regions with situational austerity (such as the NDMS system).
- Wilderness EMS systems may be federally funded, locally funded, or nonprofit. Some wilderness EMS organizations operate as schools or commercial ventures providing wilderness medical training.
- Numerous options are available to the EMS provider interested in obtaining or providing additional training in wilderness EMS and in providing patient care in diverse practice environments.
- Numerous challenges also exist to the growth of wilderness EMS as a field: federal funding, disparities in EMS funding relative to other public service entities, a reliance nationally on volunteer service, and an ongoing debate regarding the appropriateness and source of funding for rescues and wilderness medical care.
- Given the rapid growth of wilderness activities and a corresponding demand for wilderness medical care, these challenges are expected to be addressed and wilderness EMS will continue to grow as an important EMS subspecialty.

SHORT ANSWER

1. What is wilderness medicine?

_____
_____
_____
_____

2. What is a wilderness EMS system?

_____
_____
_____
_____

3. What similarities between the wilderness environment and disaster environments lead to disaster medicine sometimes being considered a part of wilderness medicine?

_____
_____
_____
_____

4. Describe the differences in practice environments between traditional EMS and wilderness EMS.

_____

_____

_____

_____

5. Describe the differences in protocols between traditional EMS and wilderness EMS.

_____

_____

_____

_____

6. Describe differences in certification and training between traditional EMS and wilderness EMS.

_____

_____

_____

_____

7. Describe the differences in equipment between traditional EMS and wilderness EMS.

_____

_____

_____

_____

8. Describe differences in resources between traditional EMS and wilderness EMS.

_____

_____

_____

_____

9. Describe the differences in team interfaces between traditional EMS and wilderness EMS.

_____

_____

_____

_____

10. Identify four agencies within the federal government of the United States that can provide wilderness EMS.

_____

_____

_____

_____

11. Identify four organizations that provide certification or coordination of wilderness EMS activities on a national level in the United States.

_____

_____

_____

_____

12. Identify challenges facing wilderness EMS systems.

_____

_____

_____

_____

MULTIPLE CHOICE

1. Including a physician or other healthcare provider within a group that is going into a wilderness area for an extended time is an example of what model of wilderness medicine?
   A. Disaster medicine
   B. Expedition
   C. Professional
   D. Recreational

2. What model of wilderness medicine involves individuals or groups that preplan to provide care in austere environments and then are called on to perform this duty when needed?
   A. Disaster medicine
   B. Expedition
   C. Professional
   D. Recreational

3. A paramedic with wilderness medicine training is hiking in a national park while on vacation. She finds another hiker who has fallen and sprained his ankle. The paramedic providing care to the injured hiker is an example of what model of wilderness medicine?
   A. Disaster medicine
   B. Expedition
   C. Professional
   D. Recreational

4. Which states currently provide formal certification in wilderness medicine?
   A. Hawaii and Nevada
   B. Maine and Maryland
   C. Maine and Wyoming
   D. Maryland and Colorado

5. The National Disaster Medical System includes
   _____.
   A. Disaster Medical Assistance Teams, Disaster Mortuary Response Teams, and Urban Search and Rescue Task Forces
   B. Disaster Medical Assistance Teams, Disaster Veterinary Assistance Teams, and Disaster Mortuary Response Teams
   C. Disaster Medical Assistance Teams, Disaster Veterinary Assistance Teams, and Urban Search and Rescue Task Forces
   D. National Medical Response Teams, Urban Search and Rescue Task Forces, and Disaster Medical Assistance Teams

55 Assessment-Based Management

READING ASSIGNMENT

Chapter 55, pages 616-626, in *Paramedic Practice Today: Above and Beyond*.

OBJECTIVES

After completing this chapter, you will be able to:

1. Explain how effectively assessing a patient is critical to making clinical decisions.
2. Explain the general approach, assessment, and management priorities for the following patients or conditions:
   - Chest pain
   - Medical and traumatic cardiac arrest
   - Acute abdominal pain
   - Gastrointestinal bleed
   - Altered mental status
   - Dyspnea
   - Syncope
   - Seizures
   - Environmental or thermal problem
   - Hazardous material or toxic exposure
   - Trauma or multiple-trauma patients
   - Allergic reactions
   - Behavioral problems
   - Obstetric or gynecologic problems
   - Pediatric patients
3. Explain how the paramedic's attitude affects his or her assessment of patients and decision making.
4. Explain how uncooperative patients affect the paramedic's assessment and decision making.
5. Explain strategies the paramedic can use to prevent labeling patients and having tunnel vision.
6. Develop strategies to decrease the distractions in the prehospital environment.
7. Describe how manpower considerations and staffing configurations affect the paramedic's assessment of patients and his or her decision making.
8. Synthesize concepts of scene management and choreography to simulated calls.
9. Explain the roles of the team leader and the patient care person.
10. List and explain the rationale for carrying in the essential patient care items.
11. When given a simulated call, list the appropriate equipment to take to the patient.
12. Explain the general approach to the emergency patient.
13. Describe how to communicate information effectively face to face, over the telephone, by radio, and in writing.

CHAPTER SUMMARY

- Assessment-based management requires that you treat the patient and not simply follow the protocol.
- With the information you gathered from your assessment of the scene, the patient's SAMPLE history, and physical examination findings, you must realize that deviation from protocol may be necessary to treat your patient appropriately.
- Use everything at your disposal to help form your assessment: your senses, the patient's signs and symptoms, medical history, and environment. Then treat your patient.
- Do not get tunnel vision. Horrific injuries, children who are sick or injured, and situations that stress your ability to perform can cause you to focus on only one aspect of the patient's care instead of care of the whole patient.
- Learn how to choreograph the scene. Preplan with your partner, practicing what you would do in any situation.
- An accurate verbal report provides the physician and receiving facility staff with a description of what you saw, what you did, and how the patient is at this point in your care.

SHORT ANSWER

1. What is assessment-based management?
   _____
   _____
   _____
   _____

137

2. Why should paramedics take an assessment-based approach to patient management rather than just following their physician-approved protocols?

_____

_____

_____

_____

3. What is pattern recognition?

_____

_____

_____

_____

4. What is the role of pattern recognition in assessment-based management?

_____

_____

_____

_____

5. What sources of information should a paramedic use to practice assessment-based management?

_____

_____

_____

_____

6. What is pattern response?

_____

_____

_____

_____

7. What is the relationship between pattern recognition, pattern response, and assessment-based management?

_____

_____

_____

_____

8. Why is accurate, effective patient presentation an essential skill for paramedics practicing assessment-based management?

_____

_____

_____

_____

9. What is tunnel vision?

_____

_____

_____

_____

10. Why does tunnel vision interfere with effective assessment-based patient management?

_____

_____

_____

_____

11. What is the inverted pyramid approach to clinical reasoning?

_____

_____

_____

_____

12. Why is the inverted pyramid approach to clinical reasoning useful in avoiding tunnel vision?

_____

_____

_____

_____

13. List factors that can affect assessment and clinical decision making.

_____

_____

_____

_____

14. What is assessment by committee? Why is assessment by committee not an effective practice?

_____

_____

_____

_____

15. List the sequence of steps in the general approach to the emergency patient.

_____

_____

_____

_____

16. What are the roles of the team leader during patient assessment and management?

_____

_____

_____

_____

17. What are the roles of the patient care provider during patient assessment and management?

_____

_____

_____

_____

18. How often should the ongoing assessment be performed on a stable patient?

_____

_____

_____

_____

19. How often should the ongoing assessment be performed on an unstable patient?

_____

_____

_____

_____

CASE STUDIES

Part one

For each of the following patients, indicate whether a focused or more detailed (head-to-toe) physical examination would be most appropriate and state the reason for your decision.

1. A 25-year-old female lacerated her left palm with a kitchen knife while preparing dinner. She is awake and alert. Respirations are 18 breaths/min, regular. Radial pulses are 106 beats/min strong, regular. Bleeding was controlled quickly by using direct pressure with a loss of approximately 50 mL of blood.

_____

_____

_____

_____

2. A 17-year-old female lost control of her vehicle and struck a tree at a speed of approximately 55 miles per hour. Extensive frontal damage occurred to the vehicle. The patient was wearing a lap belt and shoulder harness. An airbag deployed during the collision. The patient is awake and alert. Respirations are 22 breaths/min, regular. Radial pulses are 110 beats/min strong, regular. The patient has abrasions on her forearms and is complaining of pain in her right ankle, which is swollen and discolored.

_____

_____

_____

_____

3. A 55-year-old male complains of squeezing substernal chest pain radiating to his jaw bilaterally that began 15 minutes ago while he was eating dinner. He is awake, alert, and very anxious. Respirations are 24 breaths/min shallow, regular. Radial pulses are 134 beats/min strong, regular.

_____

_____

_____

_____

4. A patient was found in an abandoned building. He is unresponsive to verbal and painful stimuli. His respirations are shallow at 8 breaths/min per minute. Radial pulses are 62 beats/min strong, regular. His skin is pale, cool, and dry.

_____

_____

_____

_____

Chapter **55** Assessment-Based Management

Part two

For each of the following patient presentations, use pattern recognition to identify the most likely field diagnosis.

1. A 72-year-old male complains of difficulty breathing that awakened him from his sleep. He has a history of hypertension and a previous myocardial infarction. Physical examination reveals bilateral crackles, pedal edema, and a third heart sound (S_3). He takes hydrochlorothiazide, digoxin, and a potassium supplement.

    _____
    _____
    _____
    _____

2. A 45-year-old male complains of substernal chest pain that radiates to his left shoulder and down the inside of his left arm. He also complains of nausea and mild shortness of breath. He has a history of smoking and of elevated serum lipid levels. His skin is pale, cool, and moist.

    _____
    _____
    _____
    _____

3. A 25-year-old female developed the "worst headache of her life," which was accompanied by nausea and sensitivity to bright light. She rapidly lost consciousness and before EMS arrived experienced about 1 minute of generalized tonic-clonic seizure activity. She has a slow, bounding pulse; rapid, deep respirations; unresponsiveness to painful stimuli; and unequal pupils.

    _____
    _____
    _____
    _____

4. A 22-year-old male was the unrestrained driver of a vehicle involved in a frontal collision. He suffered blunt chest trauma by striking the steering column of his vehicle. A large bruise is present over the sternum. He has tachycardia, hypotension, distended neck veins, muffled heart sounds, and a narrow pulse pressure.

    _____
    _____
    _____
    _____

5. A 19-year-old female who is 24 weeks pregnant complains of a severe headache, spots before her eyes, and pain in the right upper abdominal quadrant. She has been experiencing swelling of her hands and face and has gained 12 lb over the last 2 weeks.

    _____
    _____
    _____
    _____

6. A 16-year-old male who was stabbed in the left lateral chest at the level of the sixth rib presents with tachycardia, hypotension, distended neck veins, and absent breath sounds on the left.

    _____
    _____
    _____
    _____

7. Your initial assessment reveals an anxious, restless patient who has pale, cool skin; a weak, rapid pulse; flat neck veins in the supine position; and dilated, sluggish pupils.

_____
_____
_____
_____

8. A patient thrown from a horse presents with bradycardia; hypotension; pale, cool, moist skin on the face and upper extremities; dry, flushed skin on the abdomen and lower extremities; and absence of sensation and motion in the lower extremities.

_____
_____
_____
_____

9. A 64-year-old male presents with a history of sudden onset of shortness of breath 10 minutes ago following an episode of coughing. The patient has a barrel chest and hypertrophied respiratory accessory muscles. He purses his lips when he exhales. Breath sounds are diminished on the left side of the chest.

_____
_____
_____
_____

10. A 22-year-old female experienced a sudden onset of severe shortness of breath about 15 minutes ago. Her right leg is in a cast secondary to surgery she had 5 days ago to correct an avulsion fracture and tendon damage in the ankle from a skiing accident. She was discharged from the hospital 2 days ago. She takes birth control pills and smokes one-half pack of cigarettes a day. Breath sounds are present and equal bilaterally.

_____
_____
_____
_____

Part three

Your patient is a 45-year-old male who complains of substernal chest pain that began approximately 20 minutes ago while he was watching television. The patient states that the pain is "squeezing" in quality, radiates to his left shoulder, and has a severity of 10/10. He also is experiencing mild shortness of breath and nausea. His past history includes elevated cholesterol levels, for which he takes simvastatin (Zocor), and asthma, for which he uses an albuterol metered-dose inhaler. His father and uncle died of acute myocardial infarctions in their late 40s. An older brother suffered an acute myocardial infarction at age 46. The patient also admits to using unprescribed sildenafil (Viagra) to facilitate sexual intercourse 8 hours ago. He states that he has no known drug allergies.

The patient is awake, alert, and very anxious. His respirations are rapid, shallow, and regular. Scattered wheezes are present throughout the lung fields. The skin is pale, cool, and moist. Capillary refill time is 3 seconds. Radial pulses are rapid, regular, and weak. The patient's neck veins are distended when he is placed in a semisitting position. The lung fields are clear. Vital signs are: BP—104/86 mm Hg; R—24 breaths/min shallow, regular; P—136 beats/min weak, regular.

Monitoring leads show a sinus tachycardia. A 12-lead ECG shows ST segment elevation in leads II, III, and aV_F. Right-sided precordial leads show ST segment elevation in V_{4R}.

Your protocol for cardiac chest pain specifies use of the following therapies:
1. Oxygen by nonrebreather mask
2. Monitor ECG
3. Establish IV at tko rate

4. Administer 325 mg of aspirin by mouth.
5. Administer 0.4 mg of nitroglycerin SL; repeat twice every 5 minutes if systolic BP > 90 mm Hg
6. Administer 2 mg of morphine sulfate IV; repeat every 5 minutes until patient is pain free to a maximum of 10 g
7. Administer 5 mg of metoprolol; repeat twice every 5 minutes IV if heart rate is above 120 beats/min

1. Using the principles of assessment-based management, determine which portions of the protocol require consultation with medical control about modifications.

_____

_____

_____

_____

_____

_____

_____

_____

56 Clinical Decision Making

READING ASSIGNMENT

Chapter 56, pages 627-635, in *Paramedic Practice Today: Above and Beyond*

OBJECTIVES

After completing this chapter, you will be able to:
1. Compare medical care in the prehospital environment with medical care in other settings.
2. Distinguish critical life-threatening, potentially life-threatening, and non–life-threatening patient presentations and the paramedic's decision-making process for each.
3. Evaluate the benefits and shortfalls of protocols, standing orders, and patient care algorithms.
4. Define the parts, stages, and sequences of the critical thinking process that the paramedic uses.
5. Describe the effects of the "fight or flight" response and the positive and negative effects it has on a paramedic's decision-making process.
6. Summarize the six *R*'s of "putting it all together": *r*ead the patient, *r*ead the scene, *r*eact, *r*eevaluate, *r*evise the management plan, and *r*eview performance.

CHAPTER SUMMARY

- Clinical decision making is the cornerstone of effective paramedic practice. It involves all clinical education, both formal and informal.
- The paramedic must work in difficult environments, and under pressure from various sources. You must also deal with patients with acute and emergent life-threatening conditions as well as those with nonacute, nonemergent, and non–life-threatening conditions.
- The paramedic's clinical decision-making process generally is governed by protocols, standing orders, and patient care algorithms either from state regulating bodies or by local medical control or a combination. You must recognize that protocols, standing orders, and patient care algorithms do not address all conditions or multiple conditions that may present in the field.
- Critical thinking involves fundamental elements. These include an adequate fund of knowledge, the ability to focus on specific and multiple elements of data, the ability to gather and organize data into workable concepts, the ability to identify and deal with medical ambiguity, the ability to distinguish relevant from irrelevant data, the ability to analyze and compare similar or contrary situations, and the ability

to provide rational decision-making reasoning and construct logical arguments concerning what you have done.
- Clinical decision making mandates that you read the scene and the patient. In addition, you must react and reevaluate the scene, the patient, and his or her reaction. Next, you must revise your treatment plan as necessary. Finally, you must review your performance to ensure quality patient care.

SHORT ANSWER

1. Compare the factors influencing medical care in the out-of-hospital environment to other medical settings.
   _____
   _____
   _____
   _____

2. Define *patient acuity*.
   _____
   _____
   _____
   _____

3. What are the three general classes of patient acuity in the prehospital environment?
   _____
   _____
   _____

4. What are the benefits of using protocols, standing orders, and patient care algorithms?
   _____
   _____
   _____
   _____

5. What are the disadvantages of using protocols, standing orders, and patient care algorithms?
   _____
   _____
   _____
   _____

6. What are the positive effects of the "fight or flight" response on paramedic decision making and response to emergencies?
   _____
   _____
   _____
   _____

7. What are the negative effects of the "fight or flight" response on paramedic decision making and response to emergencies?

_____
_____
_____
_____

8. What is a reflective thinking style?

_____
_____
_____
_____

9. When is a reflective thinking style appropriate during patient management?

_____
_____
_____
_____

10. What is an impulsive thinking style?

_____
_____
_____
_____

11. When is an impulsive thinking style appropriate during patient management?

_____
_____
_____
_____

12. How does a paramedic with an anticipatory thinking style approach patient management?

_____
_____
_____
_____

13. What is the benefit to thinking under pressure of practicing technical skills until they can be performed at a pseudo-instinctive level?

_____
_____
_____
_____

14. What are the steps in the critical decision-making process?

_____
_____
_____
_____

15. What are the "six *R*'s" of the critical thinking process?

_____
_____
_____
_____
_____
_____

MULTIPLE CHOICE

1. A positive effect of the sympathetic nervous system response on clinical decision making is that this response _____.
   A. broadens the paramedic's focus of attention, thus allowing the paramedic to consider multiple issues while also attending to decision making
   B. decreases the paramedic's blood flow to the gastrointestinal system, thus improving response time to sensory input
   C. increases the paramedic's blood pressure, thus improving brain performance
   D. narrows the paramedic's focus of attention, thus improving concentration on the decision-making task

2. In medicine, the term *acuity* refers to the _____.
   A. severity of diseases but not traumatic injuries
   B. severity of the patient's condition
   C. sudden and constant nature of a set of symptoms
   D. sudden onset of a set of symptoms

3. A clinical policy that allows giving nitroglycerin to a patient with cardiac chest pain without contacting online medical control is an example of _____.
   A. an algorithm
   B. a protocol
   C. a special provision
   D. a standing order

4. Of the following, which would be categorized as the lowest acuity?
   A. A 2-year-old with a respiratory rate of 50 breaths/min
   B. A 4-year-old with a heart rate of 200 beats/min
   C. A 20-year-old ambulatory man involved in a motor vehicle crash with a heart rate of 100 beats/min
   D. A 50-year-old man who is awake but cannot recall his name or any personal information after falling off a ladder

Case one

While you are standing by at a track meet, you are asked to evaluate an athlete who has fallen and "twisted her ankle." The patient is a 17-year-old female who is awake, alert, and oriented to person, place, and time. Respirations are regular and unlabored. Radial pulses are present, strong, and very slow. Capillary refill is less than 2 seconds. Her skin is warm and moist. The patient's right ankle is swollen, tender, and discolored. No obvious deformity is present. Pulses, skin color, movement, and capillary refill distal to the injured ankle are normal. Vital signs are: P—42 beats/min strong, regular; R—12 breaths/min regular; BP—108/62 mm Hg.

1. Using the critical decision process, determine how you should manage this patient. In your answer include any additional information you would need to obtain about the patient.

   _____
   _____
   _____
   _____
   _____
   _____

Case two

A 76-year-old male was involved in a motor vehicle crash when he lost control of his vehicle on a wet street. The car skidded sideways, striking a utility pole on the driver's side. The patient is restless and anxious. His respirations are rapid and shallow. His skin is pale and cool. Radial pulses are present, and their rate is within normal limits. Capillary refill is 3 seconds. The patient complains of pain in the left upper abdominal quadrant and in his left shoulder, which does not seem to be injured. Vital signs are: P—90 beats/min weak, regular; R—22 breaths/min shallow, regular; BP—120/80 mm Hg.

1. Using the critical decision process, determine how you should manage this patient. In your answer include any additional information you would need to obtain about the patient.

   _____
   _____
   _____
   _____
   _____
   _____

145

57 Ground and Air Transport of Critical Patients

READING ASSIGNMENT

Chapter 57, pages 636-652, in *Paramedic Practice Today: Above and Beyond*

OBJECTIVES

After completing this chapter, you will be able to:
1. Describe the role that critical care ground transport plays in the care of critical patients.
2. List the responsibilities of agencies in developing staffing needs.
3. Develop an understanding of who comprises a critical care ground transport team.
4. List some of the equipment needed for critical care ground transport.
5. Describe the advantages and disadvantages of air medical transport.
6. Identify criteria for working as a member of an air medical flight crew.
7. Identify the conditions and situations for which air medical transport should be considered.
8. Describe various considerations for preparing for air medical transport.

CHAPTER SUMMARY

- The training and availability of the critical care paramedic have allowed agencies to provide critical care ground units.
- Critical care ground transport may be appropriate for the critical care patient who requires transport to another medical facility.
- Critical care ground transports are conducted by a multidisciplinary team of healthcare professionals.
- The patient compartment of a critical care ground unit should be equipped with all standard equipment found on a mobile intensive care unit.
- The beginning of aeromedical services dates back to the 1940s and continues to present day, with approximately 350,000 rotor-wing and 100,000 fixed-wing transports annually.
- Fixed-wing and rotor-wing aircraft are used to transport ill or injured people to appropriate medical care.
- Fixed-wing aircraft have been used for almost 90 years for medical transport. These transports typically are from facility to facility.
- Rotor-wing aircraft, or helicopters, although sometimes used for facility-to-facility transport, are better known for scene-to-facility transport.
- Flight crew criteria apply to nurses, paramedics, and other members of the flight team.

- Transport physiology includes multiple factors that should be considered before and during the transport of the patient.
- Gas laws govern the body's physiologic response to variables of temperature, pressure, volume, and the relative mass of a gas.
- Boyle's law presumes that if the temperature is constant, the volume of gas is inversely proportional to its pressure.
- Dalton's law, the law of partial pressure, states that "the total partial pressure of the gas mixture is equal to the sum of partial pressures."
- Charles' law expresses that the volume of a fixed mass of gas held at a constant pressure varies directly with absolute temperature.
- Gay-Lussac's law is sometimes combined with Charles' law because it deals with the relation between pressure and temperature.
- Henry's law is associated with decompression sickness.
- Graham's law describes how gases move from a higher pressure or concentration to an area of lower pressure or concentration.
- Seven stressors have been identified that may be caused by air transport.
- The treatment for hypoxia or hyperventilation includes administering 100% oxygen, initiating positive-pressure ventilation, regulating breathing and watching for hyperventilation, checking equipment, and descending.
- Barometric pressure changes can cause several effects during ascent and descent.
- Patients who are already ill or injured can have difficulty maintaining their body temperature. Changes in ambient air temperature during transport can affect the patient.
- Humidity is the concentration of water vapor in the air; changes can require the provider to modify patient care.
- Noise affects the ability of the flight crew to communicate, alters the hearing of the patient, and can promote varying levels of fatigue.
- Vibration is defined as the motion of an object in relation to a reference point, which usually is the object at rest.
- Fatigue is the end product of all the exposures that can occur while a person is in an aircraft.
- The criteria for patient transport are the conditions required for the use of an aircraft for transport.
- Medical patients who are critically ill may require transport by fixed- or rotor-wing aircraft based on defined criteria.
- Trauma patients who have been injured may meet the established criteria for transport by rotor- or fixed-wing aircraft.

147

- Other considerations, such as weather conditions, may prevent the use of aircraft for transporting patients.
- Patient preparation includes actions to be taken before placing the patient in the aircraft.
- Hospital-to-hospital transport typically is done by fixed-wing aircraft but depends on a variety of factors.
- Scene-to-hospital transport typically is done by rotor-wing aircraft and more commonly involves trauma patients.
- The landing site preparation includes the following factors: size, location, obstructions, surface conditions, night operations, communication, and general safety.

MATCHING

1. Match the name of the gas law with the effect it describes.

_____ At a constant temperature, the volume of a gas is directly proportional to its pressure

A. Boyle's law
B. Charles' law
C. Dalton's law
D. Henry's law

_____ At a constant pressure, the volume of a gas is inversely proportional to its temperature

_____ The amount of gas dissolved in a liquid is proportional to the partial pressure of the gas

_____ The total pressure of a gas mixture is the sum of the partial pressures of the gases making up the mixture

SHORT ANSWER

1. What are the advantages air-medical transport?

_____
_____
_____
_____

2. What are the disadvantages of air-medical transport?

_____
_____
_____
_____

3. List seven factors that add to stress experienced by patients and crewmembers during air-medical transport.

_____
_____
_____
_____
_____
_____
_____
_____

4. What change in a patient's mental status usually occurs with early hypoxia?

_____
_____
_____
_____

5. What areas of the body are most likely to be affected by changes in atmospheric pressure as an aircraft changes altitude?

_____
_____
_____
_____

6. What is barosinusitis?

_____
_____
_____
_____

7. How is barosinusitis managed?

_____
_____
_____
_____

8. A patient who had a bowel resection with creation of a colostomy 6 hours ago is about to be transferred by air. What precautions should be taken to manage the effects that changes in atmospheric pressure will have on this patient?

_____
_____
_____
_____

9. What steps should be taken to manage the effects of noise on a patient during air transport? If a specific piece of equipment is used to manage noise effects on the patient, what should flight crewmembers remember to do for the patient during descent?

_____
_____
_____
_____

10. What effects can vibration of aircraft have on a patient's physiology?

_____
_____
_____
_____

11. Describe how a helicopter landing zone should be marked at night.

_____
_____
_____
_____

12. You have requested a helicopter to transport a critically injured patient from a motor vehicle crash. You have the helicopter in sight and are attempting to tell the pilot the location of the landing zone. What is the best way to provide this information to the pilot?

_____
_____
_____
_____

13. From what direction should you approach a helicopter? Why?

_____
_____
_____
_____

14. Where is the area of greatest danger when you are working around an operating helicopter?

_____
_____
_____
_____

15. If the landing zone's surface consists of dirt, what technique can be used to limit the dust cloud created by the helicopter's rotorwash?

_____
_____
_____
_____

MULTIPLE CHOICE

1. A landing zone for a helicopter should be _____.
   A. 25 by 25 feet
   B. 50 by 50 feet
   C. 75 by 75 feet
   D. 100 by 100 feet

2. Where should the landing zone be located in relation to the patient care area?
   A. 50 to 100 feet downwind
   B. 50 to 100 feet upwind
   C. 100 to 200 feet downwind
   D. 100 to 200 feet upwind

3. What is the minimum clearance that should be established between the landing zone and any bystanders, livestock, or motor vehicles?
   A. 50 feet
   B. 100 feet
   C. 200 feet
   D. 500 feet

4. What is the maximum slope for the surface of a helicopter landing zone?
   A. 5 degrees
   B. 10 degrees
   C. 15 degrees
   D. 20 degrees

5. Which statement about the relationship between altitude and humidity is correct?
   A. As air cools it holds less moisture; therefore as altitude increases, humidity decreases.
   B. As air cools it holds less moisture; therefore as altitude increases, humidity increases.
   C. As air cools it holds more moisture; therefore as altitude increases, humidity decreases.
   D. As air cools it holds more moisture; therefore as altitude increases, humidity increases.

6. Civilian use of helicopters for medical transport grew out of benefits demonstrated by the military during _____.
   A. Operation Desert Storm
   B. Operation Just Cause
   C. the Korean War
   D. World War II

7. When are fixed-wing aircraft generally used for patient transport?
   A. When a regional airport is readily accessible
   B. When helicopters are unavailable
   C. When transport distances exceed 100 miles
   D. When weather conditions make helicopter flight unsafe

8. The first step taken to manage a patient who develops signs and symptoms of hypoxia during flight should be to _____.
   A. administer a $beta_2$ agonist using a small-volume nebulizer
   B. administer high-concentration oxygen
   C. begin positive-pressure ventilation with a bag-mask device
   D. request that the pilot decrease the aircraft's altitude

58 EMS Deployment and System Status Management

READING ASSIGNMENT

Chapter 58, pages 654-666, in *Paramedic Practice Today: Above and Beyond*.

OBJECTIVES

After completing this chapter, you will be able to:
1. Define *system status management*.
2. Describe how resource planning and deployment methods affect response times.
3. Outline two primary ambulance deployment strategies.
4. Compare the advantages and disadvantages of different deployment strategies.
5. Define *unit hour utilization*.
6. Explain how system coverage costs and employee satisfaction can be balanced.

CHAPTER SUMMARY

- Deployment methods can significantly affect clinical, operational, and financial aspects of an EMS system.
- Key deployment strategies include (1) fixed-station deployment, (2) a mix of geographic and demand deployment when the system is busy, and (3) fully deployed systems that frequently use street corner posts.
- Response times, hours of coverage required to achieve response time, employee satisfaction, and cost are each considered advantages and disadvantages associated with different deployment strategies.
- Flexible deployment, or system status management (SSM), is the art and science of matching the production capacity of an ambulance system to the changing patterns of demand placed on that system.
- Unit hour utilization (UhU) is an indicator of ambulance service productivity and staff work load.
- A variety of factors must be considered when determining the best deployment strategy for a particular community. These include anticipated call demand, supply or availability of units, funding, and employee satisfaction.

SHORT ANSWER

1. What is system status management (SSM)?

2. What are the two primary ambulance deployment strategies?

3. Describe fixed station (static) deployment as a system status management strategy.

4. What are the disadvantages of fixed station deployment?

5. Describe full (flexible) deployment as a system status management strategy.

6. What are the advantages of full (flexible) deployment?

7. What are the disadvantages of full (flexible) deployment?

_____

_____

_____

_____

8. What is a unit hour?

_____

_____

_____

_____

9. What is unit hour utilization (UhU)?

_____

_____

_____

_____

10. Explain how system coverage costs and employee satisfaction can be balanced.

_____

_____

_____

_____

MULTIPLE CHOICE

1. An EMS system has five fully equipped and staffed ambulances available during a 24-hour shift from five stations. During an average shift, the system responds to 60 calls and transports 36 patients. What deployment strategy is this system using?
   A. Fixed
   B. Flexible
   C. Full
   D. Mixed

2. How many unit hours does the system have available to it during a 24-hour shift?
   A. 5
   B. 12
   C. 120
   D. 180

3. What is the unit hour utilization-transport (UhU-T) during a 24-hour shift for the EMS system described in the previous question?
   A. 0.30
   B. 0.33
   C. 0.40
   D. 0.50

4. What is the unit hour utilization-response (UhU-R) during a 24-hour shift for the EMS system described in question 2?
   A. 0.30
   B. 0.33
   C. 0.40
   D. 0.50

5. During a 12-hour shift, a crew operating in a system that uses flexible deployment responds to 4 calls, transports 3 patients, and changes post 4 times. What is the UhU-T for this crew?
   A. 0.20
   B. 0.25
   C. 0.33
   D. 0.66

6. What is the UhU-R for the crew in the previous question?
   A. 0.20
   B. 0.25
   C. 0.33
   D. 0.66

7. What is the unit hour utilization–time deployed (UhU-TD) for the crew described in question 5?
   A. 0.20
   B. 0.25
   C. 0.33
   D. 0.66

59 Crime Scene Operations

READING ASSIGNMENT

Chapter 59, pages 667-677, in *Paramedic Practice Today: Above and Beyond*.

OBJECTIVES

After completing this chapter, you will be able to:
1. Explain how EMS providers often are mistaken for the police.
2. Describe warning signs of potentially violent situations.
3. Explain specific techniques for risk reduction when approaching highway encounters, violent street incidents, residences, and dark houses.
4. Explain emergency evasive techniques for potentially violent situations, including threats of physical violence, firearms encounters, and edged-weapon encounters.
5. Explain EMS considerations for the following types of violent or potentially violent situations:
   - Gangs and gang violence
   - Clandestine drug labs
   - Interpersonal violence
6. Explain the following techniques: field contact and cover procedures during assessment and care, evasive tactics, and concealment techniques.
7. Describe police evidence considerations and techniques to assist in evidence preservation.

CHAPTER SUMMARY

- Your first priority at any crime scene is your own safety.
- Scene safety starts by identifying and responding to dangers before they threaten (*p*eople, *p*laces, *t*imes, *t*hings). If the scene is known for violence, stage at a safe distance until it is secured by law enforcement.
- EMS personnel must look for warning signs of violence during a response to a residence and retreat from the scene if danger is evident.
- Responding to highway encounters may present danger from violence as well as traffic and extrication.
- Monitor for warning signs of danger in violent street incidents and retreat as necessary.
- EMS personnel often look like law enforcement officers, so always be extremely cautious about personal safety when working in gang areas.
- Clandestine drug laboratories can produce explosive and toxic gases. Additional risks include booby traps that can maim or kill.
- When responding to scenes of interpersonal violence, be aware that acts of violence may be directed toward you.

- Safety tactics include retreat, cover and concealment, distraction and evasion, contact and cover, and warning signals and communication.
- Patient care in the hot zone requires special training, authorization, body armor, and equipment.
- Your observations at a crime scene are important and should be carefully documented. Evidence protection can be performed while caring for the patient by not unnecessarily disturbing the scene or destroying evidence.

SHORT ANSWER

1. Why is shutting down the siren and lights a few blocks from the location of a call a good safety tactic?

   _____
   _____
   _____
   _____

2. You arrive at a call for "breathing difficulty" in a residential area at 0330 hours. The house is dark with no signs of activity. The 9-1-1 system confirms the call is originating from this address. What should you do?

   _____
   _____
   _____
   _____

3. When responding to a call involving a suspicious vehicle on a highway or street, where should you spot the ambulance for greatest safety? Why?

   _____
   _____
   _____
   _____

4. What is concealment?

   _____
   _____
   _____
   _____

5. What is cover?

   _____
   _____
   _____
   _____

6. What is the only portion of the ambulance that provides cover?

_____
_____
_____
_____

7. Where should you stand when knocking on the door of a structure? Why?

_____
_____
_____

8. If a door is located in a position that requires you to stand directly in front of it to knock, what should you do?

_____
_____
_____
_____

9. What are the "contact" and "cover" responses during a structure approach and entry?

_____
_____
_____
_____

10. You have entered a residence on a response to "a possible heart attack." The person who met you at the door says, "He's in the back bedroom. It's through that door right there." What should you do? Why?

_____
_____
_____
_____

11. Why are domestic disputes particularly dangerous calls for police and EMS personnel?

_____
_____
_____
_____

12. What agency has primary responsibility for dealing with domestic disputes and violence?

_____
_____
_____
_____

13. If a party to a domestic dispute wants to leave your sight, what should you do?

_____
_____
_____
_____

14. If you feel a domestic dispute has deteriorated to the point where violence may occur, what should you and your partner do?

_____
_____
_____
_____

15. If a patient refuses to leave the scene of a call where you feel violence may occur, what should you and your partner do?

_____
_____
_____
_____

16. If you and your partner leave a scene and request police backup, what should you do?

_____
_____
_____
_____

17. What is evidence?

_____
_____
_____
_____

18. What is the fundamental principle of crime scene investigation?

_____
_____
_____
_____

19. What is a crime scene? Why is it important for EMS personnel to understand this definition?

_____
_____
_____
_____

20. If you have to remove a crime victim's clothing, what should you do with it?

_____
_____
_____
_____

21. If a patient reports having scratched an assailant, what should you do?

_____
_____
_____
_____

22. Why should blood- or fluid-soaked clothing not be placed in airtight containers?

_____
_____
_____
_____

23. What should you tell a sexual assault victim who wants to wash or use the toilet? Why?

_____
_____
_____
_____

24. Why is it important for EMS to note and record first statements made by victims or witnesses?

_____
_____
_____
_____

25. Why is controlling the amount of debris you leave on a crime scene important?

_____
_____
_____
_____

26. You have found a patient in a clandestine drug laboratory. He has localized acid burns on one of his arms. How should you manage this situation?

_____
_____
_____
_____

27. A patient was injured in an explosion of a clandestine drug lab. He is burned over 35% of his body surface area and has penetrating trauma to the chest and abdomen from glass shards. His radial pulses are absent, and the carotid pulse is weak and thready. How should you manage this situation?

_____
_____
_____
_____

28. After any acutely ill or injured persons have received care, what is the primary role of EMS during emergency operations at a clandestine drug laboratory?

_____
_____
_____
_____

MULTIPLE CHOICE

1. Which of the following statements about cover and concealment is correct?
   A. Cover will hide the rescuer, but not stop bullets; concealment will stop bullets; the box of the ambulance provides concealment; the ambulance engine block provides cover.
   B. Cover will hide the rescuer, but not stop bullets; concealment will stop bullets; the box of the ambulance provides cover; the ambulance engine block provides concealment.
   C. Cover will stop bullets; concealment will hide the rescuer, but not stop bullets; the box of the ambulance provides concealment; the ambulance engine block provides cover.
   D. Cover will stop bullets; concealment will hide the rescuer, but not stop bullets; the box of the ambulance provides cover; the ambulance engine block provides concealment.

2. When you knock on the door of a residence or apartment, the best place to stand is _____.
   A. directly in front of the door unless there is a window through which you can be observed
   B. to the side of the door unless this puts you in front of a window; then directly in front of the door
   C. to the side of the door, on the same side as the hinges (opposite the doorknob)
   D. to the side of the door, opposite the hinges (the doorknob side)

3. During a response to a call involving domestic violence, one of the combatants insists on going into an adjacent room. Your best response to this situation should be to _____.
   A. follow him or her to ensure that he or she does not return with a weapon
   B. leave the scene immediately if the patient is willing to go, but remain with him or her otherwise since leaving in this situation would be abandonment
   C. leave the scene immediately whether or not the patient is willing to go with you.
   D. physically restrain him or her because force is authorized to prevent potential injury to yourself, your partner, and your patient

4. You have responded to a report of an injured person at a single-family residence. The patients are a 21-year-old male who has superficial and partial-thickness burns on his arms and a 19-year-old female who is also at the scene. Both patients seem to be very nervous and are reluctant to provide complete information about what has happened. You notice that all of the windows of the residence have been covered from the inside. There is a strong odor like that of rotten garbage. As you begin to examine the male patient, you notice that he and the female patient are both covered with a fine white powder. At this point the best course of action would be to _____.

A. immediately remove the patients to the ambulance, transport, and request that the HAZMAT team respond to the hospital to begin decontamination when you arrive

B. move the patients to a safe distance from the structure but not to the ambulance, call for a fire department hazardous materials team response, and remain on the scene until the HAZMAT team arrives

C. remain with the patients while your partner enters the structure to determine the nature of the material to which they have been exposed

D. remove the patients to the ambulance, call for a fire department hazardous materials team response, and remain on the scene until the HAZMAT team arrives

5. The patient is a 15-year-old male who has been cut with a knife on both arms and his abdomen. The wounds seem to be superficial. The patient is awake and alert. His skin is pale and cool. Respirations are 18 breaths/min deep, regular. Radial pulses are 96 beats/min strong, regular. There are a number of other males in their teens on the scene who all are wearing matching purple polka dot shirts and bandanas like the ones worn by the patient. They are quite agitated and very concerned about their friend's condition. An appropriate strategy for managing this situation would be to _____.

A. firmly and assertively order the bystanders to stand back or leave the scene; move the patient to the ambulance immediately, transport, assess, and treat the patient en route to the hospital; avoid cutting the patient's shirt or bandana if at all possible

B. firmly and assertively order the bystanders to stand back or leave the scene; move the patient to the ambulance immediately and continue your assessment and treatment there before transporting; cut the patient's shirt or bandana away as needed to assess and treat

C. show respect to the bystanders and acknowledge their concern for the patient; move the patient to the ambulance immediately and continue your assessment and treatment there before transporting; avoid cutting the patient's shirt or bandana if at all possible

D. show respect to the bystanders and acknowledge their concern for the patient; move the patient to the ambulance immediately, transport, assess, and treat the patient en route to the hospital; avoid cutting the patient's shirt or bandana if at all possible

60 Dispatch Activities

READING ASSIGNMENT

Chapter 60, pages 678-690, in *Paramedic Practice Today: Above and Beyond.*

OBJECTIVES

After completing this chapter, you will be able to:

1. Explain how the communications center fits into the overall EMS system.
2. List the standard functions of the emergency medical dispatch center.
3. Explain the difference between a primary 9-1-1 center and a secondary 9-1-1 center.
4. Describe the common challenges of address verification.
5. List the five elements of an effective emergency medical dispatch program.
6. Explain the role of states in an emergency medical dispatch program.
7. Explain the basics of a continuing education program.
8. Describe the difference between a protocol and guidelines and telephone aid.
9. Describe the conditions, benefits, public expectations, and legal implications of prearrival instructions.
10. Describe how best practices are achieved in an emergency medical dispatch center.
11. Explain the basics of call triage and prioritization.
12. Identify patient conditions that would trigger a high-priority, intermediate-priority, and low-priority response.
13. Identify the primary objectives of a response assignment plan.
14. Identify the common response types in a response assignment plan.
15. Explain how a response assignment plan is consistently applied.
16. Identify the four goals of a quality improvement program.
17. Identify the importance of a physician medical director.
18. Explain the need for case evaluation and feedback.
19. Explain the role of the quality improvement unit.
20. Describe the factors in choosing a random sample for case audits.
21. Identify the key clinical performance indicators and the significance of each.
22. Define the call processing time.
23. Identify some common controllable and uncontrollable factors that determine call processing time.
24. Identify the need for differentiated call processing times.
25. Identify the different components of call processing.
26. Describe the process of unit selection and incident tracking.
27. Identify the process of nonemergency call taking.
28. Describe a performance-based EMS response system.
29. Explain a demand-based unit deployment process.
30. Describe the primary technology components of a state-of-the-art communications center.
31. Explain how dispatch agencies can get useful information for public health authorities on a contagious disease outbreak.

CHAPTER SUMMARY

- Emergency medical dispatch (EMD) communications centers have rapidly evolved into complex operations with sophisticated technology, requiring staffing by highly skilled emergency medical dispatchers.
- The communications center is the starting point for EMS care in a community, serving as a critical link between patients in need and EMS responders, including paramedic crews.
- Dispatchers are now widely accepted as full EMS professionals with specific training, certification, quality improvement, and continuing education requirements.
- Federal, state, and local governments, as well as numerous professional organizations, have produced both binding and nonbinding standards that define the roles of the dispatcher and the EMS communications center.
- Included in those roles are the use of patient assessment protocols, call typing, response prioritization, and the provision of prearrival instructions.
- New technologies that provide automation of previously manual processes, reliable and rapid geographic information, and better communication links with responders and other public safety agencies have replaced less-efficient systems and made the dispatch center the focal point of all information moving through the EMS system.

SHORT ANSWER

1. How does the communications center fit into the overall EMS system?

_____

_____

_____

_____

2. List the standard functions of the emergency medical dispatch center.

_____
_____
_____
_____

3. What is the difference between a primary 9-1-1 center and a secondary 9-1-1 center?

_____
_____
_____
_____

4. What is an ANI/ALI system?

_____
_____
_____
_____

5. What are the most common challenges to address verification?

_____
_____
_____
_____

6. What are the five elements of an effective emergency medical dispatch program?

_____
_____
_____
_____
_____

7. What is the role of accreditation in emergency medical dispatch?

_____
_____
_____
_____

8. What are the two primary objectives of a response assignment plan?

_____
_____

9. What are the four goals for emergency medical dispatch quality control and improvement programs?

_____
_____
_____
_____

10. List the emergency medical dispatch clinical performance indicators.

_____
_____
_____
_____

11. List the components of emergency medical dispatch call processing.

_____
_____
_____
_____

12. Describe a performance-based response system.

_____
_____
_____

13. How can dispatch agencies provide useful information to public health authorities on a contagious disease outbreak?

_____
_____
_____
_____

MULTIPLE CHOICE

1. Which of the following statements best describes the differences between an emergency medical dispatch protocol and emergency medical dispatch guidelines?
   A. A guideline a predictable, reproducible process for addressing a medical problem; a protocol is a less-structured, more subjective process.
   B. A protocol is a predictable, reproducible process for addressing a medical problem; a guideline is a less-structured, more subjective process.
   C. Protocols are established by local medical directors; guidelines are established by state law.
   D. Protocols are established by state law; guidelines are established by local medical directors.

2. Which of the following types of calls would trigger the highest priority response?
   A. Diabetic patient with high blood sugar
   B. Minor trauma with injured ankle
   C. Sudden cardiac arrest
   D. Motor vehicle crash with injury

3. Which of the following types of calls would trigger an intermediate-priority response?
   A. Chest pain with cardiac history
   B. Minor trauma with injured ankle
   C. Sudden cardiac arrest
   D. Unknown problem

4. Which of the following types of calls would trigger a low-priority response?
   A. Chest pain with cardiac history
   B. Minor trauma with injured ankle
   C. Traffic accident with injury
   D. Unknown problem

5. Which of the following response assignment plans would be appropriate for a high-priority call?
   A. ALS ambulance responding with lights and siren
   B. ALS ambulance responding without lights and siren
   C. BLS ambulance responding without lights and siren
   D. Engine, ALS ambulance, Quick response ALS unit, and defibrillator equipped police all responding with lights and siren

6. Which of the following response assignment plans would be appropriate for an intermediate-priority call?
   A. ALS ambulance responding with lights and siren
   B. ALS ambulance responding without lights and siren
   C. BLS ambulance responding without lights and siren
   D. Engine, ALS ambulance, Quick response ALS unit, and defibrillator equipped police all responding with lights and siren

7. Which of the following response assignment plans would be appropriate for a low-priority call?
   A. ALS ambulance responding with lights and siren
   B. BLS ambulance responding without lights and siren
   C. Engine, ALS ambulance responding with lights and siren
   D. Engine, ALS ambulance, quick response ALS unit, and defibrillator-equipped police all responding with lights and siren

8. The National Institutes of Health recommends auditing what percent of each emergency medical dispatcher's cases?
   A. 2% to 5%
   B. 7% to 10%
   C. 12% to 15%
   D. 17% to 20%

9. Call processing time is the elapsed time from the moment an emergency call is received at the 9-1-1 center until the _____.
   A. closest available responders have been notified with all information necessary to respond
   B. closest available responders reach the scene
   C. dispatcher is providing appropriate prearrival instructions to the caller
   D. emergency medical dispatcher finishes obtaining all information needed to assign a correct response priority

10. Which of the following factors affecting call processing time is under the control of the EMS communications center?
    A. Caller state of mind
    B. Language barriers
    C. Caller knowledge of event location
    D. Proper use of dispatch protocols

61 Emergency Vehicle Operations

READING ASSIGNMENT

Chapter 61, pages 691-704, in *Paramedic Practice Today: Above and Beyond*.

OBJECTIVES

After completing this chapter, you will be able to:
1. Identify current local and state standards that influence ambulance design, equipment requirements, and staffing of ambulances.
2. Identify and discuss the benefits and drawbacks of the three types of ambulances.
3. Identify local and state standards for ambulance marking.
4. Discuss the importance of regular vehicle cleaning and maintenance.
5. Identify the potential liability for the paramedic as it pertains to vehicle maintenance and operation.
6. Discuss the importance of completing a daily emergency vehicle equipment and supply checklist.
7. Discuss the factors to be considered when determining ambulance stationing within a community.
8. Discuss the importance of district familiarization and route planning.
9. List factors that contribute to safe vehicle operations.
10. Describe the considerations that should be given to the following:
    ■ Using escorts
    ■ Working in adverse environmental conditions
    ■ Using lights and siren
    ■ Proceeding through intersections
    ■ Parking at an emergency scene
11. Discuss the concept of due regard for the safety of all others while operating an emergency vehicle.
12. Differentiate proper from improper body mechanics for lifting and moving patients in emergency and nonemergency situations.
13. Describe the advantages and disadvantages of air medical transport and identify conditions and situations in which air medical transport should be considered.

CHAPTER SUMMARY

■ The importance of safe and proper operation of the ambulance and its equipment cannot be overstressed. It can mean the difference between arriving safely and timely versus not arriving at all.

■ The timely and appropriate care of the patients served by paramedics depends on the emergency vehicle being in good operating condition, well stocked, and clean.
■ Paramedics must remember that they are liable for the condition of their emergency vehicle and the way it is operated.

MATCHING

1. Match the type of ambulance with its description:
   ____Type I   A. Standard van, integral cab/body
   ____Type II   B. Truck-cab chassis/modular body
   ____Type III C. Specialty van, integral cab/body

SHORT ANSWER

1. What are the four privileges granted to operators of authorized emergency vehicles by most state and local traffic codes?

   _____
   _____
   _____
   _____

2. To exercise these privileges, what must the operator of the vehicle do?

   _____
   _____
   _____
   _____

3. What are three questions the operator of an authorized emergency vehicle can ask himself or herself to determine whether the vehicle is being operated with due regard for the safety of others?

   _____
   _____
   _____

4. What is the most common location for collisions involving ambulances?

   _____
   _____
   _____
   _____

5. List reasons why the most common type of collision involving ambulances occurs.

_____

_____

_____

_____

6. How can the risk of the most common form of collision involving ambulances be minimized?

_____

_____

_____

_____

7. What are the risks associated with police vehicles escorting ambulances?

_____

_____

_____

_____

8. Identify 10 medical equipment items on the ambulance that should be tested regularly.

_____

_____

_____

_____

_____

_____

_____

_____

_____

_____

9. What is a tiered response system?

_____

_____

_____

_____

10. List factors that affect deployment of ambulances within an EMS system's service area.

_____

_____

_____

_____

MULTIPLE CHOICE

1. What is the most common location or situation in which ambulances are involved in collisions?
   A. In parking lots
   B. In intersections
   C. On controlled access highways
   D. While driving in reverse gear

2. While making an emergency response, you come up behind a school bus that is stopped at the side of the road with its red lights flashing. You should _____.
   A. pass cautiously, using your lights and siren
   B. pull into the opposing lanes to pass with a larger safety margin
   C. stop and wait until the bus driver signals you on
   D. turn your lights and siren off until the bus driver turns his lights off

3. When operating with lights and sirens, an ambulance may _____.
   A. disregard regulations governing direction of travel if proper caution is used
   B. exceed the posted speed limit without liability
   C. pass an off-loading school bus, even when its red warning lights are flashing
   D. pass other vehicles without signaling or "clearing" the passing lane

4. Which of these statements about multiple vehicle responses is correct?
   A. Multiple vehicle responses are extremely hazardous and extreme care should be used when proceeding through an intersection in which another emergency vehicle has passed.
   B. Other emergency vehicles should be followed as closely as possible so motorists cannot pull between it and the ambulance.
   C. The safety of both vehicles' operators and passengers is decreased if there is too much distance between the ambulance and the other responding vehicles.
   D. Use of multiple vehicle responses increases the safety of both vehicles' operators and passengers.

5. The federal agency that establishes guidelines for ambulance equipment and design that are related to infection control is the _____.
   A. Centers for Disease Control and Prevention
   B. Environmental Protection Agency
   C. Occupational Safety and Health Administration
   D. U.S. Department of Transportation

6. Which of the following is a factor you should consider when using the siren during an emergency response?
   A. Motorists are more likely to yield if the siren tone is never changed.
   B. Use of a siren is unlikely to save a significant amount of time during most emergency responses.
   C. Use of a siren is unlikely to significantly affect a patient's condition.
   D. Use of a siren is unlikely to cause the driver of the ambulance to increase his or her speed.

7. The federal guidelines that specify ambulance design and manufacturing requirements are issued by the _____.
   A. Federal Highway Administration
   B. General Services Administration
   C. U.S. Department of Health and Human Services
   D. U.S. Department of Transportation

8. If no fire or escaping liquids or fumes are present, what is the minimum distance the ambulance should be parked from the site of a motor vehicle collision?
   A. 25 feet
   B. 50 feet
   C. 75 feet
   D. 100 feet

9. If a fire is present, what is the minimum distance the ambulance should be parked from the site of a motor vehicle crash?
   A. 50 feet
   B. 100 feet
   C. 150 feet
   D. 500 feet

CASE STUDIES

For each of the following motor vehicle crash scenes, indicate the location where you would park the ambulance.

Case one

1. Your unit is the first emergency services vehicle to arrive on the scene. You are approaching from the direction indicated by the arrow.

1. A police unit has arrived first and is in the position indicated by the star. You are approaching from the direction indicated by the arrow.

_____

_____

_____

_____

_____

62 EMS Operations Command and Control

Chapter 62, pages 705-717, in *Paramedic Practice Today: Above and Beyond*.

OBJECTIVES

After completing this chapter, you will be able to:
1. Explain the need for the incident management system or incident command system in managing EMS incidents.
2. Compare command procedures used at small-, medium-, and large-scale medical incidents.
3. Define the term *multiple-casualty incident*.
4. Explain the local or regional threshold for establishing command and implementation of the incident management system, including threshold multiple-casualty incident declaration.
5. Define the term *disaster management*.
6. Describe the functional components of the incident management system in terms of command, finance, logistics, operations, and planning.
7. Describe the role of the paramedic and EMS system in planning for multiple-casualty incidents and disasters.
8. Describe the role of table-top exercises and small and large drills in preparation for multiple-casualty incidents.
9. List the physical and psychological signs of critical incident stress.
10. Describe the role of critical incident stress management sessions in multiple-casualty incidents.
11. Describe the role of command.
12. Compare singular and unified command and describe when each is most applicable.
13. Describe the methods and rationale for identifying specific functions and leaders for these functions in the incident command system.
14. Describe the role of command posts and emergency operations centers in multiple-casualty incidents and disaster management.
15. Describe the need and procedures for transfer of command.
16. Describe essential elements of scene size-up when arriving at a potential multiple-casualty incident.
17. Describe modifications of telecommunications procedures during a multiple-casualty incident.
18. List and describe the functions of the following groups and leaders in an incident command system as they pertain to EMS incidents:
    - Safety
    - Logistics
    - Rehabilitation
    - Staging
    - Treatment
    - Triage
    - Transportation
    - Extrication or rescue
    - Disposition of deceased (morgue)
    - Communications
19. Describe the role of the physician at multiple-casualty incidents.
20. Describe the need for and techniques used in tracking patients during multiple-casualty incidents.
21. Describe techniques used to allocate patients to hospitals and track them.
22. List and describe the essential equipment to provide logistical support to multiple-casualty incident operations, including airway, respiratory and hemorrhage control; burn management; and patient immobilization.
23. Define and describe the principles of triage.
24. Given a list of 20 patients with various multiple injuries, determine the appropriate triage priority with 90% accuracy.
25. Define *primary* and *secondary triage*.
26. Describe when primary and secondary triage techniques should be implemented.
27. Describe the START method of initial triage.
28. Given color-coded tags and numeric priorities, assign the following terms to each: immediate, delayed, hold, and deceased.

CHAPTER SUMMARY

- Basic elements of the incident command system (ICS) include command, finance, logistics, operations, planning, and safety.
- The incident commander's role includes triage, treatment, transportation, staging, rehabilitation, safety, and logistics.
- Critical components to any ICS include a uniform, a consistent set of rules, and a common language.
- The most important component to any ICS is communications.
- The incident commander is responsible for or delegates the creation of an action plan and manages the event at the highest level by establishing strategic objectives and tactical priorities.
- The finance officer is responsible for providing accurate accounting and monitoring of all costs associated with the incident.

- The planning officer supports the operation by providing the incident commander with past, present, and future information about the incident.
- The incident commander places responsibility and accountability of achieving tactical objectives with the sector officer.
- The logistics officer is responsible for providing required equipment, materials, and supplies to the scene of an incident.
- The triage officer is responsible for conducting a thorough assessment of the scene, identifying all injured and ill patients, and categorizing them by severity.
- The treatment officer is responsible for coordinating the treatment of all injured and ill patients and ensuring each patient is delivered to the transport area.
- The movement of patients to medical facilities is the responsibility of the transportation officer.
- In an effort to prevent bottlenecks and congestion at the incident scene, a staging area and a staging officer should be identified. The staging officer should track the arrival and departure of units in the staging area.
- A rehabilitation area is a place where workers are provided hydration, nourishment, and medical monitoring.
- The safety officer institutes safety practices and stops unsafe acts from taking place during EMS events.
- Principles and techniques of triage are applied in two stages in large-scale incidents.

SHORT ANSWER

1. What is a multiple-casualty incident (MCI)?

   _____
   _____
   _____
   _____

2. What are the four phases of emergency management?

   _____
   _____
   _____
   _____

3. What types of activities occur in each of the phases of emergency management?

   _____
   _____
   _____
   _____

4. What are the essential elements of a scene size-up when arriving at a potential MCI?

   _____
   _____
   _____
   _____

5. What distinguishes a closed (stable) incident from an open (unstable) incident?

   _____
   _____
   _____
   _____

6. What are the principal roles of each of the following components of the incident management system (IMS)?
   Command:_____

   _____

   Finance-administration:_____

   _____

   Logistics: _____

   _____

   Operations:_____

   _____

   Planning:_____

   _____

7. What is the function of each of the following special staff officers in the IMS?
   Information: _____

   _____

   Safety:_____

   _____

   Liaison:_____

   _____

8. What is the difference between single and unified incident command, and when is each system most applicable?

   _____
   _____
   _____
   _____

9. What are the roles of the first arriving EMS personnel at an MCI?

   _____
   _____
   _____
   _____

10. What is the role of each of the following groups during management of an MCI?

Staging: _____

_____

Extrication/rescue: _____

_____

Triage: _____

_____

Treatment: _____

_____

Transport: _____

_____

Rehabilitation: _____

_____

Morgue: _____

_____

11. What is the function of a command post?

_____

_____

_____

_____

12. What is the function of an emergency operations center (EOC)?

_____

_____

_____

_____

13. What are the principal roles of physicians in the out-of-hospital setting during an MCI?

_____

_____

_____

_____

14. Define *primary* and *secondary triage*.

_____

_____

_____

_____

15. Where do primary and secondary triage take place during the management of a mass-casualty incident?

_____

_____

_____

_____

16. What are the steps in performing triage using the START system?

_____

_____

_____

_____

17. What is the difference between a division and a group in the IMS?

_____

_____

_____

_____

18. What is the significance of each of the following color codes during triage?

Red: _____

Yellow: _____

Green: _____

Black: _____

19. Describe procedures for allocating patients to hospitals during an MCI.

_____

_____

_____

_____

20. Describe procedures for tracking patients during an MCI.

_____

_____

_____

_____

21. Describe modifications of communications procedures during MCIs.

_____

_____

_____

_____

22. A tornado struck a community, creating a damage track that was 3 miles long and approximately ½ mile wide. (A diagram of the track is shown below.) As EMS commander, how could you organize the response to an incident of this size while maintaining an optimum span of control? Your response can be an organizational chart with appropriate markings on the diagram below.

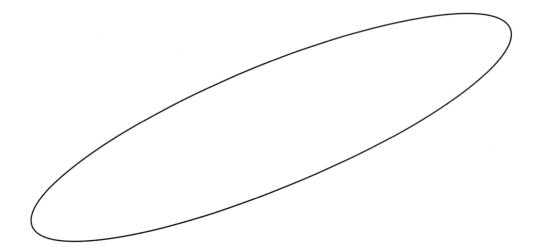

23. On the following chart, fill in the general and special staff officer positions of the incident management system that report to the incident commander.

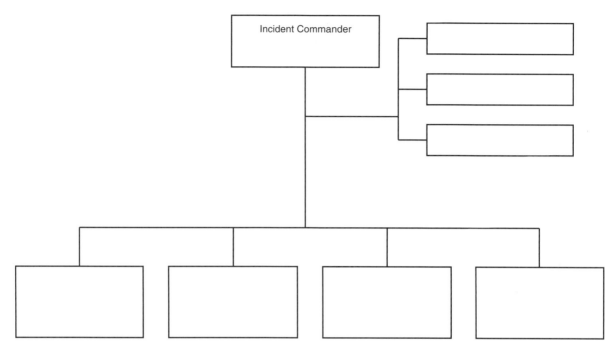

MULTIPLE CHOICE

1. Under the START triage system, the first distinction is based on the patient's ability to _____.
   A. walk
   B. breathe spontaneously at < 30 breaths/min
   C. follow a simple command
   D. tell you his or her name

2. During triage, the best way to assess perfusion quickly and accurately is to _____.
   A. assess mental status
   B. check capillary refill time
   C. palpate a carotid pulse
   D. palpate a radial pulse

3. The optimum number of subordinates that one supervisor can manage effectively during an incident is _____.
   A. 1
   B. 3
   C. 5
   D. 10

4. The safety officer has the authority to _____.
   A. activate the EOC
   B. bypass the chain of command if necessary
   C. disseminate public information
   D. interact with outside agency representatives

5. Under the IMS, the person responsible for EMS on the scene usually will report to the
   A. incident commander
   B. logistics section chief
   C. operations section chief
   D. staging officer

6. Under the IMS, the principal distinction between the roles of the incident commander and the operations section chief is that the _____.
   A. incident commander always is located off-site while the operations chief is located at the incident command post
   B. incident commander deals with strategic goals and objectives while the operations chief's focus is on operational and tactical concerns
   C. operations chief always is located off-site while the incident commander is located at the incident command post
   D. operations chief deals with strategic goals and objectives while the incident commander's focus is on operational and tactical concerns

7. In the IMS, the information officer is responsible for _____.
   A. bypassing the chain of command when talking to the press
   B. coordinating all incident decisions
   C. interacting with the operations officer every 30 minutes
   D. interfacing with the news media and disseminating public information

8. A staging area is a
   A. location where commanders gather to make decisions
   B. location where patients are treated and then held before transport to the hospital
   C. location where resources are held until given an assignment
   D. site where volunteers report during a large incident

169

Case one

A call came in to 9-1-1 at 1330 hours about a fire at the home improvement store located in the Highway Shopping Center at River Road and State Highway 163.

The 9-1-1 dispatcher immediately dispatched Engine Companies 4, 8, and 10; Truck 8; and District Chief 2 to the scene. Engine 4 was first to arrive on the scene followed by Engines 8 and 10 and Truck 8 within 5 minutes. Although only 8 minutes had passed since the initial 9-1-1 call, the east end of the home improvement store, where the garden center was located, was fully involved. The captain on Engine 4 established incident command. Initial size-up indicated that:

- Two employees assigned to the garden center were unaccounted for. Several other employees were suffering from smoke inhalation.
- Although the sprinkler system had activated, many of the combustibles could not be suppressed with water.
- The garden center contained an undetermined amount of fertilizers and other toxic substances. The warehouse, located at the rear of the store, contained 12 pallets of fertilizer and additional toxic substances ranging from aerosol cans to butane canisters for use with camp stoves. Other toxic substances were located throughout the store.
- Winds are blowing from the north at 12 miles per hour, and the fire is spreading quickly. The fire threatens adjacent buildings, including a shoe store, a walk-in medical clinic, and a supermarket.

1. Engines 4, 8, and 10 are each staffed with one officer and two firefighters. Truck 8 is staffed with one officer and three firefighters. Has the incident commander's optimum span of control been exceeded, and if so at what point?

   _____
   _____
   _____
   _____

2. Which of the command staff positions should the incident commander have established immediately?

   _____
   _____
   _____
   _____

3. The incident commander has established an incident command post (CP) in a parking lot on the northwest side of and across the street from the shopping center. What critical factor must be monitored as the incident progresses to determine whether there is a need to relocate the CP?

   _____
   _____
   _____
   _____

4. When District Chief 2 arrives at the scene, how should he interact with the captain on Engine 4?

   _____
   _____
   _____
   _____

5. Responders have arrived from law enforcement, EMS, public works, and the health department. Additionally, mutual aid agreements with neighboring communities have been activated to obtain additional fire suppression and EMS support. What type of command structure should be established?

_____

_____

_____

_____

Case two

1. Triage each of the following patients using the START method. Indicate whether a patient is categorized as green, yellow, red, or black.

   A. Walk: no. Respirations: 26 breaths/min. Circulation: no radial pulses. Mental status: unconscious. Injuries: lacerations/abrasions of face, arms, chest; fractured ribs on left side with bruising.

   _____

   _____

   _____

   _____

   B. Walk: yes. Respirations: 20 breaths/min. Circulation: radial pulse present left arm. Mental status: conscious and oriented. Injuries: abrasions/contusions on face, bloody nose, deformity right forearm.

   _____

   _____

   _____

   _____

   C. Walk: no. Respirations: 0 breaths/min initial, 0 breaths/min on reopening of airway. Circulation: no pulses. Mental status: unconscious. Injuries: large bruise/hematoma on anterior neck; facial lacerations, bruises; cyanosis.

   _____

   _____

   _____

   _____

   D. Walk: no. Respirations: 16 breaths/min. Circulation: <2 seconds. Mental status: conscious, oriented. Injuries: open fracture right tibia/fibula; facial cuts/bruises; abrasions of palms.

   _____

   _____

   _____

   _____

   E. Walk: no. Respirations: 32 breaths/min. Circulation: <2 seconds. Mental status: conscious and crying. Injuries: deformity of right tibia; abrasions and bruises on legs, face.

   _____

   _____

   _____

   _____

   F. Walk: no. Respirations: 0 breaths/min initial, 0/min on reopening of airway. Circulation: no radial pulses. Mental status: unconscious. Injuries: lacerations, hematomas, bruising of head; periorbital ecchymosis; cyanosis.

   _____

   _____

   _____

   _____

171

G. Walk: no. Respirations: 0 breaths/min initial, 26 breaths/min on reopening of airway. Circulation: radial pulses present. Mental status: unconscious. Injuries: Battle's sign; clear, colorless fluid draining from right ear.

_____

_____

_____

_____

63 Vehicle Rescue and Rescue Awareness Operations

READING ASSIGNMENT

Chapter 63, pages 718-765, in *Paramedic Practice Today: Above and Beyond.*

OBJECTIVES

After completing this chapter, you will be able to:

1. Define the term *rescue*.
2. Explain the medical and mechanical aspects of rescue situations.
3. Explain the role of the paramedic in delivering care at the rescue site and continuing through the rescue process to definitive care.
4. Describe the three levels of skills for responders to a technical rescue incident and how they differ.
5. Describe in order the priorities for safety in any rescue.
6. Describe the phases of a rescue operation.
7. List the three capabilities that situational awareness gives the emergency responder.
8. List and describe the types of personal protective equipment needed to operate safely in the rescue environment, including head protection, eye protection, hand protection, personal flotation devices, thermal protection and layering systems, high-visibility clothing, and specialized footwear.
9. Integrate the principles of rescue awareness and operations to rescue patients from highway incidents.
10. Have a working knowledge of various technologic improvements found on vehicles today that can affect emergency medical, safety, and extrication and rescue operations at motor vehicle incidents.
11. Explain supplemental restraint and airbag systems as well as methods to neutralize them.
12. Describe the necessary practices and procedures to resolve concerns presented by a hybrid gasoline and electric vehicle involved in a fire, crash, or extrication incident.
13. List and describe the major categories of safety hazards related to EMS personnel working at vehicle crash, fire, and rescue incidents.
14. Describe the electrical hazards (above and below ground) commonly found at highway incidents.
15. List the four phases of rescue for dealing with entrapment and extrication at a crash scene and describe the individual extrication tasks that comprise each phase of the process.
16. Explain typical door anatomy and methods to access stuck doors.
17. Develop specific skills in emergency stabilization of vehicles and access procedures and an awareness of specific extrication strategies.
18. Explain assessment procedures and modifications necessary when caring for entrapped patients.
19. Explain the differences in risk between moving water and flat water rescue.
20. Given a picture of moving water, identify and explain the features and hazards associated with hydraulics, strainers, and dams and hydroelectric sites.
21. Explain the effects of immersion hypothermia on the ability to survive sudden immersion and self-rescue.
22. Explain the phenomenon of the cold protective response in cold water drowning situations.
23. Given a list of rescue scenarios, identify the victim survivability profile and differentiate rescue versus body recovery situations.
24. Explain specific methods for assessment and spinal stabilization.
25. Explain why water entry techniques are methods of last resort.
26. Explain the rescue techniques associated with "talk, reach, throw, row."
27. Explain the self-rescue position if unexpectedly immersed in moving water.
28. Given a series of pictures, identify which would be considered confined spaces and potentially oxygen deficient.
29. Identify the hazards associated with confined spaces and risks posed to potential rescuers, including oxygen deficiency, chemical or toxic exposure or explosion, engulfment, machinery entrapment, and electricity.
30. Identify the poisonous gases commonly found in confined spaces, including hydrogen sulfide, carbon dioxide, carbon monoxide, low and high oxygen concentrations, methane, ammonia, and nitrogen dioxide.
31. Identify components necessary to ensure site safety before confined space rescue attempts.
32. Explain the hazard of cave-in during trench rescue operations.
33. Define *low angle, high angle, belay, rappel,* and *scrambling.*
34. Explain the different types of rescue litters and the advantages and disadvantages associated with each.
35. Describe the procedure for basket litter packaging for low-angle evacuations.

36. Develop proficiency in patient packaging and evacuation techniques that pertain to hazardous or rescue environments.
37. Explain the procedures for low-angle litter evacuation, including anchoring, litter and rope attachment, and lowering and raising procedures.
38. Explain nontechnical high-angle rescue procedures with an aerial apparatus.

CHAPTER SUMMARY

- Rescue is a patient-driven event, so you must continue to relate to the patient throughout the rescue both physically and emotionally.
- A rescue must combine both technical and medical skills. Everyone involved in a rescue must be aware of the rescue's effect on the patient. You must be aware of the situation of the rescue and the hazards for both paramedic and patient.
- Rescue often involves a patient needing medical care. This means careful preparation and realistic training. At a rescue, you must understand the hazards, know when it is safe or unsafe to access the patient, and have the necessary skills.
- The three levels of skills for responders to a technical rescue incident are awareness, operations, and technician.
- The priorities for safety in any rescue are personal safety, rescue team safety, safety of bystanders, and patient safety, in that order.
- The phases of a rescue operation are arrive and size-up the scene, establish command and conduct scene assessment, determine number of patients and triage if necessary, determine if the situation is search and rescue or body recovery, conduct a risk versus benefit analysis, request additional resources, establish ICS as command/control mechanism, and estimate time to access and evacuate.
- Phase 1 activities are those in which responding crew members would initially be involved on arrival: scene safety, vehicle stabilization, patient access, and initial medical care.
- Phase 2 is a disentanglement phase to remove the sidewall on one side of the vehicle, giving EMS providers maximal room for patient care and sufficient space to package and remove the patient.
- Phase 3 activities remove the vehicle roof.
- Phase 4 requires movement of the dashboard, instrument panel, and firewall structure of the vehicle away from the front seat passengers.
- You must maintain situational awareness throughout the rescue by being aware of everything happening in the environment.
- Patient packaging prepares the patient for transport and involves physically stabilizing the patient to prevent additional injury.
- Personal protective equipment (PPE) includes clothing and equipment to protect the wearer from injury and death and may include helmets, hearing protection, hand protection, foot protection, and protective clothing.

- A downed electrical wire should never be moved by responders. The preferred action is to secure the scene, communicate with any stranded occupants of the vehicle, and await the arrival of professional utility company personnel.
- Airbags that have not deployed present responders with obvious safety concerns for both the responders and their patient.
- Recommended vehicle crash procedures applicable to hybrid vehicles include hybrid vehicle identification, vehicle stabilization, access to passenger compartment, shift gear selector lever, turning ignition off and placing key on dash, checking that dash light indicating an energized hybrid vehicle system goes out, and shutting down hybrid vehicle's 12-volt electrical system at the battery.
- Because of the forces it creates, moving water is dangerous to individuals and rescuers. Hydraulics and strainers create particularly dangerous hazards.
- Water causes heat loss 25 times faster than air, and water temperature less than 98° F will cause hypothermia.
- Cold protective response can result in individuals surviving extended periods of submersion. A patient is never cold and dead—only warm and dead.
- Individuals who accidentally fall into cold water should use basic tactics to survive, including such techniques as HELP and huddle.
- Spinal immobilization in water requires special training, and only trained water rescue responders should attempt rescue, including in-water immobilization.
- The basic principles of water rescue include the following: never underestimate the power of moving water, do not enter water without specialized training and equipment, and always wear a personal flotation device (PFD). The basic rescue model for untrained rescuers is talk, reach, throw, and row. For their own safety, rescuers need a PFD, a helmet, knife, and thermal protection. For victim safety, they need flotation along with equipment for immobilization, extrication, and thermal protection.
- Confined spaces are particularly dangerous for rescuers. OSHA has defined confined space (permit space). Among the hazards in confined spaces are atmospheric dangers, fire and explosion, engulfment, electricity, structural hazards, and fall hazards. OSHA requires a permit process before a rescuer can enter a confined space.
- Among the first actions for EMS personnel at a confined space emergency are to establish a safe perimeter, prevent additional entry to the space, assist in remote retrieval, and determine from the permit or entry supervisor the type of work being done at the time of the accident.
- Trench collapse is one of the most dangerous calls for EMS personnel. The first steps are to secure the scene, initiate command, and secure a perimeter.
- Rescue in hazardous terrain can be challenging and dangerous and requires specialized training for the individual and team.

- A rescue often involves transporting the patient in a litter. Rescuers must know which litters are appropriate, how to package and secure and protect the patient, and how to arrange medical equipment for use during transport.
- Among the skills needed in low-angle or high-angle evacuation are knowledge of placing anchors, rope-lowering systems, braking systems, and hauling systems.
- In working with helicopters, rescuers must understand helicopter limitations, ground safety, and air safety. Among the helicopter rescue techniques are one-skid landing, hovering, short haul, and sling load.

SHORT ANSWER

1. Define *rescue*.

   _____
   _____
   _____
   _____

2. What is the role of the paramedic during a rescue operation?

   _____
   _____
   _____
   _____

3. What are the phases of a rescue operation?

   _____
   _____
   _____
   _____

4. What are the types of personnel protective equipment needed to operate safely in the rescue environment?

   _____
   _____
   _____
   _____

5. What is the purpose of the "patient access" phase of a rescue operation?

   _____
   _____
   _____
   _____

6. What steps must be taken before the "patient access" phase begins?

   _____
   _____
   _____
   _____

7. What position in the IMS (other than incident commander) must be filled during every rescue operation?

   _____
   _____
   _____
   _____

8. Describe techniques used to improve safety at highway incidents.

   Apparatus placement:_____
   _____
   _____
   _____
   _____

   Headlights and emergency vehicle lighting: _____
   _____
   _____
   _____
   _____

   Cones, flares: _____
   _____
   _____
   _____
   _____

   Reflective and high visibility clothing: _____
   _____
   _____
   _____
   _____

9. Describe hazards associated with these vehicle components and methods of controlling them.

   Airbag/supplemental restraint devices: _____
   _____
   _____
   _____
   _____

   Conventional fuel systems: _____
   _____
   _____
   _____
   _____

   Alternate fuel systems: _____
   _____
   _____
   _____
   _____

10. Where are the A, B, C, and D posts of a motor vehicle located?

   _____
   _____
   _____
   _____

11. Describe common electrical hazards found at highway incidents.

_____

_____

_____

12. Describe the difference between tempered and safety glass, common locations of each in a vehicle, and how to break each type safely.

_____

_____

_____

_____

13. What effect will immersion hypothermia have on ability to survive sudden immersion?

_____

_____

_____

_____

14. Describe the phenomenon of cold protective response in cold water drowning situations. How does this response affect decision making in resuscitation situations?

_____

_____

_____

_____

15. What risks are associated with low-head dams?

_____

_____

_____

_____

16. What is a recirculating current?

_____

_____

_____

_____

17. What is a strainer?

_____

_____

_____

_____

18. Explain the rescue techniques associated with "reach-throw-row-go."

_____

_____

_____

_____

19. Why are water entry rescue techniques the method of last resort?

_____

_____

_____

_____

20. What is the self-rescue position used if you fall into moving water during a rescue operation?

_____

_____

_____

_____

21. What is the heat-lessening escape position (HELP)?

_____

_____

_____

_____

22. Why does HELP decrease heat loss?

_____

_____

_____

_____

23. What are common hazards associated with confined space rescue attempts?

_____

_____

_____

_____

24. List hazardous gases commonly found in confined spaces.

_____

_____

_____

_____

25. Describe procedures necessary to ensure site safety before confined space rescue attempts.

_____

_____

_____

26. Describe procedures used during trench rescue operations, including techniques needed to ensure rescuer safety.

_____

_____

_____

27. Define the following terms:
    Low angle: _____
    _____

    High angle: _____
    _____

    Belay: _____
    _____

    Rappel: _____
    _____

    Scrambling: _____
    _____

    Hasty rope slide:_____
    _____

28. Discuss methods of pain control for entrapped patients and risks associated with these methods.
    _____
    _____
    _____
    _____

29. Discuss the need for and techniques of providing thermal control for entrapped patients.
    _____
    _____
    _____
    _____

30. Describe the pathophysiology and management of crush syndrome.
    _____
    _____
    _____
    _____

MULTIPLE CHOICE

1. Your ambulance is the first unit to arrive at a report of a person trapped by the collapse of a ditch at a construction site. Your initial action should be to _____.
   A. enter the ditch and attempt to uncover the patient's face
   B. properly shore the ditch so no further slides or collapses occur
   C. remove the loose soil with your hands so the victim will receive no further injuries
   D. secure the perimeter and request a specialized trench rescue team

2. You are responding to a "vehicle collision with injuries" on a steep highway in mountainous terrain west of your city. Arriving on the scene, you see an ominous set of fresh skid marks leading to a splintered guardrail. Approximately 200 feet down the embankment, you see an automobile resting on its side. In the distance, you can hear the siren of a back-up ambulance from a neighboring city. As you and your partner reach the car, you see the patient lying partially out of a broken window. He has a deep wound on his forehead from which blood mixed with clear fluid is flowing. His respirations are shallow and gasping with gurgling sounds. As your first priority, you should _____.
   A. ensure that the vehicle is stable
   B. ensure that the vehicle's ignition is off and that the airbag system is disarmed
   C. open the airway with cervical spine control using a jaw thrust maneuver
   D. stop the bleeding without applying pressure, because a skull fracture may be present

3. You respond to a call to find two cars have been involved in a head-on collision. As you approach the scene, you notice that the passengers and driver of car No. 1 are out of the vehicle, walking around and talking to bystanders. The passenger from car No. 2 appears to be in severe distress. The driver of car No. 2 appears to be dead. All of the doors of car No. 2 are jammed, the windows are closed, and the passenger is too confused to cooperate in opening a door. You should gain access to the patient by _____.
   A. breaking the side window
   B. breaking the windshield
   C. cutting through the roof
   D. prying the door open

4. During a rescue attempt, you fall into swift water. You should try to _____.
   A. float on your back with your feet pointed downstream
   B. float on your back with your feet pointed upstream
   C. pull yourself into a fetal position and face downstream
   D. pull yourself into a fetal position and face upstream

5. During a water rescue, what personnel should wear personal flotation devices?
   A. Anyone involved in the rescue whose responsibilities require them to work in, on, or near the water
   B. Only those personnel who physically enter the water to rescue or treat the patient
   C. Personnel who enter the water to rescue the patient and personnel who support those rescuers either in boats or on the shore
   D. Personnel who enter the water to rescue the patient or who support those personnel from boats

6. The most common hazard associated with rescue in confined spaces is _____.
   A. oxygen deficiency
   B. physical instability and risk of collapse
   C. presence of sharp or otherwise hazardous objects
   D. presence of toxic or caustic substances

7. Which of the following statements about rescue from automobiles is correct?
   A. In newer model vehicles, the safest method for displacing a steering column may be to push the A-post and the dash forward.
   B. The glass in an automobile's windshield can be broken with a sharp blow to one of its corners.
   C. The roof of unibody construction vehicles can be flapped or cut away without affecting the structural integrity of the rest of the vehicle.
   D. The steering column of front-wheel drive vehicles can be safely displaced by attaching a chain to it an pulling it upward and forward using the Hurst tool or a come-along tool.

8. A 9-year-old girl fell through the ice of a frozen pond. It took the fire department about 40 minutes to locate her. The patient is unresponsive, pulseless, and apneic. The ECG monitor shows asystole. You should _____.
   A. request a response by the police and the medical examiner
   B. start CPR immediately and transport
   C. start CPR immediately, transport, and begin aggressive rewarming in the ambulance
   D. transport without performing CPR

9. What is the primary function of paramedics during the disentanglement phase of extrication?
   A. Assessing and monitoring the condition of the patient
   B. Determining who was responsible for the collision
   C. Ensuring the vehicle is stable
   D. Initiating traffic control measures when necessary

CASE STUDY

It is 1600 hours on a Friday afternoon. The temperature is 95° F, and the humidity is 80%. It has not rained for some time. Construction company employees are installing a sanitary sewer line in a new industrial complex located in an area on the outskirts of your community. A backhoe is digging a 5-foot–wide by 15-foot–deep trench in sandy soil. The backhoe operator is in a bit of a hurry and is piling the soil too close to the trench. Two workers are in the trench driving home lengths of pipe. Because of the heat and humidity, they are working without shirts, and they are not wearing hard hats. The trench has not been shored in an attempt to save time.

An 18-wheeler with a load of crushed rock to be used as bedding for the pipe enters the construction site. As the truck backs over the dry earth, the ground shakes and the unstable soil slides into the trench. One worker is completely buried. The other is pinned against the wall of the trench by dirt that reaches up to his chest. The pressure of the dirt makes his breathing difficult.

At 1603 you are dispatched to the accident site, which is approximately 5 minutes away. En route, you are advised that the fire department is responding with an engine company, a truck company, and a district chief.

1. What additional resources should be requested?

   _____
   _____
   _____
   _____

2. What protective equipment should be used by the rescuers?

   _____
   _____
   _____
   _____

3. What hazards should be managed?

   _____
   _____
   _____
   _____

4. What is the most appropriate strategy for gaining access to the patients?

_____

_____

_____

_____

5. What special medical considerations exist during the management of this incident for both the patients and the rescuers?

_____

_____

_____

_____

6. Are there any special considerations for patient evacuation and transport?

_____

_____

_____

_____

64 Response to Hazardous Materials Incidents

READING ASSIGNMENT

Chapter 64, pages 766-802, in *Paramedic Practice Today: Above and Beyond.*

OBJECTIVES

After completing this chapter, you will be able to:
1. Identify training regulations regarding EMS and hazardous materials response and contact agencies that may provide additional information.
2. Identify commonly used recognition and identification clues.
3. Identify the international and U.S. Department of Transportation hazard classes.
4. Use physical properties to assess the movement of hazardous material.
5. Use chemical properties to determine a chemical's hazard potential.
6. Identify the properties used to determine a chemical's toxicity.
7. Identify written and verbal resources that can be accessed to obtain chemical information.
8. Determine the safest way to approach a hazardous materials incident.
9. Identify the exclusion (hot), contamination reduction (warm), and support (cold) zones at a hazardous materials or weapon of mass destruction incident and describe the EMS actions performed in each zone.
10. Identify the types of personal protective equipment that should be used by EMS responders at a hazardous materials incident.
11. List the four Environmental Protection Agency designated levels of protection and discuss the use and limitations of each.
12. Identify the procedures necessary for proper responder monitoring and rehabilitation at a hazardous materials incident.
13. Describe responder decontamination procedures.
14. Discuss the need for patient decontamination and explain how it is carried out.
15. Describe how effective mass casualty decontamination may be carried out.
16. Identify the proper treatment for commonly encountered hazardous materials.
17. Discuss the need for early scene-to-hospital communication.
18. Identify ways to reduce secondary exposure risk during patient transportation.
19. Identify the procedures that must take place at the end of the incident.

CHAPTER SUMMARY

- A hazardous materials incident is one of the most challenging emergencies that EMS face. Hazardous materials responses involve out-of-the-norm activities such as the use of personal protective equipment (PPE) and decontamination.
- Responders must be able to recognize the presence of hazardous materials at an incident.
- Responders must be able to use available references and understand the importance of chemical and physical properties when assessing the hazards at an incident involving hazardous materials.
- Proper approach and scene management practices are essential to responder safety at hazardous materials incidents.
- Special training is required before responders may operate at this type of emergency.
- EMS personnel must be able to select and use proper PPE if they will operate in the warm or hot zones of a hazardous materials incident.
- EMS responders should be able to provide the hazardous materials team with medical support and responder rehabilitation at a hazardous materials incident.
- Proper decontamination of both responders and patients is essential to limit harm and the chance of secondary contamination.
- EMS responders should have an understanding of the proper treatment practices for commonly encountered hazardous materials.
- Responders must understand the need for interaction with local hospitals and the need for proper transport procedures when transporting patients from the scene of a hazardous materials incident.
- Post-incident procedures such as debriefing, analysis, and review are vital pieces of a hazardous materials response.

SHORT ANSWERS

1. What are objectives of hazardous materials awareness training?

   _____
   _____
   _____
   _____

2. What is primary contamination?

   _____
   _____
   _____
   _____

3. What is secondary contamination?

_____

_____

_____

4. Define each of the following toxicologic principles.
Acute toxicity:_____

_____

_____

Delayed toxicity:_____

_____

_____

Route of exposure:_____

_____

_____

Local effects:_____

_____

_____

Systemic effects:_____

_____

_____

Dose response:_____

_____

_____

Synergistic effects:_____

_____

_____

5. Define and discuss the importance to the risk assessment process of each of these toxicologic terms:

Threshold limit value/time-weighted average (TLV/TWA):_____

_____

_____

Threshold limit value/short-term exposure limit (TLV/STEL):_____

_____

_____

Threshold limit value/ceiling level (TLV/CL):_____

_____

_____

50% Lethal concentration (LC50):_____

_____

_____

50% Lethal dose (LD50):_____

_____

_____

Parts per million (ppm):_____

_____

_____

Parts per billion (ppb):_____

_____

_____

Immediately dangerous to life and health (IDLH):

_____

_____

6. Discuss how the substance and the route of exposure/contamination alter triage and decontamination methods.

_____

_____

_____

_____

7. Discuss the common signs, symptoms, and management for exposures to the following substances:

Corrosives (acids/alkalis):_____

_____

_____

_____

_____

Pulmonary irritants:_____

_____

_____

_____

_____

Pesticides (carbamates/organophosphates):_____

_____

_____

_____

_____

Chemical asphyxiants (cyanide/carbon monoxide):

_____

_____

_____

Hydrocarbon solvents (xylene/methylene chloride):

_____

_____

_____

8. Define and discuss the importance to the risk assessment process of each of the following:

Boiling point:_____

_____

_____

_____

Flash point:_____

_____

_____

_____

Upper and lower flammable limits:_____

_____

_____

_____

Ignition temperature:_____

_____

_____

_____

Specific gravity:_____

_____

_____

_____

Vapor density:_____

_____

_____

_____

_____

Vapor pressure:_____

_____

_____

_____

Water solubility:_____

_____

_____

_____

Alpha, beta, gamma radiation:_____

_____

_____

_____

9. Sketch the organization of the scene of a hazardous materials incident. Indicate the positions of each of the following: Hot Zone, Warm Zone, Cold Zone, Access Corridor, Victim Decontamination Corridor, Rescuer Decontamination Corridor, Treatment Area, Medical Monitoring Area, Rehab Area, Transport Area, and Command Post.

10. Describe the procedure for decontaminating a nonambulatory patient including discussion of areas of the body that are difficult to decontaminate.

_____
_____
_____
_____

11. Explain medical monitoring procedures for HAZMAT team members.

_____
_____
_____
_____

12. Identify and discuss factors that influence the level of heat stress experienced by HAZMAT team members.

_____
_____
_____
_____

13. Discuss documentation necessary for HAZMAT medical monitoring and rehabilitation operations.

_____
_____
_____
_____

MULTIPLE CHOICE

1. A product with a high vapor pressure will _____.
   A. evaporate less rapidly than a product with a low vapor pressure
   B. evaporate more rapidly than one with a low vapor pressure
   C. have a higher flash point than a product with a low vapor pressure
   D. have a lower flash point than one with a low vapor pressure

2. A product involved in a hazardous materials incident has a flash point of 10° F. The ambient temperature at the scene is 86° F. This means that the product _____.
   A. is likely to have completely vaporized and therefore presents no fire or explosion hazard
   B. is unable to ignite as long as the environmental temperature exceeds 10° F
   C. probably will be releasing enough vapors to ignite since the ambient temperature exceeds the flash point
   D. probably will not release enough vapors to ignite since the ambient temperature exceeds the flash point

3. A product involved in a hazardous materials incident has a vapor density of 1.5. You should anticipate that the product would tend to _____.
   A. ignite less readily than products with low vapor densities
   B. remain in a relatively small area immediately surrounding the container
   C. rise and disperse readily
   D. sink and accumulate in low-lying areas around the site of the release

4. A vapor cloud is escaping from a tank truck involved in a collision. Using binoculars, you can tell that the diamond-shaped placards on the truck are green. Based on this information, you can determine that the product is a nonflammable gas that _____.
   A. must be identified more specifically before any action is taken
   B. presents no fire or explosion hazards
   C. presents no fire, explosion, or reactivity hazards
   D. presents no fire, explosion, or toxicity hazards

5. A product has a specific gravity of 0.8. Based on this information, you know that the material will _____.
   A. tend to float on water
   B. tend to rise in air
   C. tend to sink in air
   D. tend to sink in water

6. Which of the following statements about decontamination is correct?
   A. Decontamination of equipment usually is not necessary.
   B. Immediate decontamination of casualties is part of their emergency medical care.
   C. The decontamination area is set up after HAZMAT team members have entered the hot zone.
   D. The decontamination area should be set up in the cold zone.

7. Which statement about the DOT placarding system is correct?
   A. A placard for each hazard being transported must be placed on both sides and both ends of the transport vessel.
   B. Placards are required on all shipments of hazardous materials.
   C. Shipments of certain classes of materials must be placarded regardless of the quantity of material being shipped.
   D. The DANGEROUS placard indicates that the material is a respiratory hazard.

8. In a HAZMAT situation, the most common route of exposure is _____.
   A. gastrointestinal ingestion
   B. parenteral injection
   C. respiratory inhalation
   D. topical absorption

9. Structural firefighting equipment provides what level of HAZMAT protection?
   A. Level A
   B. Level B
   C. Level C
   D. Level D

10. A train derailment has resulted in the release of several chemicals that are reacting with one another to produce a visible purple vapor cloud. From the train consist and the waybills, you have been able to identify the individual products. At this point, a call to CHEMTREC will be unable to provide you with _____.
    A. activation of specialized response teams from the shippers of the products
    B. information from the CHEMTREC communicator on the probable nature and properties of the products of reactions between the spilled chemicals
    C. more detailed information about the properties and hazards of each of the products involved
    D. referrals to employees of the chemicals' manufacturers who are specialists in their behavior

11. The transportation warning placard for a flammable gas will have _____.
    A. a red color, a ball-on-fire symbol, and a hazard class "3" number.
    B. a red color, a flame symbol, and a hazard class "2" number.
    C. a yellow color, a ball-on-fire symbol, and a hazard class "5" number.
    D. an orange color, a flame symbol, and a hazard class "2" number.

12. The most hazardous type of radiation is _____.
    A. alpha radiation
    B. beta radiation
    C. delta radiation
    D. gamma radiation

65 Tactical EMS

Chapter 65, pages 803-823, in *Paramedic Practice Today: Above and Beyond*.

OBJECTIVES

After completing this chapter, you will be able to:
1. List the types of missions to which civilian special weapons and tactics teams respond.
2. Define *tactical EMS*.
3. List at least five duties of a tactical EMS medic.
4. Describe the three sides of the tactical EMS triangle.
5. Recognize the difference between cover and concealment.
6. Define *tactical casualty care*.
7. List the three most common causes of preventable death on the battlefield.
8. List the priorities of tactical casualty care.
9. Match the tactical casualty care stages of care to the incident command system hot, warm, and cold zones and describe the appropriate care in each stage.
10. Identify the appropriate training for the tactical EMS medic.
11. Formulate an inventory of tactical EMS equipment, including tactical medical equipment, prioritized into four distinct lines.
12. Discuss the advantages and disadvantages of arming the tactical EMS medic.

CHAPTER SUMMARY

- Civilian special operations teams, most commonly referred to as special weapons and tactics (SWAT) teams, respond to unusually hazardous threats. These threats are beyond the capabilities of normal law enforcement. They include snipers, barricaded armed suspects, hostage situations, felony warrants on well-armed suspects, weapons of mass destruction, and other extraordinary deployments.
- Tactical emergency medical services (TEMS), or more appropriately tactical medicine, is defined as "the comprehensive out-of-hospital medical support for law enforcement's tactical teams during training and special operations."
- Although TEMS medics provide tactical casualty care on the inner perimeter of SWAT missions, their duties usually are much broader. They include medical threat assessments before missions, remote assessment of downed casualties during missions, health maintenance of team members, and assessment before incarceration of suspects.

- TEMS providers should be experienced paramedics who maintain numerous patient contacts each year and are well rounded in all parts of the TEMS triangle, including tactical skills, medical skills, and personal fitness.
- TEMS medics should wear proper person protection equipment. In addition, they should have a working knowledge of cover, which is protection from enemy fire, and concealment, which is defined as protection from enemy observation.
- Tactical combat casualty care (TCCC) represents the field care portion of battlefield medicine. It directly applies to the care given to casualties incurred on the inner perimeter of civilian SWAT operations.
- The most common causes of preventable death on the battlefield are (1) exsanguination from external bleeding (60%), (2) tension pneumothorax (33%), (3) airway compromise (6%), and (4) all other causes (1%).
- The priorities of TCCC are (1) fire superiority (suppress the threat), (2) prevent further casualties (get out of the line of fire), (3) triage, and (4) treat the life threats.
- TCCC under fire is comparable to the incident command system hot zone. All efforts are made to get the casualty out of the line of fire, and the only appropriate care rendered should be stopping exsanguinating bleeding with a quick-draw tourniquet.
- TCCC tactical field care is comparable to the incident command system warm zone. Casualties are protected until a clear route to medical transport is secured, and emergency care is rendered in a tactical manner without putting anything down or giving away the position.
- TCCC medical and casualty evacuation is comparable to the incident command system cold zone. Casualties are en route to a hospital or await transport in the outer perimeter.
- TEMS medics should participate in all appropriate and authorized tactical law enforcement and medical training. Most importantly, they should train with the tactical team they serve and provide self-aid and buddy aid training to their tactical operators in case of mass-casualty catastrophes.
- TEMS medics should stage their equipment so that all care under fire and tactical field care equipment can be quickly drawn with one hand without looking and without setting anything down.
- No right or wrong answer exists regarding whether TEMS medics should be armed. It is a matter of the needs and policies of the tactical team they serve.

187

MATCHING

1. Match the incident command system zones with the stage of tactical combat casualty care that should be rendered in each zone.
   ____ Cold zone   A. Care under fire
   ____ Hot zone   B. MEDEVAC/CASEVAC
   ____ Warm zone   C. Tactical field care

2. Match each list of equipment with the appropriate line of care.
   ____ First line
   ____ Fourth line
   ____ Second line
   ____ Third line

   A. Additional tourniquet and dressing, roller gauze, chest decompression needles, surgical airway kit
   B. Tactical tourniquet, tactical battle dressing
   C. Extrication collar, endotracheal intubation kit, SAM splints, BP cuff, and stethoscope
   D. Oxygen cylinders and delivery supplies, ECG/Spo$_2$ monitor, full spinal immobilization supplies

SHORT ANSWER

1. Define *tactical emergency medical services*.

2. List nine missions to which civilian SWAT teams respond.

3. List at least five duties of a tactical medic.

4. What are the three parts of the tactical EMS triangle?

5. What are the three most common causes of preventable death on the battlefield?

6. Define *tactical casualty care*.

7. What are the priorities of tactical combat casualty care?

8. What is concealment?

9. What is cover?

10. List the advantages of tactical medics carrying firearms during operations.

11. List the disadvantages of tactical medics carrying firearms during operations.

MULTIPLE CHOICE

1. The most common cause of preventable death in combat situations is _____.
   A. airway obstruction
   B. exsanguination from extremity wounds
   C. head trauma
   D. tension pneumothorax

2. When treatment is provided according to tactical combat casualty care guidelines, the highest patient care priority is _____.
   A. controlling hemorrhage from extremity wounds
   B. ensuring adequate oxygenation and ventilation
   C. maintaining an open airway
   D. preventing excessive movement of the cervical spine

3. Once fire superiority has been established, appropriate treatment in the hot zone would include _____.
   A. applying a tactical dressing to control extremity hemorrhage
   B. applying a tourniquet to control extremity hemorrhage
   C. decompressing a tension pneumothorax
   D. inserting a dual-lumen airway

4. The sequence of priorities in tactical combat casualty care is _____.
   A. achieve fire superiority, prevent further casualties, triage, treat according to TCCC guidelines
   B. achieve fire superiority, triage, prevent further casualties, treat according to TCCC guidelines
   C. prevent further casualties, achieve fire superiority, triage, treat according to TCCC guidelines
   D. triage, achieve fire superiority, prevent further casualties, treat according to TCCC guidelines

5. Equipment that should be readily accessible in pockets of the tactical medic's vest or body armor includes _____.
   A. one tactical tourniquet and one tactical battle dressing
   B. tactical tourniquet, tactical battle dressing, roller gauze, chest seals, chest decompression needles, epinephrine autoinjector
   C. tactical tourniquet, tactical battle dressing, roller gauze, chest seals, chest decompression needles, SAM splints, flex cuff restraints
   D. tactical tourniquet, tactical battle dressing, roller gauze, chest seals, chest decompression needles, dual-lumen airway, trauma shears

6. Which of the following statements best describes cover?
   A. Cover prevents an enemy from seeing you and can be provided by a vehicle's engine block.
   B. Cover prevents an enemy from seeing you and can be provided by walls of structures.
   C. Cover provides protection from enemy fire and can be provided by walls of structures.
   D. Cover provides protection from enemy fire and can be provided by a vehicle's engine block.

7. Medical equipment that every member of the tactical team should carry and be trained to use includes _____.
   A. one tactical tourniquet and one tactical battle dressing
   B. one tactical tourniquet, one tactical battle dressing, and a chest seal or occlusive dressing
   C. one tactical tourniquet, one tactical battle dressing, and a hemostatic dressing or granules (QuikClot or HemCon)
   D. one tactical tourniquet, one tactical battle dressing, and roller gauze

8. The problem most commonly managed by tactical medics is _____.
   A. blunt trauma produced by bullets striking ballistic vests
   B. burns from distraction devices and other pyrotechnics
   C. minor injuries or illnesses during training evolutions or extended missions
   D. penetrating extremity injuries

9. When critical injuries occur during a tactical operation, the first medical priority is to immediately assess _____.
   A. any injured suspect, regardless of potential injuries that may have occurred to tactical officers
   B. any injured tactical officer, regardless of potential injuries that may have occurred to suspects
   C. patients with hemorrhage from extremity injuries, regardless of whether they are tactical officers or suspects
   D. patients with trauma to the face or chest, regardless of whether they are tactical officers or suspects

66 Disaster Response and Domestic Preparedness

READING ASSIGNMENT

Chapter 66, pages 826-848, in *Paramedic Practice Today: Above and Beyond.*

OBJECTIVES

After completing this chapter, you will be able to:
1. Explain the importance of disaster response preplanning and preparedness.
2. Describe the purpose of the National Response Plan.
3. Describe the federal medical resources available from the National Disaster Medical System.
4. Discuss the need for and the use of an incident command system.
5. Describe the role of EMS in the incident command system.
6. Identify the different types of natural disasters and the emergency medical needs associated with each.
7. Identify chemical weapons of mass destruction agents that should be of concern to first responders.
8. Identify the five classes of chemical warfare agents and give examples from each class.
9. Identify the epidemiologic clues that may indicate an act of bioterrorism is occurring.
10. List the biologic agents considered the most critical threats.
11. Identify particular concerns that exist with large-scale radiologic events.
12. Explain why explosive and incendiary devices are used most often by terrorists.
13. Describe blast injuries and the human response.

CHAPTER SUMMARY

■ A response to a disaster tests every part of the EMS system. These situations mandate that the paramedic use skills usually practiced only in drills and exercises.
■ The response to a natural disaster may force medical personnel to operate for extended periods in an austere environment.
■ The response to technologic disasters may place the paramedic in an unsafe situation.
■ The threat of weapons of mass destruction (WMD) is always present.

■ Responders must be able to recognize these events and respond appropriately.
■ Responders should have a working knowledge of the different types of WMD expected to be used.

MATCHING

1. Match the primary functional area of the incident command system with its description.

_____ Collects and evaluates information about incident and response	A. Command
	B. Finance
	C. Logistics
_____ Directs, orders, and controls all resources used to manage an incident	D. Operations
	E. Planning
_____ Locates and organizes facilities, services, and materials needed to manage an incident	
_____ Manages all tactical operations at an incident	
_____ Tracks incident costs	

2. Match the chemical agents with their class.

_____ Chlorine, anhydrous ammonia, phosgene	A. Pulmonary agents
_____ CS, CNB	B. Blister agents
_____ Cyanide, cyanogens, chloride	C. Riot control agents
_____ Sulfur mustard	D. Blood agents
_____ Tabun, sarin, soman, VXE	E. Nerve agents

3. Match the types of blast injuries with their descriptions.

_____ Trauma from flying debris	A. Primary
_____ Trauma from patient being thrown by blast	B. Secondary
_____ Trauma from pressure wave	C. Tertiary

191

SHORT ANSWER

1. Why is preplanning of disaster response necessary?

2. What is the purpose of the National Response Plan?

3. What are emergency service functions (ESFs)?

4. What federal agency coordinates the Public Health and Medical Services emergency services function?

5. What federal agency administers and coordinates the National Disaster Medical System (NDMS)?

6. What is a Disaster Medical Assistance Team (DMAT)?

7. What are National Medical Response Teams for Weapons of Mass Destruction (NMRT-WMD)?

8. What are Disaster Mortuary Operations Teams (DMORTs)?

9. List 10 indicators that a disease outbreak is an act of biologic terrorism rather than a natural event.

10. What is an EMP? What is the effect of EMP?

11. Why have most terrorist attacks involved the use of explosive or incendiary devices rather than chemical, biologic, or radioactive materials?

MULTIPLE CHOICE

1. You are responding to a scene where the incident management system already has been put into effect. Unless otherwise directed, on arrival you should report to the _____.
   A. incident commander
   B. logistics chief
   C. operations chief
   D. staging area manager

2. The optimum number of subordinates that one supervisor can manage effectively during an incident is _____.
   A. 5
   B. 1
   C. 10
   D. 3

3. The safety officer has authority to _____.
   A. activate the emergency operations center
   B. bypass the chain of command to prevent unsafe acts
   C. disseminate information to the media to ensure public safety
   D. interact with outside agency representatives

4. Under the incident management system (IMS), the person responsible for EMS on the scene usually will report to the _____.
   A. incident commander
   B. logistics section chief
   C. operations section chief
   D. staging officer

192

5. Under the IMS, the principal distinction between the roles of the incident commander and the operations section chief is that the _____.
   A. incident commander always is located off-site while the operations chief is located at the incident command post
   B. incident commander deals with strategic goals and objectives while the focus of the operations chief is on operational and tactical concerns
   C. operations chief always is located off-site while the incident commander is located at the incident command post
   D. operations chief deals with strategic goals and objectives while the focus of the incident commander is on operational and tactical concerns

6. In the incident management system, the information officer is responsible for _____.
   A. bypassing the chain of command when talking to the press
   B. coordinating all incident decisions
   C. interacting with the operations officer every 30 minutes
   D. interfacing with the news media and disseminating public information

7. A staging area is a _____.
   A. location where commanders gather to make decisions
   B. location where patients are treated and then held before transport to the hospital
   C. location where resources are held until given an assignment
   D. site where volunteers report during a large incident

8. Which of the following is a special staff function under the IMS rather than a primary functional area?
   A. Finance and administration
   B. Logistics
   C. Planning and intelligence
   D. Public information

9. What is the one position in the incident management system that always is established at every incident?
   A. Incident commander
   B. Logistics chief
   C. Operations chief
   D. Safety officer

10. The chemical agent that has a faint odor of bitter almonds is _____.
    A. cyanide
    B. phosgene
    C. sarin
    D. sulfur mustard

11. Which of the following best describes the odor of phosgene?
    A. Bitter almonds
    B. Bleach
    C. Freshly cut grass or hay
    D. Window cleaner

12. Why is cyanide toxic?
    A. It binds to hemoglobin, preventing oxygen transport.
    B. It is metabolized to thiocyanate, causing metabolic acidosis and renal failure.
    C. It paralyzes the respiratory center in the medulla, causing respiratory arrest.
    D. It prevents use of oxygen in cellular metabolism, stopping ATP production.

13. What are the antidotes to cyanide?
    A. Amyl nitrite, sodium nitrite, and sodium thiosulfate
    B. Atropine, naloxone
    C. Atropine, pralidoxime
    D. Sodium nitroprusside, sodium thiosulfate

14. A patient who is exposed to phosgene will develop _____.
    A. a rapid onset of pharyngeal edema that can cause airway obstruction
    B. cellular hypoxia from inhibition of electron transport
    C. pulmonary edema 2 to 24 hours after exposure
    D. tissue hypoxia secondary to phosgene binding to hemoglobin

15. Nerve agents are toxic because they _____.
    A. bind to acetylcholine receptor sites at the neuromuscular junction, causing paralysis and respiratory arrest
    B. inhibit the action of the enzyme that breaks down acetylcholine
    C. prevent reabsorption of acetylcholine by the neurons of the parasympathetic nervous system
    D. stimulate opiate receptors in the central nervous system, causing respiratory depression, constricted pupils, and bradycardia

16. Deaths from nerve agent toxicity usually result from _____.
    A. aspiration of excessive secretions in the upper airway
    B. electrolyte imbalance caused by vomiting
    C. hypovolemia from increased gastrointestinal fluid loss
    D. weakness or paralysis of the respiratory muscles

17. Which of the following biologic agents is classified by the Centers for Disease Control and Prevention as a category B pathogen?
    A. Anthrax
    B. Botulism
    C. Encephalitis
    D. Tularemia

18. How can the lesions of smallpox be distinguished from those caused by chickenpox?
    A. As the infection progresses, all lesions from chickenpox remain at the same stage.
    B. As the infection progresses smallpox lesions include a combination of vesicles, scabs, and pustules.
    C. The lesions of chickenpox occur primarily on the face, arms, and legs, including the palms and soles.
    D. The lesions of smallpox occur primarily on the face, arms, and legs, including the palms and soles.

19. Which of the following statements about plague is correct?
   A. All three forms of plague present initially with fever, chills, and myalgia.
   B. Bubonic plague is the most severe form of this disease.
   C. Pneumonic plague is the most common form of this disease.
   D. Septicemic plague develops secondary to untreated pneumonic plague.

20. Which of the following statements about tularemia is correct?
   A. Patients must be exposed to a large number of the bacteria to develop this disease.
   B. The disease can progress to a pulmonary syndrome that includes sore throat, nonproductive cough, and bronchitis.
   C. Tularemia is easily spread from person to person.
   D. Use of an N-95 mask is recommended when care is being provided to a patient with pulmonary tularemia.

21. Which statement about simple radiologic devices is correct?
   A. Simple radiologic devices typically are gamma radiation sources.
   B. Exposure to a simple radiologic device requires in-hospital treatment with a chelating agent or pharmacologic blocker to prevent serious long-term effects.
   C. Patients exposed to simple radiologic devices can become radioactive themselves.
   D. Patients exposed to simple radiologic devices present a risk of secondary contamination unless properly handled.

22. What is a "dirty bomb"?
   A. A combination of a radioactive source and a conventional explosive designed to spread large amounts of radioactive contaminates
   B. A nuclear device designed to generate large amounts of alpha- and beta-emitting fallout
   C. A weapon designed to concentrate a large amount of its energy into neutrons and x-rays
   D. A weapon that produces a large amount of radioactive contamination but requires very sophisticated nuclear technology skills to build

23. The cells that are affected the most by exposure to radiation are found in _____.
   A. the bone marrow and gastrointestinal tract
   B. the cardiovascular system and respiratory system
   C. the central nervous system and reproductive system
   D. the respiratory system and endocrine system

24. A patient who was near an explosive device when it detonated has shortness of breath. Breath sounds are absent on the left side of her chest, which is hyperresonant to percussion. What type of trauma has this patient suffered?
   A. Primary
   B. Secondary
   C. Tertiary
   D. Type IV (quaternary)

25. What type of weapon of mass destruction most commonly is used as a secondary device by terrorists?
   A. Biologic
   B. Chemical
   C. Explosive
   D. Radiologic

CASE STUDIES

Case one

You have been dispatched to a report of a large number of "sick people" at a government office building. The patients are complaining of abdominal pain, vomiting, diarrhea, urinary incontinence, heavy salivation, diaphoresis, and watery eyes. They also are complaining that their vision is "dim" and that it is difficult to see even in bright light. Auscultation of their chests reveals wheezing and rhonchi. Several patients also are beginning to experience muscle twitching and weakness.

1. What type of toxin was used?

   _____
   _____
   _____
   _____

2. What is the mechanism of toxicity of these poisons?

   _____
   _____
   _____
   _____

194

Chapter **66** **Disaster Response and Domestic Preparedness**

3. What is the drug used in the short-term treatment for these poisons, and how is it effective?

_____

_____

_____

_____

4. What is the definitive antidote for these poisons and how does it work?

_____

_____

_____

_____

Case two

You have been dispatched to a report of a large number of "sick people" at a shopping mall. The patients are complaining of headache, light-headedness, nausea, vomiting, and difficulty breathing. Several of the more seriously affected patients have begun to seize. Pulse oximetry indicates that several of the patients are saturating at 100% on room air, and the venous blood from attempted IVs is bright red. A security guard tells you he thought he smelled almonds just before people began to become ill.

1. What toxin was used?

_____

2. What is the mechanism of toxicity of this poison?

_____

_____

_____

_____

3. Why do the patients have high SpO_2 readings and bright red venous blood?

_____

_____

_____

_____

4. What are the antidotes for this toxin that are included in the Taylor or Lilly antidote kits?

_____

_____

_____

_____

5. How do the antidotes reverse the effects of this toxin?

_____

_____

_____

_____

6. Do these patients need to be decontaminated?

_____

_____

_____

_____

Chapter **66** **Disaster Response and Domestic Preparedness**

Answer Keys

CHAPTER 35: OBSTETRICS AND GYNECOLOGY

SHORT ANSWER

1. Spontaneous abortion
   Criminal abortion
   Therapeutic abortion
   Missed abortion
   Incomplete abortion
   (Objective 6)
2. __4__ Cervix
   __3__ Uterus
   __2__ Fallopian tube
   __5__ Vagina
   __1__ Ovary
   (Objective 2)
3. Mittelschmerz is pain that occurs near the middle of the menstrual cycle associated with ovulation. (Objective 3)
4. The endometrium is the lining of the uterus. If a fertilized ovum does not implant in the endometrium, it is sloughed and expelled from the uterus during the menstrual period. (Objective 1)
5. Infection of retained tissue resulting in sepsis. Inability of the uterus to contract completely resulting in severe hemorrhage and hypovolemic shock. (Objective 6)
6. Tubal ectopic pregnancy. (Objective 6)
7. When was your last normal menstrual period? (Objective 6)
8. The patient is suffering from supine hypotensive syndrome. When she lies in a supine position, her uterus compresses the inferior vena cava, decreasing venous return to the heart. This leads to a drop in cardiac output and blood pressure. Supine hypotensive syndrome can be prevented by having the patient lie on her left side. In this position, gravity shifts the uterus away from the vena cava. (Objective 9)
9. Patients in late-term pregnancy should be transported on their left sides to avoid compression of the inferior vena cava by the uterus, resulting in supine hypotensive syndrome. (Objective 9)
10. Magnesium sulfate is given to prevent eclamptic seizures. (Objective 9)
11. Magnesium toxicity can produce hypotension, respiratory depression, and cardiac dysrhythmias. A patient receiving magnesium sulfate should have her ECG monitored. Her respiratory effort should be monitored closely, and her blood pressure should be checked frequently. The patellar tendon reflex should be checked frequently. A decreased patellar tendon reflex in a patient receiving magnesium sulfate is an indication of impending toxicity. (Objective 9)
12. Calcium will antagonize the toxic effects of magnesium. (Objective 9)
13. Prolapsed umbilical cord. Breech birth in which the head does not deliver within 3 minutes of the body. (Objective 24)
14. Ensuring that the infant's airway and breathing are adequate. (Objective 21)
15. Uterine massage, which promotes uterine contraction and control of bleeding. Infusion of oxytocin (Pitocin), which promotes uterine contraction and control of bleeding. Allowing the infant to breastfeed, which triggers release of oxytocin from the mother's posterior pituitary and promotes uterine contraction and control of bleeding. (Objective 19)
16. Using a gloved hand, push the vaginal wall away from the baby's mouth and nose to make an airway. (Objective 24)
17. A prolapsed umbilical cord is present when the umbilical cord comes out of the vagina before the infant. As labor progresses, the infant's head compresses the umbilical cord against the mother's pelvis, obstructing blood flow through the cord. The mother should be put in either the knee-chest position or an exaggerated shock position with her hips elevated. High-concentration oxygen should be administered. A gloved hand should be inserted into the vagina and used to lift the infant's head away from the umbilical cord. The mother and infant should be transported rapidly while pressure is maintained to keep the infant's head away from the umbilical cord. (Objective 24)
18. The infant's head should be guided downward gently to help free it from under the mother's pubic bone. (Objective 24)
19. The placenta should be transported to the hospital so it can be examined to ensure it is intact. Placental fragments retained within the uterus can cause postpartum hemorrhage. (Objective 20)
20. The sac should be torn with a clamp and removed from the infant so the baby can breathe. (Objective 24)
21. The mother's sensation of needing to move her bowels and the bulging of the vaginal area indicate that the infant's head is in the vagina, which means that labor is in the second stage. (Objective 10)

22. Braxton Hicks contractions are intermittent uterine contractions that occur during the later stages of pregnancy. They sometimes are referred to as "false labor." Braxton Hicks contractions can be distinguished from true labor in the following ways: (1) They occur at irregular intervals and do not increase in duration over time. (2) They occur primarily in the lower abdomen and groin area rather than in the upper abdomen and back. (3) They do not occur more frequently when the patient walks. (4) They are not associated with discharge of a mucous plug mixed with blood from the cervix (bloody show). (Objective 7)

23. Shoulder dystocia is a life-threatening obstetric emergency in which the infant's shoulders are too wide to pass through the mother's pelvis. Shoulder dystocia is characterized by "turtle sign" in which the infant's head appears at the vaginal opening during a contraction but retracts into the vagina between contractions. Shoulder dystocia is managed by having the mother flex her knees and abduct her thighs (McRoberts maneuver), while firm pressure is applied just above the pubic bone. (Objective 24)

24. Inversion of the uterus through the vagina usually occurs as a result of traction being applied to the umbilical cord in an attempt to speed placental delivery. The following actions should be employed if uterine inversion occurs: (1) Do not detach the placenta if it remains in place because this can result in severe bleeding. (2) Make one attempt to return the uterus to its normal position by pressing on the uterine attachment to the cervix. (3) If the uterus will not return to its normal position in one attempt, cover it with moist sterile dressings. (4) Treat the mother for shock by administering oxygen and infusing isotonic crystalloid solution. (5) Transport to the hospital. (Objective 24)

25. Gently attempt to slip the loop of umbilical cord from around the neck. If the cord is too tightly wound around the neck to slip it free, clamp and cut it. (Objective 24)

26. This is a limb presentation. A limb presentation can indicate that the infant is lying transversely across the pelvis and will not deliver vaginally without being repositioned. If a limb presentation is present, the mother should be transported immediately. (Objective 24)

27. Blood clots. Amniotic fluid. (Objective 24)

28.

12 (day of LMP) + 7 (days) = 19 (date of delivery)

5 (month of LMP) − 3 (months)
= 2 (delivery month)

Add 1 year.

Therefore the estimated date of confinement is February 19, 2009. (Objective 7)

29. The uterine fundus reaches the umbilicus at approximately 20 weeks' gestation. It usually gains 1 cm in height above the fundus each week after the twentieth week of gestation. (Objectives 7, 8)

30. A tocolytic agent is a drug that stops labor. Ritodrine and terbutaline are beta$_2$ agonists. Beta$_2$ agonists relax smooth muscle. Since the uterus is made of smooth muscle, beta$_2$ agonists can stop preterm labor. (Objective 9)

MULTIPLE CHOICE

1. A. To deliver the anterior shoulder, you should gently guide the infant's head downward. (Objective 18)

2. A. The second stage of labor begins with full cervical dilation and ends with the delivery of the infant. (Objective 10)

3. C. At approximately 20 weeks, the fundus may be located at the level of the umbilicus. (Objectives 7, 8)

4. D. Terbutaline has been given because it will relax uterine smooth muscle, interrupting preterm labor. (Objectives 24, 25)

5. B. Calcium will reverse the magnesium toxicity this patient is developing. (Objective 9)

6. D. A limb presentation has occurred. The patient should be transported to the hospital immediately because delivery of the infant in the field will not be possible. (Objective 24)

7. C. The patient has signs and symptoms of preeclampsia. She is in danger of having a seizure. If a seizure occurs, her preeclampsia will have progressed to eclampsia. (Objective 9)

8. C. The second stage of labor begins with complete dilation of the cervix and ends with delivery of the infant. The bulging of the vaginal area and the mother's sensation of needing to move her bowels indicate the infant's head is in the vagina; therefore the second stage of labor is in progress. *Crowning* would be the term used to describe the outward bulging of the vaginal area, but crowning is not a stage of labor. (Objective 10)

9. B. The patient probably has a ruptured ectopic pregnancy. Ruptured ectopic pregnancy is characterized by a rapid onset of lower abdominal pain and/or signs of hypovolemic shock in a woman of childbearing age who typically has missed a menstrual period. Uterine rupture is a problem that occurs in the last trimester of pregnancy. Spontaneous abortion is characterized by cramping pain, heavy vaginal bleeding, and possible passage of tissue. Acute appendicitis typically begins with loss of appetite and pain in the periumbilical area and progresses to right lower quadrant pain accompanied by fever. (Objective 9)

10. A. This patient probably has a placental abruption. Typical signs and symptoms of placental abruption are severe abdominal pain; a rigid, tender uterus; and signs of shock out of proportion to any obvious bleeding. Placenta previa is characterized by

painless, heavy, bright red bleeding during the last trimester of pregnancy. Spontaneous abortion occurs before the twentieth week of pregnancy. Uterine rupture presents with severe, tearing pain; rapid progression of shock; and palpable changes in the shape and continuity of the uterus. (Objectives 9, 15)

11. B. This patient probably has placenta previa. Placenta previa is characterized by heavy, painless, bright red vaginal bleeding during the last trimester of pregnancy. Uterine rupture and abruptio placentae both present with pain. A spontaneous abortion occurs before the twentieth week of pregnancy. (Objectives 9, 15)

12. A. This patient has pelvic inflammatory disease. (Objective 4)

13. D. During a breech delivery, if the infant's head does not delivery within 3 minutes of the body, you should push the vaginal wall away from the infant's nose and mouth to form an airway and transport immediately. (Objective 24)

14. C. Your first priority following the birth of an infant is to ensure the infant's airway and breathing are adequate. (Objective 21)

15. C. If an infant is born still enclosed in the amniotic sac, you should puncture or tear the bag and remove it from around the infant. (Objectives 21, 24)

16. D. The only circumstances in which a paramedic may insert his or her hand into the vagina of a pregnant patient are prolapsed umbilical cord and breech birth when the head does not deliver within 3 minutes of the body. (Objective 24)

17. B. The placenta should be transported to the hospital so it can be examined to ensure all of it has been expelled. (Objective 20)\

18. D. The first stage of labor is the period from onset of contractions until the cervix is fully dilated. (Objective 10)

19. C. If heavy or excessive bleeding is present following delivery, you should raise the lower extremities, give oxygen, and gently massage the lower abdomen. Uterine massage will promote contractions that will help control bleeding. Packing the vagina will not stop bleeding that is coming from within the uterus. (Objective 24)

20. D. If the placenta has not delivered soon after the infant, you should transport without delay. Pulling on the umbilical cord or overly aggressive uterine massage can cause uterine inversion. (Objectives 20, 24)

21. B. The area between the vagina and the anus is the perineum. (Objective 1)

22. A. The spine board should be positioned so the patient is tilted toward her left side. This position will move the uterus off of the inferior vena cava and avoid decreasing venous return to the heart. (Objective 9)

23. B. When vital signs are taken on the patient in the previous question, you would anticipate that pregnancy would result in her heart rate being faster and her blood pressure being lower. (Objective 7)

24. C. Management of the patient in the previous question should include oxygen via nonrebreather mask. The nasal cannula will not deliver a high enough concentration of oxygen to meet the needs of a patient who is in shock. The patient's tidal volume and respiratory rate are adequate, so she does not need to be assisted with a bag-mask or demand valve. (Objective 24)

CASE STUDIES

Case One

1. Heavy, painless, bright-red vaginal bleeding during the last trimester of pregnancy is most likely caused by placenta previa. (Objective 9)

2. Administer oxygen by nonrebreather mask at 10 to 15 L/min. Place the patient on her left side to avoid interfering with venous return to the heart. Establish two large-bore IVs with isotonic crystalloid solution and infuse fluid rapidly. If the patient's blood pressure does not respond to fluid infusion, consider applying the pneumatic antishock garment and inflating the legs only. (Objective 9)

3. The physician should be reminded that in placenta previa the placenta lies partly or completely over the os cervix. A vaginal examination can result in perforation of the placenta with massive vaginal bleeding. A better strategy would be to perform an abdominal ultrasound to determine whether or not placenta previa is present. (Objective 9)

Case Two

1. Severe abdominal pain; a tender, rigid uterus; and signs of shock out of proportion to any obvious bleeding during the third trimester of pregnancy suggest abruptio placentae. (Objective 9)

2. The placenta has separated from the uterine wall, and bleeding is occurring at the point of separation. The dizziness and weakness are a result of hypoperfusion secondary to volume loss. (Objective 9)

3. These are signs of increased sympathetic tone that is attempting to compensate for the blood loss that is occurring in the uterus. (Objective 9)

4. Bleeding from the site of a placental abruption irritates the uterus and causes it to spasm. (Objective 9)

5. Older women who have had multiple births are at increased risk for placental abruption because the uterus loses its ability to attach firmly to the placenta. (Objective 9)

6. Hypertension can lead to rupture of vessels within the placenta, which triggers bleeding, which begins the process of separating the placenta from the uterine wall.

7. Administer oxygen by nonrebreather mask at 10 to 15 L/min. Place the patient on her left side to avoid interfering with venous return to the heart. Establish two large-bore IVs with isotonic crystalloid solution and infuse fluid rapidly. If the patient's blood pressure does not respond to fluid infusion, consider applying the pneumatic anti-shock garment and inflating the legs only. (Objective 9)

Case Three

1. The patient probably has a tubal ectopic pregnancy. Tubal ectopic pregnancy is characterized by a sudden onset of lower abdominal pain and/or signs and symptoms of shock in a woman of childbearing age who usually has missed a menstrual period. (Objective 9)

2. Ectopic pregnancy refers to any pregnancy that occurs outside of the uterine cavity. Most tubal ectopic pregnancies occur in the fallopian tube because this is the site of fertilization. If a fertilized ovum does not implant in the uterine cavity, the next most likely site of implantation is in the fallopian tube. (Objective 9)

3. After implantation, the zygote releases a hormone, human chorionic gonadotropin (HCG), that sustains the corpus luteum that has formed on the ovary at the site of ovulation. In return, the corpus luteum produces progesterone, which maintains the stability of the endometrium. As the tubal ectopic pregnancy begins to outgrow the fallopian tube, its production of HCG falls. Without HCG, the corpus luteum begins to die, and progesterone levels fall. As progesterone levels fall, the endometrium begins to slough off, and a small amount of vaginal bleeding occurs. (Objective 9)

4. An intrauterine device (IUD) prevents pregnancy by interfering with implantation of a fertilized ovum in the uterine cavity. By interfering with implantation in the uterine cavity, the IUD increases the probability of implantation in the fallopian tube. (Objective 9)

5. Tubal ectopic pregnancy can lead to rupture of the fallopian tube and life-threatening bleeding within the pelvic cavity. (Objective 9)

6. The changes in the vital signs suggest that the patient is hypovolemic. (Objective 9)

7. The increase in pulse rate and fall in blood pressure when the patient moves to a sitting position is called a positive tilt test. (Objective 9)

8. Administer oxygen by nonrebreather mask at 10 to 15 L/min. Establish two large-bore IVs with isotonic crystalloid solution and infuse fluid rapidly. If the patient's blood pressure does not respond to fluid infusion, consider applying the pneumatic anti-shock garment. (Objective 9)

CHAPTER 36: NEONATOLOGY

SHORT ANSWER

1. Complete the following chart.

	0	1	2
Appearance	Blue, pale	Body pink, extremities blue	Completely pink
Pulse	Absent	Below 100 beats/min	Above 100 beats/min
Grimace	No response	Grimaces	Cries
Activity	Limp	Some extremity flexion	Active motion
Respirations	Absent	Slow and irregular	Strong cry

(Objective 12)

2. 1. Dry, warm, position, suction, stimulate
   2. Oxygen
   3. Bag-mask ventilation
   4. Chest compressions
   5. Intubation
   6. Medications
   (Objectives 8, 14)

3. Ensuring the infant's airway and breathing are adequate. (Objectives 4, 5)

4. Infants and small children have a large body surface to volume ratio. This causes them to lose heat more rapidly than older children or adults. (Objective 16)

5. A newborn's heart rate is the principal sign that should guide resuscitation. A newborn's heart rate is an excellent indicator of the quality of oxygenation. (Objective 9)

6. Supplemental oxygen should be given by blow-by. If possible the oxygen should be warmed and humidified. Blowing cold oxygen directly onto the area around a newborn's mouth and nose can cause the heart rate to decrease. (Objective 8)

7. Pulmonary surfactant is a compound produced by the type II pneumatocytes that breaks the surface tension of the water on the inner surface of the alveoli. This keeps the surface tension from collapsing the alveoli. (Objective 17)

8. Surfactant production begins between 28 and 32 weeks' gestation. Infants born before 32 weeks' gestation typically develop infant respiratory distress syndrome because of inadequate surfactant production. (Objective 17)

9. An infant born before surfactant is produced in the lungs must overcome the surface tension of the alveoli to expand the lungs on each breath. The increased work of breathing quickly leads to exhaustion and respiratory failure. These infants must be endotracheally intubated so their breathing can be assisted with a bag-mask. (Objective 17)

200

Answer Keys

10. A newborn's ventilations should be assisted with a bag-mask if the heart rate is less than 100 beats per minute. (Objective 8)
11. Chest compressions should be performed on a newborn infant if the heart rate is less than 60 beats per minute. (Objective 8)
12. Chest compressions on a newborn infant should be performed at a rate of 120 compressions per minute. Using a ratio of 3 compressions to 1 ventilation, this will result in 120 events—90 compressions and 30 ventilations—occurring per minute. (Objectives 8, 13, 14)
13. The compression to ventilation ratio for a newborn infant should be 3 to 1. (Objectives 8, 13, 14)
14. Palpate the umbilical artery at the base of the umbilical cord or stump. Use a stethoscope to count the heartbeats by listening over the precordium. Apply a cardiac monitor and use the rate meter to count the heart rate. If methods 2 or 3 are used, a peripheral pulse must be palpated regularly to ensure the heartbeats being counted are producing blood flow in the periphery. (Objectives 8, 9)
15. Meconium is a dark green material that makes up an infant's first bowel movement. Meconium consists of mucus mixed with cells that sloughed off of the wall of the gastrointestinal tract during gestation. (Objective 17)
16. If particulate meconium is present in the amniotic fluid, the action taken is determined by how active the infant is following delivery. If the infant is active with good respiratory effort, no action is needed. If the infant is depressed with absent or poor respiratory effort, a significant amount of meconium has been aspirated. The infant should be intubated and the infant's airway should be suctioned using a meconium aspirator until meconium no longer is returned, until the infant begins breathing effectively, or until a falling heart rate indicates the need to support the infant's respirations with a bag-mask. (Objective 18)
17. Acrocyanosis is cyanosis of the hands and feet. Acrocyanosis is a common observation in newborn infants. It is the result of sluggish peripheral circulation following delivery and does not indicate inadequate oxygenation of the blood. (Objectives 9, 10)
18. The tongue and oral mucosa are the best locations for evaluating for the presence of central cyanosis in a newborn. (Objectives 9, 10)
19. Vascular access in a newborn infant is most easily achieved by placing a catheter into the umbilical vein. (Objectives 8, 10)
20. The initial drug of choice for bradycardia in a newborn is oxygen. If oxygen is not effective, epinephrine should be used to stimulate the myocardium. (Objective 18)
21. Meningomyelocele is herniation of the spinal cord and meninges through a defect in the spinal column. (Objective 6)

22. The infant should be placed in a lateral position. The exposed tissue should be covered with sterile gauze dressings soaked in warm saline solution and then covered with a plastic bag to decrease water and heat loss. (Objective 7)
23. An omphalocele is a congenital hernia at the umbilicus that allows a portion of the abdominal contents to become extruded from the abdominal cavity. (Objective 6)
24. The exposed organs should be covered with sterile gauze dressings soaked in warm saline solution and then covered with a plastic bag to decrease water and heat loss. (Objective 7)

MULTIPLE CHOICE

1. B. A neonate is an infant from the time of birth to 1 month of age. (Objective 1)
2. B. *Newborn* or *newly born infant* is a term used to describe a neonate during the first few hours of life. (Objective 1)
3. C. A newborn infant's respiratory rate should be 40 to 60 breaths/min. (Objective 9)
4. B. The infant has aspirated meconium. You should intubate the infant's trachea and apply direct suction to the ET tube. (Objective 18)
5. A. Although meconium is present, the infant is breathing adequately. Acrocyanosis is a normal finding and does not indicate inadequate oxygenation. You should dry the infant thoroughly and wrap it in warm blankets. (Objective 18)
6. D. The first-line medication for newborn resuscitations is oxygen. (Objectives 9, 10)
7. A. *Acrocyanosis* refers to a bluish discoloration of the peripheral extremities. Acrocyanosis is not a sign of inadequate oxygenation. (Objectives 9, 10)
8. D. Cyanosis of the extremities is common, but central cyanosis is abnormal. (Objective 9)
9. C. Your next step will be to begin bag-mask ventilation. The infant's respirations clearly are inadequate, so administration of blow-by oxygen is unlikely to be effective. Chest compressions are not indicated because the heart rate is greater than 60 beats/min. Epinephrine is given only after oxygen, assisted ventilations, and chest compressions have been ineffective. (Objectives 8, 10)
10. C. The 1-minute Apgar score is 3.
    *A*ppearance: central cyanosis = 0; *p*ulse rate of 78 beats/min = 1; *g*rimace absent = 0; *a*ctivity = weak flexion = 1; *r*espirations slow and gasping = 1. (Objective 12)
11. D. The first priority following the birth of an infant is ensuring the infant's airway and breathing are adequate. (Objectives 9, 10)
12. D. If an infant does not cry or breathe within 30 seconds after birth, you should stimulate the infant by tapping the soles of its feet or rubbing its back. (Objectives 8, 9, 10)

201

13. D. The need for intervention with ventilation and CPR in a newborn is determined by apnea and insufficient pulse rate after stimulation, suction, and oxygen. If an infant is depressed, there is no need to delay resuscitation to obtain a Apgar score. (Objectives 8, 9, 10)

14. C. If a newborn's heart rate is less than 100 beats/min, you should ventilate the lungs with a bag-mask and oxygen for 30 seconds and then reevaluate the heart rate. (Objectives 8, 9, 10)

15. C. If a newborn infant has adequate respirations and heart rate, but its arms and legs are cyanotic, you should give oxygen by blow-by and observe for improvement. Ventilations should be performed if the respirations are inadequate or the heart rate is less than 100 beats/min. Chest compressions should be given if the heart rate is less than 60 beats/min. (Objectives 8, 9, 10)

16. D. The infant probably will suffer respiratory depression following delivery but should not be given naloxone since a withdrawal reaction might occur. Infants of mothers who are narcotic addicts also are addicted. Giving naloxone to these infants can produce narcotic withdrawal, which in infants is a life-threatening problem. (Objective 19)

17. D. At approximately 30 minutes postpartum, you should check the infant's blood glucose level because the infant is at risk for developing hypoglycemia. (Objectives 17, 18)

18. A. Central cyanosis unresponsive to bag-mask ventilation; a small, flat abdomen; absent breath sounds over the left lung field; and displacement of the heart sounds to the right indicate the presence of a diaphragmatic hernia. (Objective 6)

19. B. Appropriate management for the infant in the previous question would include positioning her head and thorax higher than her abdomen and feet, placing a nasogastric or orogastric tube, and withholding further bag-mask ventilation until an endotracheal tube is placed. Using a bag-mask to ventilate an infant with a diaphragmatic hernia can cause distention of the stomach. Because the stomach may be displaced into the thoracic cavity, this could put pressure on the heart and lungs. An endotracheal tube should be placed so the airway can be ventilated directly. A gastric tube should be inserted to remove any air that may have entered the stomach. (Objective 7)

20. B. The Apgar score is 3. *A*ppearance: completely cyanotic = 0; *p*ulse rate below 100 beats/min = 1; *g*rimace: frowns when stimulated = 1; *a*ctivity: limp = 0; *r*espirations: slow, irregular = 1. (Objective 12)

21. A. Appropriate methods for stimulating a newborn include flicking the soles of the feet or gently rubbing the back. (Objective 10)

22. B. "Milking" or stripping the umbilical cord following delivery is contraindicated because it produces polycythemia and increases blood viscosity. (Objective 10)

23. C. Chest compressions should be performed on a newborn if the heart rate is less than 60 beats/min. (Objectives 8, 14)

24. B. The correct technique for giving chest compressions and ventilations to a newborn infant is a rate of 120 per minute with a compression-to-ventilation ratio of 3:1. (Objectives 8, 14)

25. C. A premature newborn is an infant born before 37 weeks' gestation or with a weight less than 2.2 kg. (Objective 17)

26. A. A newborn suspected of being hypovolemic should be given 10 mL/kg of Ringer's lactate or normal saline. (Objective 18)

27. C. Fever in a neonate should be considered a sign of a life-threatening infection until proven otherwise. (Objective 17)

28. B. When you suction a newborn's airway you should suction the mouth first so there is nothing there to aspirate if the infant gasps when the nose is suctioned. (Objective 10)

CASE STUDIES

Case One

1. This material is meconium. (Objective 17)

2. The presence of meconium in the amniotic fluid indicates the fetus is stressed, most probably from hypoxia. The fetus also is at risk of meconium aspiration. (Objective 17)

3. The infant will not yet be producing surfactant. Therefore it will not be able to ventilate adequately.

4. The infant will need to be intubated and have its ventilations assisted with a bag-mask. (Objective 17)

5. Because the infant is apneic and cyanotic, its respirations should be assisted immediately using a bag-mask. (Objectives 8, 10, 18)

6. Chest compressions should be performed at a rate of 120 per minute using a compression-to-ventilation ratio of 3:1. (Objectives 8, 10, 18)

7. Chest compressions should be discontinued. Ventilations should be continued using the bag-mask. Because of the high probability this infant will develop infant respiratory distress syndrome, an endotracheal tube should be placed. (Objectives 8, 10, 18)

8. The infant probably is hypovolemic because of the placental abruption. (Objectives 8, 10, 18)

9. Vascular access should be obtained and 10 mL/kg fluid boluses should be given until perfusion improves. (Objectives 8, 10, 18)

10. Because the infant is small and was physiologically stressed, it also could be hypoglycemic. A blood glucose level should be checked. If hypoglycemia is present, $D_{10}W$ should be given. (Objectives 8, 10, 18)

Case Two

1. Dry, warm, position, suction, and stimulate the infant. (Objectives 8, 10, 18)
2. Neonates have a high surface to volume ratio. Therefore they will lose heat quickly and develop hypothermia. (Objectives 8, 10, 18)
3. Administer oxygen by blow-by if respirations appear adequate or assist ventilations with oxygen if respirations are absent or inadequate. (Objectives 8, 10, 18)
4. The oral mucosa and tongue. (Objective 9)
5. If respirations are absent or inadequate or if the heart rate is less than 100 beats per minute. (Objectives 8, 10, 18)
6. The heart rate. (Objective 9)
7. By palpating the umbilical artery at the base of the umbilical stump. (Objective 9)
8. Chest compressions should be performed if the heart rate is less than 60 beats per minute. (Objectives 8, 10, 18)
9. In neonates cardiac output is entirely rate dependent because a small heart cannot significantly vary its stroke volume. Chest compressions are necessary to augment the heart rate and maintain an adequate cardiac output. (Objectives 8, 10, 18)
10. Chest compressions on a neonate should be performed at a rate of 120 compressions per minute. (Objectives 8, 10, 18)
11. The compression depth should be one third the diameter of the chest. (Objectives 8, 10, 18)
12. The compression-to-ventilation ratio should be 3:1. (Objectives 8, 10, 18)
13. If the neonate does not respond to compressions and ventilations, an endotracheal tube should be placed. (Objectives 8, 10, 18)
14. Epinephrine is the first medication given after oxygen during neonatal resuscitation. (Objectives 8, 10, 18)
15. Epinephrine can be given by the endotracheal or intravenous routes.
16. 0.01 to 0.03 mg/kg. (Objectives 8, 10, 18)
17. 0.01 mg/kg. (Objectives 8, 10, 18)
18. By placing a catheter into the umbilical vein. (Objectives 8, 10, 18)
19. Volume should be given to a newborn infant if the infant is pale or has weak peripheral pulses in a situation where there was possible blood loss from the maternal-fetal unit. (Objectives 8, 10, 18)
20. 10 mL/kg. (Objectives 8, 10, 18)
21. Administration of glucose to a newborn should be based on a blood glucose level measurement. The need to measure a blood glucose level and give glucose to a newborn should be anticipated in situations where:
    - There is a maternal history of diabetes.
    - The infant's weight is greater than 9 lb.
    - The infant is premature or is small for gestational age.
    - The infant required resuscitation.
    - The infant was physiologically stressed.
    - The infant became hypothermic. (Objectives 8, 10, 18)
22. If administration of glucose to a newborn is indicated, $D_{10}W$ should be used. $D_{25}W$ and $D_{50}W$ are highly concentrated solutions that can cause damage to a newborn's veins and that can trigger undesirable fluid shifts into the vascular space. Hypertonic solutions can cause intracranial hemorrhages in newborns and can lead to osmotic diuresis and hypovolemia. (Objectives 8, 10, 18)
23. 4 mL/kg of $D_{10}W$. (Objectives 8, 10, 18)
24. Naloxone should be given to a newborn if narcotics were given to the mother to control pain during labor and delivery and the newborn now has depressed respirations. (Objective 19)
25. 0.1 mg/kg repeated every 2 to 3 minutes as needed. (Objective 19)
26. If you suspect the infant's mother is a narcotics abuser, the neonate should not receive naloxone. If the mother is addicted to narcotics, the infant also will be addicted. Giving naloxone to a newborn who is addicted to narcotics can trigger narcotic withdrawal, which in an infant is life-threatening. (Objective 19)

CHAPTER 37: PEDIATRICS

SHORT ANSWER

1.

	Asthma	Bronchiolitis
Age group affected:	Older than 2 years	Younger than 2 years (most less than 1 year)
History of allergies:	Yes	No
History of low-grade fever:	No, unless asthma trigger is infection	Yes

(Objective 18)

2.

	Croup	Epiglottitis
Etiology (bacterial or viral):	Viral	Bacterial
Age groups affected:	6 months to 6 years	3 to 7 years
Speed of onset:	Gradual, several days	Rapid, hours
Pain on swallowing:	None or very mild	Severe, cannot swallow
Presence of drooling:	Absent	Present
Fever:	Low grade	Hight

(Objective 16)

3. Hypovolemic shock is the most common form of shock in pediatric patients. (Objective 20)
4. The fontanels are soft spots in the infant's skull that allow for rapid growth of the brain during the first year of life. (Objectives 3, 4)
5. The fontanel of a dehydrated infant becomes sunken below the surrounding skull. (Objectives 3, 4)
6. Status asthmaticus is a severe asthma attack that will not respond to treatment with beta$_2$-adrenergic agonists. (Objective 18)
7. Status asthmaticus is managed with oxygen, continued administration of nebulized beta$_2$-adrenergic agonists, assisted ventilations, correction of dehydration and acidosis, possible subcutaneous administration of beta$_2$-adrenergic agonists, and possible endotracheal intubation. Other therapies that may be ordered for status asthmaticus include aminophylline, magnesium sulfate, and terbutaline by continuous infusion. (Objective 18)
8. During an asthma attack, patients have increased respiratory water loss and decreased fluid intake. Therefore they are at risk of becoming dehydrated. Dehydration will worsen an asthma attack by thickening the mucus in the lower airways, causing plug formation. (Objective 18)
9. First, patients experiencing a severe asthma attack may have abused their metered dose inhalers and may be suffering from an overdose of beta$_2$ agonists. Second, some patients who overuse their metered dose inhalers develop a resistance to the effects of their usual bronchodilator. Trying a different agent may be useful. (Objective 18)
10. One of the features of an asthma attack is overproduction of mucus in the lower airway. Because medical oxygen contains no moisture, administration of unhumidified oxygen during as asthma attack can produce drying of the mucus in the lower airway and cause plug formation. (Objective 18)
11. Croup is managed by giving humidified oxygen and nebulized racemic epinephrine. (Objective 16)
12. The principal danger associated with epiglottitis is complete airway obstruction. (Objective 16)
13. Sudden infant death syndrome is a disease process of unknown etiology that results in the sudden, unexpected death of an infant during the first year of life. In SIDS, a complete postmortem examination reveals no identifiable cause for the infant's death. (Objective 37)
14. The most common cause of cardiac arrest in children is respiratory failure. (Objective 25)
15. The principal cause of death from seizures is hypoxia resulting from loss of the airway. (Objective 27)
16. Status epilepticus is present when a patient has two or more seizures without regaining consciousness. (Objective 27)

17. Status epilepticus is treated with benzodiazepines. Diazepam (Valium) is the drug used most commonly in the prehospital setting. However, some pediatricians prefer lorazepam (Ativan). (Objective 27)
18. Hypovolemia in pediatric patients is treated using boluses of IV fluid. This technique is used to avoid producing volume overload. (Objective 21)
19. (Age of child + 4)/4. If the age of the child is not known, pick the endotracheal tube closest in size to the child's little finger. (Objective 7)
20. In children less than 8 years old, the cricoid cartilage is the narrowest point in the airway. When an endotracheal tube of the proper size is inserted, the cricoid cartilage forms a functional cuff that seals the airway, making a cuff unnecessary. Because the airways of children are smaller than adult airways, placing a cuff on a pediatric endotracheal tube would decrease the lumen of the tube to a point where it would be difficult to adequately ventilate. (Objective 7)
21. The largest paddles that completely contact the chest wall without touching each other should be used. For most children over 10 kg (approximately 1 year of age), adult-sized paddles are appropriate. (Objective 24)
22. The initial defibrillator energy setting for pediatric patients should be 2 J/kg. The energy used for repeat shocks should be 4 J/kg. (Objective 24)
23. The dose of atropine for pediatric patients is 0.02 mg/kg. The patient must receive at least a minimum dose of 0.1 mg. Giving less than 0.1 mg of atropine can result in slowing of the heart rate, a phenomenon known as paradoxical bradycardia. (Objective 24)
24. Intravenous, intraosseous, and endotracheal. (Objective 24)
25. Oxygen is the first drug used in management of symptomatic bradycardia in pediatric patients. If oxygen and assisted ventilations do not increase the heart rate, epinephrine is the second-line drug for pediatric bradycardia. (Objective 24)
26. 0.01 mg/kg (0.1 mL/kg) of the 1:10,000 solution. (Objective 24)
27. 0.1 mg/kg (0.1 mL/kg) of the 1:1000 solution. (Objective 24)

MULTIPLE CHOICE

1. D. Children and infants who are burned are more likely to suffer significant fluid loss than adults because their body surface area is larger in proportion to body volume. (Objective 31)
2. C. Management of this patient should include infusion of 20 mL/kg of isotonic crystalloid and blood glucose determination. The history of prolonged vomiting and diarrhea suggests hypovolemia. Because the child has not been able to retain anything in the gastrointestinal tract for 2 days,

hypoglycemia also may be present. The rhythm should not be cardioverted because it is sinus tachycardia. (Objective 20)

3. A. The peak incidence for sudden infant death syndrome is in the 1- to 6-month age group. (Objective 37)

4. C. "Jitteriness" and trembling in a pediatric patient with hypoglycemia are caused by the body's activation of the sympathetic nervous system resulting in the liver releasing additional glucose. Epinephrine release associated with increased sympathetic tone stimulates glycogenolysis and the release of sugar stored in the liver. (Objectives 26, 28)

5. C. If the blood glucose level cannot be determined in a patient who has signs and symptoms of hypoglycemia, dextrose should be administered. The most appropriate therapy following management of the ABCs and obtaining IV access is to give oxygen and give $D_{25}W$ at a dose of 2 to 4 mL/kg. (Objectives 26, 28)

6. B. In children, cardiac output is most dependent upon heart rate. Small hearts cannot significantly vary their stroke volume. (Objective 23)

7. D. The first-line medication for all pediatric resuscitations is oxygen. Most pediatric cardiac arrests are caused by hypoxia produced by respiratory failure or arrest. (Objectives 24, 25)

8. D. Inspiratory stridor, pain on swallowing, high fever, and drooling would be most typical of a patient with epiglottitis. Seal bark cough occurs in croup. Rales (crackles) occur in lower airway disease and are not associated with epiglottitis. (Objective 16)

9. C. Common nontraumatic causes of shock in the pediatric patient include sepsis and volume depletion. Hypovolemia is the most common cause of shock in children. The second most common cause of pediatric shock is sepsis. Cardiogenic shock in children is rare. (Objective 20)

10. B. Hypotension and bradycardia are late signs of shock in the pediatric patient. Tachypnea and pallor are early signs of shock in children. (Objective 20)

11. C. Sinus tachycardia is the most common cardiac dysrhythmia in pediatric patients. Causes of sinus tachycardia in children include volume depletion, fever, pain, and anxiety. (Objective 23)

12. B. Croup is most common from 6 months to 6 years of age. (Objective 16)

13. B. Management of a child with croup and mild to moderate respiratory difficulty would include blow-by oxygen, nebulized saline, and nebulized racemic epinephrine. The alpha$_1$ effects of racemic epinephrine are useful in reducing the subglottic inflammatory edema present in croup. Subcutaneous epinephrine is administered to patients with bronchospasm, because of epinephrine's beta$_2$ effects. (Objective 16)

14. D. The leading cause of death in children and young adults is trauma. (Objective 31)

15. C. The most likely initial skin color finding in a child with compensated shock is pallor. Mottling is present in the later stages of shock. (Objective 20)

16. D. Surgical cricothyrotomy is indicated in a 14-year-old child with an obstructed airway that does not respond to abdominal thrusts. A patient who is coughing has a partial airway obstruction and should be encouraged to cough up the foreign body. Surgical cricothyrotomy is not recommended in children under the age of 8. Because the cricoid cartilage is the narrowest portion of the pediatric airway, surgical cricothyrotomy in younger children is a difficult procedure that can lead to acute loss of the airway or to chronic complications caused by scar tissue formation if the patient survives. In younger children, needle cricothyrotomy is the preferred procedure. (Objective 6)

17. A. Your next step to perform or direct to be performed is to begin chest compressions. Because the chest is rising with bag-mask ventilations, the airway obstruction has been relieved. However, the infant's heart rate is 50 beats/min. If an infant or child's heart rate is less than 60 beats/min, chest compressions should be performed. (Objectives 24, 25)

18. C. A narrow complex tachycardia with a rate greater than 180 beats/min in a child with no history of volume loss, fever, or trauma probably is supraventricular tachycardia. (Objectives 22, 23)

19. B. Fever is the most common cause of seizures from 3 months to 5 years of age. (Objective 28)

20. C. Tachycardia with bounding pulses; warm, flushed skin; slow capillary refill; and irritability are likely findings in a pediatric patient with early septic shock. (Objective 20)

21. B. This child has croup. Epiglottitis is characterized by a rapid onset, drooling, and high fever. Bronchiolitis usually occurs in children under 1 year old and causes wheezing. Foreign body airway obstruction is suspected in situations where a previously healthy, afebrile child rapidly develops signs and symptoms of respiratory distress. (Objective 16)

22. A. Observations of a child you make from across the room before initial contact should include muscle tone, interaction, skin color, respiratory effort and rate. Assessment of airway and capillary refill requires contact with the patient. (Objective 3)

23. A. This patient has epiglottitis. He is suffering from a life-threatening emergency because he may experience complete airway obstruction. (Objective 16)

24. A. This patient has croup. Treatment would include humidified oxygen and nebulized racemic epinephrine. (Objective 16)

25. C. This infant has signs and symptoms of bronchiolitis. The initial treatment would be to administer humidified oxygen. Subcutaneous epinephrine or nebulized racemic epinephrine is not indicated. Nebulized albuterol may be considered. (Objective 18)

26. D. A 2-year-old child would be intubated using a Miller blade and an uncuffed tube. Straight blades are preferred for small children because they allow better control of the epiglottis, which tends to be long and "floppy." Uncuffed tubes are used in children less than 8 years old because the narrow cricoid cartilatge forms a functional cuff around the tube. (Objective 7)

27. C. You should give 0.1 mg/kg of epinephrine 1:1000 down the endotracheal tube. (Objectives 24, 25)

CASE STUDIES

Case One

1. This patient has bronchiolitis. (Objective 18)
2. The respiratory syncytial virus (RSV) causes bronchiolitis. (Objective 18)
3. RSV causes upper respiratory tract infections in adults and older children. Infants frequently acquire RSV infections from older relatives. (Objective 18)
4. RSV infection causes inflammatory edema in the bronchioles, narrowing them. Wheezing is a result of air moving through the narrowed bronchioles. (Objective 18)
5. The child should be given high-concentration, humidified oxygen. His ventilations should be assisted because he is in danger of tiring and developing respiratory failure. Administration of nebulized albuterol can be considered. However, nebulized bronchodilators often have minimal effect in bronchiolitis because the wheezing is a result of inflammatory edema, not bronchospasm. If the child requires prolonged assistance, endotracheal intubation can be performed. When the patient's ventilations are being assisted, caution should be taken to avoid air trapping, which can result from impaired expiration. Air trapping can increase intrathoracic pressure and produce diminished venous return to the heart and decreased cardiac output. (Objective 19)

Case Two

1. The dysrhythmia is supraventricular tachycardia. (Objective 23)
2. The rhythm is too fast. (Objective 22)
3. The patient is stable. (Objective 23)
4. This infant is barely compensating for the decreased cardiac output caused by his high heart rate. Feeding requires increased work. The demand for increased cardiac output created by the effort of feeding causes him to temporarily decompensate. (Objective 23)
5. Assess airway, breathing, and circulation. Give high-concentration oxygen. Provide vagal stimulation by placing ice on the bridge of the infant's nose. If vagal stimulation does not decrease the heart rate, establish an IV and give 0.1 mg/kg adenosine rapid IV push. If the heart rate does not decrease, repeat adenosine 0.2 mg/kg twice. (Objective 24)

Case Three

1. The dysrhythmia is supraventricular tachycardia. (Objective 23)
2. An increased heart rate decreases the time available between beats for the heart to fill. A very fast heart rate can decrease preload to the point where stroke volume, cardiac output, and blood pressure fall. (Objective 23)
3. Decreased cardiac output is producing systemic hypoperfusion and metabolic acidosis. Metabolic acidosis leads to stimulation of the respiratory center and an increased respiratory rate. Additionally, a high heart rate can cause blood to back up into the pulmonary circulation, producing congestion of the pulmonary vascular bed and pulmonary edema, which increases the work of breathing. (Objective 23)
4. This patient is unstable. (Objective 23)
5. Assess airway, breathing, and circulation. Assist ventilations with high-concentration oxygen. Perform synchronized cardioversion using 0.5 J/kg. If the initial cardioversion attempt is not effective, repeat synchronized cardioversion using 1.0 J/kg. (Objective 24)

Case Four

1. Yes; the history of volume loss and the child's altered mental status indicate possible hypovolemic shock. (Objective 20)
2. The child's airway, breathing, and circulation should be assessed. During the assessment of circulation, perfusion should be evaluated by checking heart rate, presence and quality of distal pulses, skin color and temperature, and capillary refill. Status of hydration should be evaluated by assessing the oral mucous membranes and the skin turgor. (Objective 20)
3. Yes; the patient is in shock. (Objective 20)
4. Altered mental status; rapid, but unlabored respirations; rapid pulse rate; cool extremities; mottled skin. (Objective 20)
5. This patient is suffering from hypovolemic shock. The dry oral mucous membranes and poor skin turgor indicate the patient is volume depleted. (Objective 20)
6. The patient is in compensated shock because he is not yet hypotensive. (Objective 20)
7. Assess airway, breathing, and circulation. Give high-concentration oxygen. Consider assisting ventilations if the child shows signs of tiring, which could lead to respiratory failure. Obtain vascular access. Give 20 mL/kg isotonic crystalloid IV fluid boluses until perfusion is adequate. Evaluate blood glucose levels. If hypoglycemia is present, give $D_{25}W$. (Objective 21)
8. Establish an introsseous line. (Objective 21)
9. You will feel a decrease in resistance as the needle passes through the cortex of the bone into the marrow space. The needle will stand by itself. You may be able to aspirate marrow through the needle. Fluid will

infuse easily without swelling at the vascular access site. (Objective 10)

10. You should give an isotonic crystalloid such as normal saline or Ringer's lactate. (Objective 21)
11. 20 mL/kg. (Objective 21)
12. The patient has metabolic acidosis secondary to hypoperfusion. (Objective 20)
13. The patient should be given high-concentration oxygen and receive fluid boluses until adequate perfusion is restored. (Objective 21)

Case Five

1. The rhythm is aystole. (Objective 23)
2. Chest compressions should be performed at a rate of 100 per minute. (Objective 39)
3. The sternum should be compressed ⅓ to ½ of the anterior-posterior diameter of the chest. (Objective 39)
4. The patient's head and neck should be kept in a neutral position while he is being intubated. Patients who drown in swimming pools should be suspected of having cervical spine fractures because they may have struck their heads on the side or the bottom of the pool. (Objective 31)
5. The patient should be given epinephrine. (Objective 24)
6. If an IV has not been established, epinephrine can be given by the endotracheal route. (Objective 24)
7. 0.1 mg/kg (0.1 mL/kg) of the 1:1000 solution should be administered. (Objective 24)

Case Six

1. The dysrhythmia is sinus bradycardia. (Objective 23)
2. Sinus bradycardia will produce slowing of the heart rate and slowing of conduction through the AV junction, leading to bradydysrhythmias and AV blocks. Slowing of the SA node associated with increased myocardial irritability can produce premature atrial, junctional, and ventricular contractions. Atrial, junctional, or ventricular tachycardia may be present. Digitalis toxicity also produces loss of appetite, gastrointestinal distress, and irritability. Patients may complain of seeing yellow-green halos around lights. Severe digitalis toxicity can produce life-threatening hyperkalemia. (Objective 23)
3. Yes; a sinus bradycardia is consistent with digitalis ingestion. (Objective 23)
4. The patient is stable. (Objective 23)
5. Children have healthy cardiovascular systems. By increasing her systemic vascular resistance, this patient is compensating from a decrease in her heart rate and cardiac output. (Objective 23)
6. Assess the patient's airway, breathing, and circulation. Administer high-concentration oxygen. Consider establishing vascular access as a precautionary measure in case the patient becomes unstable. Have an external cardiac pacemaker readily available in case the patient becomes unstable. (Objective 24)

Case Seven

1. The rhythm is sinus tachycardia. (Objective 23)
2. Because the patient is unconscious, pulseless, and apneic, he has pulseless electrical activity. (Objective 23)
3. Hypoxia, hypovolemia, acidosis, cardiac tamponade, and tension pneumothorax. (Objective 23)
4. Epinephrine always is the first IV medication given during cardiac arrest. (Objective 24)
5. 0.01 mg/kg (0.1 mL/kg) of the 1:10,000 solution. (Objective 24)
6. 0.01 mg/kg (0.1 mL/kg) of the 1:10,000 solution. (Objective 24)

Case Eight

1. The dysrhythmia is ventricular fibrillation. (Objective 23)
2. Ventricular fibrillation is an uncommon rhythm of pediatric cardiac arrest. For ventricular fibrillation to sustain itself, a critical mass of the myocardium must be fibrillating. This critical mass does not decrease as the heart's size decreases. Therefore below a certain size the myocardium is unable to fibrillate because the mass of myocardium needed to maintain ventricular fibrillation is greater than the total mass of the patient's heart. (Objective 23)
3. Problems that would increase myocardial irritability should be suspected. These include drug toxicity and electrolyte imbalance. (Objective 23)
4. The largest paddles that completely contact the chest wall without touching should be used. (Objective 24)
5. The defibrillator paddles should be placed on the anterior and posterior surfaces of the patient's chest. (Objective 24)
6. The initial energy setting should be 2 J/kg. (Objective 24)
7. All subsequent shocks should be given at 4 J/kg. (Objective 24)
8. A 7-month-old child would typically require a 3.5- to 4-mm endotracheal tube. The proper size can be selected by using the tube closest to the diameter of the child's little finger. (Objective 7)
9. Breath sounds should be checked by listening at the midaxillary line. Breath sounds in infants and small children tend to transmit easily to the opposite side of the chest. Listening at the midaxillary line increases the probability that the sounds being heard are coming from the side of the chest being tested. (Objective 7)
10. Breath sounds over the epigastrium indicate the tube is in the esophagus. (Objective 8)
11. The endotracheal tube should be removed. The patient should be oxygenated and ventilated using a bag-mask. Then the patient should be reintubated. (Objective 8)
12. Epinephrine can be given at this point. (Objective 24)

13. Epinephrine constricts the peripheral circulation and dilates the blood vessels in the myocardium, lungs, and brain, improving the effectiveness of chest compressions. (Objective 24)
14. Epinephrine can be given down the endotracheal tube. (Objective 24)
15. Epinephrine given down the endotracheal tube should be given in a dose of 0.1 mg/kg (0.1 mL/kg of the 1:1000 solution) initially and in repeat doses. (Objective 24)

Case Nine

1. The patient has a head injury with increased intracranial pressure. (Objective 31)
2. The patient probably is suffering from shaken baby syndrome. (Objective 36)
3. The mechanism of the injury described by the boyfriend does not involve enough force to cause the head injury suffered by this patient. The mechanism of injury described by the boyfriend also does not account for the linear bruises on the child's arms. (Objective 36)
4. Assess the patient's airway, breathing, and circulation. Restrict motion of the patient's spine. Place an endotracheal tube. Perform controlled hyperventilation with high-concentration oxygen to reduce intracranial pressure. Transport. Establish vascular access en route. Transport to a facility with pediatric neurology/neurosurgery capabilities. (Objective 31)
5. Report your suspicions of child abuse to the personnel at the emergency department and to the appropriate law enforcement agencies. (Objective 36)

Case Ten

1. This patient has epiglottitis. (Objective 16)
2. Epiglottitis usually is caused by a bacterium, most commonly *Haemophilus influenzae*. (Objective 16)
3. Children in this age range are interacting with other children in day care or at school. This interaction increases the risk of exposure to the organism that causes epiglottitis. (Objective 16)
4. This patient is at risk of complete airway obstruction. (Objective 16)
5. The patient should be allowed to position himself to maintain his own airway. High-concentration oxygen should be given by mask if the patient will tolerate it or by blow-by if he will not. The patient should be transported to a facility with capabilities for securing the airway of a child with epiglottitis. Every effort should be made to avoid exciting or upsetting the child. (Objective 17)
6. Immunization against *Haemophilus influenzae* is decreasing the incidence of pediatric epiglottitis. The disease now is seen more commonly in newborns who have not yet been immunized and in older adults. (Objective 16)

Case Eleven

1. This child probably does not have febrile seizures. A child typically will have one febrile seizure per episode of febrile illness. Repeated seizures suggest some other cause. (Objective 27)
2. Meningitis should be a primary consideration in this child. Hypoglycemia and hypoxia should be ruled out as causes. Possible causes unrelated to the febrile illness, such as drug toxicity and head trauma, also should be considered. (Objective 27)
3. Recurrent seizures without an intervening period of consciousness are status epilepticus. (Objective 27)
4. The patient's blood glucose level should be checked. Because the brain requires a constant supply of glucose, hypoglycemia should be considered as a possible cause anytime a patient presents with altered mental status, seizures, or localizing neurologic signs. (Objective 28)
5. A benzodiazepine such as diazepam or lorazepam should be used to stop the seizure. (Objective 28)
6. Benzodiazepines will cause depressed respirations and may cause hypotension. (Objective 28)

CHAPTER 38: GERIATRICS

SHORT ANSWER

1. Aging decreases dermal thickness and blood supply. These changes delay wound healing. They also predispose the elderly to deeper burns with shorter exposure to less heat. (Objective 87)
2. Aging tends to increase the rate of bone resorption, particularly in older women. This effect makes the elderly more susceptible to fractures, including fractures of the cervical spine during sudden decelerations unlikely to injure a younger person. (Objective 61)
3. Aging decreases respiratory reserve capacity. This effect decreases the ability of older patients to compensate for chest trauma or acute respiratory disease. (Objective 19)
4. Aging decreases myocardial reserve capacity, making the elderly prone to developing fluid overload during volume resuscitation. (Objective 24)
5. In the elderly, the peripheral blood vessels lose their ability to constrict and dilate. This change decreases the ability of an older person to increase his or her systemic vascular resistance to compensate for volume loss. Loss of the ability to vasoconstrict and vasodilate also decreases the ability of older persons to tolerate hot or cold environments by adjusting the rate of heat loss through the skin surface. (Objective 25)
6. Aging decreases the filtering capacity of the kidney. As a result drugs tend to remain in the body for longer periods of time and patients are at increased risk for developing toxic effects when taking what normally would be therapeutic doses of drugs. The decreased ability of the kidneys to make urine also increases the

risk of older persons becoming volume overloaded during fluid resuscitation. (Objective 7)

7. These signs are not necessarily the result of volume depletion. Aging causes a loss of skin elasticity that can result in "tenting" of the skin when the patient is adequately hydrated. Skin turgor should be checked over an older person's forehead and sternum because these are two of the last areas where aging decreases the skin's elasticity. (Objective 15)

8. This patient's pedal edema probably is a result of increased hydrostatic pressure caused by keeping the legs in a dependent position for an extended period of time. (Objectives 15, 25, 26, 27)

9. A silent myocardial infarction is a heart attack that presents without chest pain. The elderly are prone to silent myocardial infarctions because the aging process slows nerve conduction velocity and decreases pain sensation. Diabetic clients also are prone to developing silent MIs. (Objective 27)

10. Aging causes the brain to shrink and to occupy less space inside the cranial cavity. The signs and symptoms of subdural hematoma will have a slower onset in an older person because there is more space within the skull for blood to accumulate before intracranial pressure begins to increase. (Objectives 86, 87)

11. Beta-blockers interfere with the ability to increase heart rate as a response to decreased preload. Because a steadily increasing heart rate is one of the early indicators of hypovolemia, beta-blocker use may mask the signs of shock. (Objectives 15, 73)

12. Patients taking diuretics are at risk for developing hypokalemia—low serum potassium level. Hypokalemia can produce dysrhythmias, particularly in patients who are taking digitalis. (Objective 73)

13. Aging decreases hepatic blood flow and the liver's ability to metabolize drugs. In older persons, maintenance doses of drugs frequently have to be reduced to avoid an accumulation of the drug in the body that could cause toxic effects. (Objective 7)

MULTIPLE CHOICE

1. A. The geriatric patient who is experiencing a silent myocardial infarction is most likely to present with dyspnea or abdominal pain. (Objective 27)

2. B. In the United States, the most common cause of dementia among older persons is Alzheimer's disease. (Objective 32)

3. C. The most common psychiatric disorder among geriatric patients is depression. (Objective 50)

4. B. When you are assessing or managing an older patient, you should use physical contact to compensate for loss of sight or hearing. Raising the volume of your voice can offend an older person who does not have hearing loss. Older persons may consider failure of a younger person to address

them by their last name and proper title as a sign of disrespect. Separation of an older patient from family and friends may worsen anxiety. (Objective 15)

5. C. Special problems that may be encountered when dealing with geriatric patients may include increased susceptibility to general deterioration as a result of illness. The elderly tend to have high pain thresholds, a tendency to dehydration because of decreased thirst, and decreased sensitivity of taste and smell. (Objective 15)

6. A. The edema of his ankles and feet probably is a result of prolonged immobility and the positioning of his lower extremities. The absence of neck vein distention, crackles in the lung fields, and abdominal distention suggest that the pedal edema is not a result of heart failure or liver disease. (Objectives 15, 27)

7. C. The blisters on the patient's lower extremities most likely are the result of increased hydrostatic pressure caused by right-sided congestive heart failure. The history of hypertension and multiple acute myocardial infarctions supports a field diagnosis of congestive heart failure. In older persons, congestive heart failure may present with episodes of nocturnal confusion as a result of hypoxia caused by pulmonary edema. (Objectives 15, 26, 27)

8. B. Drug overdoses, medication interactions, or electrolyte imbalances are acute etiologies that may be mistaken for "senile dementia." Brain tumors, Huntington's disease, Parkinson's disease, and Alzheimer's disease are chronic conditions that cause gradual changes in cognitive abilities and behavior. (Objective 34)

9. B. Patients taking diuretics are at risk for developing hypokalemia—low serum potassium level. (Objective 73)

10. C. Extreme weakness, syncope, loss of bladder and bowel control, and malaise would be most suggestive of an acute myocardial infarction in a geriatric patient. Jaundice, stiff neck, and headache would be unlikely to be associated with a myocardial infarction in an elderly person. (Objective 27)

11. D. The most appropriate action would be to splint the injured ankle; apply a cervical collar, spine board, and head blocks; and transport. The patient's cardiac rhythm is atrial fibrillation with a controlled rate. This rhythm does not need to be treated. (Objectives 25, 27, 89)

12. D. The most appropriate action would be to dress and bandage the abrasion, ask about tetanus prophylaxis, and determine whether transport is desired. The patient has a pacemaker that appears to be functioning appropriately. (Objectives 25, 27, 89)

13. D. The dysrhythmia is sinus rhythm with first-degree AV block. (Objectives 25, 27)

14. D. The patient in the previous question should be monitored closely because he is at risk of developing second- or third-degree AV block. (Objectives 25, 27)
15. B. The most likely underlying cause for the problem affecting the patient in the previous question is digitalis toxicity. (Objective 23)

CASE STUDIES

Case One

1. The patient probably has an abdominal aortic aneurysm. (Objectives 27, 28)
2. It is unlikely that his symptoms are caused by a spinal fracture with a spinal cord injury. The lower back pain and the neurologic deficits in his lower extremities were present before he fell. The underlying cause of the deficits was responsible for the fall rather than the fall causing an injury that produced the deficits. (Objectives 27, 28)
3. It is unlikely that the patient is having a stroke because the numbness and weakness in his extremities is bilateral. A stroke would be expected to produce a unilateral deficit that would affect the arm and leg on the same side of the body. (Objectives 27, 28)
4. The abdominal aortic aneurysm is leaking blood into his retroperitoneal space. This loss of blood is producing hypotension. Bleeding from the aneurysm is decreasing blood flow to his lower extremities, accounting for the mottling. (Objectives 27, 28)
5. The aorta is located in the retroperitoneal space adjacent to the lumbar spine. An aortic aneurysm can press against the spinal nerve roots of the lower back, producing pain that radiates down the leg. Because of this pattern of pain, abdominal aortic aneurysm frequently is misdiagnosed as lumbar disk disease. (Objectives 27, 28)
6. The aorta is located within the retroperitoneal space. Retroperitoneal organs are more likely to produce pain referred to the back rather than the abdominal pain that is associated with stretching or inflammation of the peritoneum. (Objectives 27, 28)
7. Assess airway, breathing, and circulation. Place the patient on high-concentration oxygen using a nonrebreather mask. Start two-large bore IVs using an isotonic crystalloid. Monitor the ECG. Place the pneumatic antishock garment on the patient so it can be inflated quickly if the blood pressure begins to fall. (Objective 30)

Case Two

1. The patient probably has suffered a pathologic fracture of the lumbar spine. Cancer of the prostate often metastasizes to the lumbar spine, predisposing patients to fractures in this area. (Objectives 64, 66, 65, 86)
2. The patient should be treated as if he suffered a spinal injury secondary to trauma. He should be secured to a long spine board. An IV should be established with an isotonic crystalloid. Appropriate analgesia should be given to control his pain. (Objectives 65, 66, 89)

Case Three

1. The peripheral edema and crackles could result from congestive heart failure. However, in the elderly pedal edema and crackles may be a result of the aging process. It is important to evaluate the overall clinical picture before attributing findings to a specific disease process. (Objectives 15, 25, 27)
2. The weakness and fatigue could result from congestive heart failure with pulmonary edema or acute myocardial infarction. The presence of a complete AV block in a patient who does not have an implanted pacemaker and who provides no past history of cardiac problems suggests a recent acute event affecting the heart. (Objectives 25, 27)
3. This patient possibly could have a silent myocardial infarction. (Objectives 25, 27)
4. The aging process decreases nerve conduction velocity, which decreases the ability to feel pain. Diabetes causes peripheral neuropathy, which also decreases the ability to feel pain. (Objectives 25, 27)
5. Assess airway, breathing, and circulation. Administer high-concentration oxygen using a nonrebreather mask. Establish an IV. Acquire a 12-lead ECG and evaluate for evidence of myocardial ischemia or injury. Administer aspirin and nitroglycerin. (Objective 30)

Case Four

1. The patient's rhythm is second-degree AV block, type II. (Objectives 26, 28)
2. The problem being experienced by the patient is an Adams-Stokes attack or Adams-Stokes syncope. During the period where the P waves did not conduct to the ventricles, the patient experienced a sufficient drop in her cardiac output to become symptomatic. (Objectives 26, 28)
3. The patient should be given high-concentration oxygen. An IV should be established. The ECG should be monitored. A 12-lead ECG should be obtained to evaluate the patient for myocardial ischemia or injury. The electrodes for the cardiac pacemaker should be placed as a precautionary measure. If the patient develops an extended period when P waves do not conduct to the ventricles, the external pacemaker should be used to support her heart rate and cardiac output until a permanent pacemaker can be inserted. (Objective 30)

Case Five

1. Possibilities to consider would include silent acute myocardial infarction or anemia secondary to blood loss from the gastrointestinal tract. (Objectives 26, 44, 47)
2. The patient should be asked whether she has noticed any changes in her bowel movements. In particular have they become darker than normal? (Objective 47)

CHAPTER 39: ABUSE AND ASSAULT

SHORT ANSWER

1. Male is unemployed. Male uses illegal drugs at least once per year. Partners have different religious backgrounds. Family income is below poverty level. Partners are unmarried. Either partner is violent toward children at home. Male did not graduate from high school. Male is unemployed or has a blue-collar job. Male is between 18 and 30 years old. Male saw his father hit his mother. (Objective 3)
2. Pregnancy. Forty-five percent of women suffer some form of battery during pregnancy. Substance abuse. Emotional disorders such as depression, anxiety, or suicidal behavior. (Objective 4)
3. Directly question the patient about the issue of intentional abuse. Avoid judgmental questions or attitudes. Listen carefully, and indicate you are paying attention. Encourage attempts to take control of their lives. Help the patient determine what he or she want for self and children. Do not leave without advising the patient on precautions to protect himself or herself. Remind the patient that intentional injury of another person is a crime and that the patient can seek protection and assistance from law enforcement officers. (Objective 8)
4. Increased life expectancies. Increased dependence on others. Decreased productivity in later years. Physical and mental impairments. Limited resources for long-term care. Economic factors such as strained family finances. Stress on middle-aged caregivers responsible for their children and their parents. (Objective 14)
5. Domestic abuse of elders being cared for in home-based settings. Institutional abuse of elders being cared for by a person with a legal or contractual responsibility to provide care. (Objective 15)
6. Physical, emotional, or sexual mistreatment of or neglect of a person from infancy to 18 years of age. (Objective 13)
7. A history of physical or emotional abuse as a child. Use or abuse of drugs and/or alcohol. Immaturity and preoccupation with self. Lack of obvious feeling for the child. Apparent lack of concern for the child's injury, treatment, or prognosis. Open criticism of the child. Little identification with the child's physical or emotional pain. (Objective 12)
8. Passive behavior in children under age 6; aggressive behavior in children over age 6. Crying hopelessly during treatment or not crying at all. Avoiding parents or showing little concern for their absence. Unusual wariness or fearfulness of physical contact. Apprehensiveness or constant alertness for danger. Sudden behavioral changes. Absence of nearly all emotions. Neediness. (Objective 12)
9. Multiple soft tissue injuries in different places on the body in different stages of healing. Burns or scalds, particularly of the soles of the feet, the palms, the back, or the buttocks. Burns or soft tissue injuries with shapes that suggest the object used to cause the injury. Injuries inconsistent with the mechanism that was reported to have caused them. Fractures, particularly rib fractures. Head injuries. Shaken baby syndrome. Abdominal injuries. (Objective 12)
10. Shaken baby syndrome is a neurologic injury that occurs when a caregiver reacts to frustration with a crying baby by picking it up and shaking it vigorously. The shaking causes movement within the skull that can result in subdural hematomas and diffuse cerebral edema. Shaking also can cause injuries to the spine and to the retina. (Objective 12)
11. Malnutrition. Severe diaper rash. Diarrhea and/or dehydration. Hair loss. Untreated medical conditions. Inappropriate, dirty, torn clothing or lack of clothing. Tired or listless affect. Near constant demands for physical contact and attention. (Objective 12)
12. Provide a safe environment for the patient. Protect the patient's privacy. Be nonjudgmental and supportive. Avoid questioning about the specifics of the assault. Limit history taking to information needed to provide care. Limit physical examination to what is necessary to provide care. Provide the patient with as much control over the situation as possible. (Objective 17)
13. Encourage patients to not urinate, defecate, douche, bathe, eat, drink, or smoke. Collect contaminated items of clothing not being worn by the patient in paper bags. If the patient reports scratching the assailant, cover his/her hands with paper bags secured loosely at the wrists. Ensure any evidence you collect passes directly into the custody of a law enforcement officer. Provide the officer with your name and unit number and include his/her name and badge number in your report. (Objective 18)

MULTIPLE CHOICE

1. B. Institutional abuse may include acts of omission, such as failing to address hygiene adequately. The incidence of abuse is expected to increase over the next 20 to 30 years. Elders with limited resources are more likely to be abused. Adult children are more likely than any other relatives to be elder abusers. (Objective 15)

2. A. The belief that the abuser will change is a common factor in cases of abuse going unreported. (Objective 5)
3. D. Withholding medication from a child who refuses to finish eating dinner would be abusive. (Objective 12)
4. D. Provide a safe environment, while nonjudgmentally attempting to obtain details of the event. (Objective 8)
5. B. Fractures are the second most common injuries in child abuse, following soft tissue injuries. Intentional scald injuries are more likely to take the form of stocking or glove burns. Rib fractures are uncommon in children and frequently indicate child abuse. Abdominal trauma occurs rarely in child abuse, but typically is serious. (Objective 13)
6. A. Apprehension and wariness are most likely to indicate an abused child. Abused children frequently show no concern about the absence of parents or caregivers. They typically do not show emotion. They often are very "needy," constantly requesting food and favors from others. (Objective 13)
7. C. Preservation of the chain of evidence may include placing paper bags over the victim's hands and collecting removed clothing for investigation. Thorough documentation is vital. Victims of sexual assault should be discouraged from cleaning themselves in order to protect evidence. EMS personnel should report any situation in which they suspect abuse. (Objective 18)
8. C. Privately report your suspicions to the emergency department staff. Confronting the parents or attempting to obtain a confession could cause them to flee with the injured child or to physically attack you. Laws that require reporting of suspected child abuse protect persons who make reports in good faith from lawsuits. (Objective 10)
9. B. May be a victim of child abuse. This burn pattern suggests intentional immersion of the legs into hot water. Burns of the feet always are considered critical injuries. Burns should be covered with dry dressings. Use of moist dressings, particularly on larger burns in children, can produce accelerated heat loss and hypothermia. (Objective 13)

CASE STUDY

1. The child appears to be a victim of child abuse, probably shaken baby syndrome, committed by the boyfriend. (Objective 13)
2. The child was under the care of a person who is not a biological parent at the time the problem began. The caregiver did not call for help, although something obviously is wrong with the child. The caregiver does not seem concerned about the situation. The history being provided is vague and does not explain the problems present. (Objective 12)
3. Encourage the mother to consent to transport of the infant. Do not openly accuse or confront the boyfriend. Protect the infant's back and neck because shaken baby syndrome frequently is associated with spinal injuries. Monitor the infant closely for signs of increased intracranial pressure during transport. (Objective 8)

CHAPTER 40: PATIENTS WITH SPECIAL CHALLENGES

SHORT ANSWER

1. Cystic fibrosis is an inherited disorder that involves the exocrine glands of the respiratory and digestive tracts and the eccrine sweat glands. Oversecretion of mucus obstructs the lower airways, pancreatic ducts, and bile ducts. Excess loss of sodium chloride occurs in sweat. (Objective 30)
2. EMS personnel are most likely to have to manage episodes of respiratory distress in patients with cystic fibrosis. Suctioning, supplemental oxygen administration, and support of ventilations may be required. (Objective 30)
3. No; many patients with athetoid and diplegic cerebral palsy are highly intelligent. Do not assume a patient with cerebral palsy is mentally retarded or cannot communicate with you. (Objective 30)
4. The guide dog should accompany its owner to the hospital, either in the ambulance or in another vehicle based on local protocol. Do not touch the dog or its harness without asking the owner's permission. (Objective 6)
5. Describe everything you are going to do. Provide appropriate information to help the patient orient him/herself during transport. If the patient is going to walk, let him/her take your arm. Guide by leading, not pushing. (Objective 6)
6. Allow the patient time to say what she needs to say; do not interrupt. Do not complete the patient's sentences for her or correct her. If necessary, provide her with paper and a writing instrument so she can write what she wishes to communicate. (Objective 9)
7. Myasthenia gravis is an autoimmune disorder in which muscles become weak and tire easily. The disorder is caused by the attack of lymphocytes on the acetylcholine receptors found on the voluntary skeletal muscle side of neuroeffector junctions. Fewer receptors are available to be stimulated, and the antibodies of the immune system often attach to the receptors, blocking them from being stimulated. When the presynaptic neuron releases acetylcholine, instead of stimulating a muscle contraction as normal, the neurotransmitter is blocked. This condition usually is an acquired immunologic disorder, but it can be caused by inherited problems of the neuroeffector junction. The cause of this disorder is believed to be related to the thymus, an endocrine gland important in the body's immunity. (Objective 30)

8. During a myasthenic crisis the muscles of respiration are involved, which can lead to respiratory failure and arrest. This can occur without associated findings other than a history of myasthenia gravis (Objective 30)

9. Postpolio syndrome affects polio survivors decades after they have recovered from the initial infection. The cause is unknown and it does not affect all survivors. It is believed that the syndrome is a result of the degeneration of the nerves in the muscles that survived the original infection as they cannot accommodate the additional stress of compensating for the lost nerves.

10. Patients affected by postpolio syndrome experience a new onset of weakness in the same muscles that were affected by the original infection, as well as muscles that did not appear to be affected at the time. Symptoms include a slow and progressive muscle weakness, generalized fatigue, easily fatigued muscles, and muscle atrophy. Weakness can be asymmetric in some cases. Pain may be present from joint degeneration. The pattern of decline in muscular function may be unpredictable and may include periods of stability in their symptoms followed by the onset of new motor dysfunction.

11. Explain to the patient that her health is your primary concern rather than the ability to pay for services. As needed discuss the following items with her:
    1. The patient's ability to pay should never be a factor in obtaining emergency healthcare.
    2. Federal law mandates that medical screening be provided, regardless of the patient's ability to pay.
    3. Payment programs for healthcare services are available in most hospitals.
    4. Government services are available to assist patients in paying for healthcare.
    5. Free (or near-free) healthcare services are available through local, state, and federally funded organizations.

12. Gowers' sign is present when a child rolls onto the stomach and then pushes themselves up using their arms to "climb their legs" in an attempt to stand. This is indicative of muscular dystrophy as the child does not have enough strength in the muscles to stand without using the arms for assistance.

13. Apraxia is a neurologic disorder that results from dysfunction of the cerebral hemispheres of the brain. This dysfunction causes an inability to execute skilled voluntary movements despite having the desire to perform the movements and being able to demonstrate normal muscular function associated with the movements.

MULTIPLE CHOICE

1. B. Have the dog accompany the patient to the hospital. (Objective 6)

2. D. Otitis media, middle ear infection, is a common etiology of conductive deafness in children. (Objective 1)

3. D. Tinnitus, ringing in the ears, is associated with aspirin toxicity and sensorineural deafness. (Objective 1)

4. C. When speaking to your hearing-impaired patient, it is best to speak slowly and in a normal voice. Yelling or using exaggerated gestures distorts your facial and body language and makes communication more difficult. (Objective 3)

5. D. Quickly and concisely write questions on a note pad. (Objective 3)

6. B. Perform an assessment before moving her, even though she denies injury. (Objective 11)

7. B. The patient's presentation is most indicative of expressive (motor) aphasia. (Objective 7)

8. D. A developmental disability can best be defined as impaired or insufficient brain development that prevents learning at the usual rate. (Objective 19)

9. B. Osteoarthritis is the type of arthritis most often encountered in the prehospital environment. (Objective 30)

10. C. Asymmetric muscle weakness and a reduced size of the affected limb are findings consistent with postpoliomyelitis syndrome. (Objective 31)

11. A. The initial management of this patient would be to assess the tracheostomy tube for possible obstruction. Before removing a tracheostomy tube, you should first attempt to clear any obstructions by suctioning the tube. (Objective 32)

CASE STUDY

1. The patient's ventriculoperitoneal shunt is not functioning properly, and he is developing increased intracranial pressure. (Objective 31)

2. The patient should be transported to the hospital rapidly so a neurosurgeon can correct the problem with the shunt. If the patient deteriorates rapidly during transport, controlled hyperventilation can be used to reduce intracranial pressure. (Objective 31)

CHAPTER 41: SOCIETAL ISSUES

SHORT ANSWER

1. Schizophrenia, bipolar disorder, and major depression are the most common psychiatric disorders affecting homeless persons. (Objective 6)

2. Chronic illness among the homeless frequently goes untreated because of lack of economic resources and barriers to healthcare access created by psychiatric illness. The physiologic stresses of homelessness created by inadequate diet, inability to maintain proper hygiene, and chronic environmental exposure can accelerate the progression of chronic disease processes. (Objective 5)

3. Be empathetic and nonjudgmental. Remain calm and professional. Respect the patient's personal space. Do not speak harshly. (Objective 5)
4. Codependence is exhibiting excessive, inappropriate caring behavior for another. (Objective 2)
5. Because codependents believe they are the only persons who understand the problems of the persons they care for, they may prevent appropriate intervention by healthcare professionals. The codependent may become a victim if the addiction or problem leads to violence. (Objective 2)

MULTIPLE CHOICE

1. C. Mortality among the homeless is four times that of the general population. Twenty-three percent of the homeless suffer from a psychiatric disorder. At least half of mentally ill homeless persons also have a substance abuse problem. The presence of multiple disease processes combined with environmental stressors and lack of economic resources produces health problems in the homeless population that are significantly different from those seen in domiciled patients. (Objective 5)
2. A. Homelessness is common in the United States and has a significant effect on EMS. (Objective 5)
3. D. The best position to stand when you are interacting with a homeless person is 3 to 4 feet away, slight turned. Standing 1 to 2 feet from another person invades the their personal space and produces a stress response. Directly facing another person can be interpreted as a sign of aggression. (Objective 5)
4. B. Codependent persons are overly caring because they typically come from dysfunctional families. (Objective 2)
5. D. The most appropriate response by EMS personnel to a suspected codependent relationship would be to share their impressions of the relationship with personnel at the receiving hospital so appropriate help can be offered. Ignoring the situation altogether can lead to inadequate management of the problems present. However, attempting to confront a codependent individual in the out-of-hospital setting can result in the individual becoming angry or defensive and interfering with attempts to provide care. (Objective 2)
6. C. The poor frequently use emergency departments and EMS as a source of primary healthcare. EMS personnel should recognize that they and their colleagues in the emergency department are the only healthcare providers to whom a significant part of the population may have access and should be willing to provide treatment and transport for nonemergency problems. Poverty impacts the middle and upper classes by increasing the taxes they must pay to fund support programs. In spite of support programs, poverty significantly reduces life expectancy. (Objective 3)

7. B. Explain the importance of early intervention in heart attack, contact the hospital by telephone, and have the patient talk to a physician. Economically disadvantaged persons, including the "working poor," often will refuse essential emergency care because of concerns about costs. Every effort should be made to encourage these patients to consider their health first. Because physicians have a perceived level of higher expertise, they may be able to convince persons refusing care to seek help when other attempts have failed. (Objective 3)

CASE STUDIES

Case One

1. These behaviors are signs of respect in the cultures of East and Southeast Asia. Understanding this cultural difference is important because persons raised in the dominant cultural tradition of the United States tend to interpret unwillingness to talk or make eye contact as indicating feelings of guilt. (Objective 1)

Case Two

1. A curandera is a Mexican folk healer. (Objective 1)
2. As long as the curandera does not interfere with your care of the patient, you should respect her and allow her to continue her rituals. Curanderas are highly respected in their communities. If EMS personnel show a curandera disrespect or interfere with her efforts to treat a patient, the patient or the patient's family may ask the EMS personnel to leave.

Case Three

1. The patient probably has a gastrointestinal hemorrhage from an ulcer caused by chronic NSAID use. (Objective 1)
2. Jehovah's Witnesses will not take blood or blood products.
3. You should inform her that you will be starting the IV with a salt-water solution and will not administer blood or blood products.

CHAPTER 42: CARE FOR THE PATIENT WITH A CHRONIC ILLNESS

SHORT ANSWER

1. The first step in managing a situation in which a home ventilator has malfunctioned is to disconnect the patient from the ventilator and ventilate him or her using a bag- mask. Only after adequate ventilations of the patient have been ensured should you attempt to correct any problems with the ventilator. (Objective 15)
2. A PICC line is a peripherally inserted central catheter. PICC lines are catheters that have been inserted into a peripheral vein and then threaded into the central venous circulation. (Objective 17)

3. The catheter should be clamped between the leak and the patient. If a clamp with teeth, such as a hemostat, is used, wrapping the tube with a gauze dressing can prevent further damage to it. (Objective 17)

4. Use of naloxone is not recommended with this patient. Because naloxone is an opiate antagonist, it will block the patient's opiate receptor sites. Although this will reverse the patient's respiratory depression, it also will remove all analgesic effects from the opiates and put the patient in severe pain that cannot be relieved. A better strategy in this situation would be to support the patient's ventilations with a bag-mask until respiratory depression caused by the opiates corrects itself. (Objective 23)

5. Patients with indwelling tubes in the gastrointestinal tract should be transported in a semi-Fowler's position. This reduces the chance that the patient will aspirate. (Objective 19)

6. The collecting bag should be kept below the level of the patient's urinary bladder to ensure the catheter drains properly. (Objective 20)

7. A central venous catheter that is opened to the atmosphere can cause an air embolism. (Objective 18)

8. The patient should be placed on his/her left side and tilted 30 degrees head down. This position will cause air that enters the heart to rise away from the outflow tract of the right ventricle, slowing the rate at which air leaves the heart and enters the pulmonary circulation. The patient should be given oxygen, and respirations should be supported as necessary. (Objective 18)

9. Contamination of the patient or his/her bedding with feces, urine, or emesis from incontinence or leaking collection bags. Improperly contained or discarded medical wastes. Draining wounds or decubitus ulcers. Sharps. Spraying of mucus from tracheostomy tubes. Danger of electrical shock from medical equipment. Fire or explosion hazards associated with the presence of oxygen. Hazards created by equipment that may trip or fall on the rescuers. (Objective 9)

10. Decubitus wounds also are known as pressure ulcers, pressure sores, decubitus ulcers, or bedsores. A decubitus wound usually is the result of prolonged pressure on a body part. The person's body weight presses on the tissue and skin over a bone, such as the spine, coccyx, hips, heels, or elbows. Blood flow to the area is decreased because the person's body weight traps the skin, soft tissue, and muscle between the bone and another surface, such as a mattress, bedrail, wheelchair, or brace. Without adequate blood flow to the area, the tissue begins to break down and eventually decays. (Objective 21)

11. Stage 1: A reddened skin area that does not disappear when you relieve pressure. No break in skin integrity is present. Treatment consists of removing pressure on the area. This usually is accomplished by frequent turning or repositioning and using soft, protective pads and cushions. Adequate nutrition is essential, including vitamin C, protein, and fluids. Stage 2: A partial-thickness break in the skin develops that may resemble a blister, an abrasion, or a shallow crater. Sludge may be present in the wound bed. Treatment involves covering, protecting, and cleaning the affected area. Stage 3: A full-thickness break in the skin that resembles a deep crater. The subcutaneous tissue is exposed. Because the wound extends through all the skin layers, it is now a potential site of serious infection. Treatment involves maintaining adequate nutrition and hydration; relieving pressure on the affected area; and cleaning, covering, and protecting the wound. Stage 4: A full-thickness break in the skin that involves underlying muscle, tendons, and bone. If it is not aggressively treated, the wound may become the source of a life-threatening infection. Relieving pressure on the affected area, and cleaning, covering, and protecting the wound are important. However, if the patient does not receive adequate nutrition and hydration, the wound will not heal. Surgery may be needed to remove decayed tissue. Amputation is sometimes necessary. (Objective 21)

MULTIPLE CHOICE

1. C. An infant or child with a gastrostomy tube should be transported sitting with the head elevated to minimize risks of aspiration. (Objective 19)

2. B. Disconnect the patient from the mechanical ventilator and assist his ventilations with a bag-mask and oxygen. Attempts to repair a malfunctioning ventilator should never be made until adequate ventilation of the patient by other means has been ensured. An oxygen mask will not support a patient who is not adequately ventilating. (Objective 15)

3. D. You should wrap the tips of a hemostat with gauze and use the hemostat to clamp the PICC line. (Objective 18)

4. B. A terminally ill patient in the home care environment experiencing respiratory distress should be given a thorough initial assessment and provided with appropriate care. (Objective 24)

5. B. In the event of a life-threatening emergency, a patient with a signed, valid do not resuscitate order should receive only comfort measures unless the advance directive specifically states otherwise. (Objective 24)

6. C. The anatomic location that would be least likely to be the site of a colostomy stoma would be in the right upper quadrant from the ascending colon. (Objective 19)

7. D. You should transport the patient to the nearest facility for further treatment. Implanted medication ports should be cannulated only with special needles

called *Huber needles* that will not damage the port. Using a conventional over-the-needle IV catheter on an implanted medication port will damage the port, making it useless and requiring it to be replaced. The only time an implanted medication port should be cannulated without a Huber needle is during a cardiac arrest when no other drug route is available. Because the patient is hypotensive, giving nitroglycerin would not be appropriate. The endotracheal route is not available for drug administration because the patient is conscious. (Objective 18)

8. C. The most common complication of urinary catheters is infection. The Texas catheter is not intended for long-term use. Internal catheters are indicated for patients who are unable to empty urine collected by the urinary bladder. Suprapubic catheters do involve invasion into the abdominal wall. (Objective 20)

9. D. If the family of a hospice patient calls EMS, the paramedics should respect the wishes of the patient and family and maintain patient dignity at all times. (Objective 24)

10. C. Your primary concern at this moment is ensuring an adequate airway even though there is a spinal injury. (Objective 12)

11. A. If a tracheostomy tube is dislodged from the stoma and cannot be replaced easily, you should insert an appropriately sized endotracheal tube into the tracheostoma. (Objective 12)

12. A. An appropriate question to ask would be, "Does the patient have a do not resuscitate order?" The presence of a valid do not resuscitate order will help guide your approach to the patient. (Objective 24)

13. B. You should assist the patient's breathing with a bag-mask and contact medical control for further orders. Although naloxone would reverse the respiratory arrest, it also would reverse the analgesic effects of the morphine, leaving the patient in uncontrollable pain. Since the patient's respiratory arrest is a result of your giving morphine rather than the natural progression of the patient's disease process, it is appropriate to support him until you can consult with medical control. (Objective 23)

14. A. While you are contacting medical control for orders, you should disconnect the ventilator and ventilate the lungs with a bag-mask device and oxygen. The first step in managing a patient whose ventilator is malfunctioning is to ensure adequate oxygenation and ventilation with a bag-mask. Once the patient's ventilations are supported, efforts can begin to correct the problem with the ventilator. (Objective 15)

15. A. A PICC line enters a peripheral vein and extends into the central venous circulation. (Objective 17)

16. A. The best position in which to place this patient would be on his left side 30 degrees head down. The patient has an air embolism. Positioning the patient on his left side 30 degrees head down will cause air to rise away from the outflow tract of the right ventricle and slow the rate at which air enters the pulmonary circulation. (Objective 18)

17. A. You should comply with the wishes of the spouse and the advance directive and do nothing. An advance directive is an expression of a patient's wishes related to receiving healthcare. The ethical principal of autonomy requires that advance directives be respected. Objective 24)

CASE STUDY

1. The patient is in compensated hypovolemic shock with a blood pressure near the lower acceptable limit for her age. She should receive volume resuscitation using an isotonic crystalloid. Since she has had no nutrient intake for 10 hours, her blood glucose level should be determined. If she is hypoglycemic, she should be given $D_{10}W$ or $D_{25}W$. (Objective 19)

2. It may be possible to treat this patient by replacing the dislodged gastric tube and using it to rehydrate her. Because children with severe developmental delays often are medically fragile, this alternative may be preferable to establishing an IV with the associated risk of infection. (Objective 19)

3. Because the feeding tube has been dislodged for an extended time period, the stoma may have begun to close. Reinsertion of the tube may be difficult. In this case a smaller tube could be inserted and used to begin rehydration. If the stoma was created recently, the opening in the stomach may not yet have adhered fully to the opening in the abdominal wall. When the tube was dislodged, the stomach and abdominal wall might have separated. If this is the case, a tube placed through the stoma might enter the peritoneal cavity rather than the stomach. (Objective 19)

CHAPTER 43: TRAUMA SYSTEMS AND MECHANISM OF INJURY

SHORT ANSWER

1. The purpose of the initial assessment (primary survey) is to immediately identify life-threatening problems involving the airway, breathing, circulation, or central nervous system. (Objective 13)

2. The patient's ventilations should be assisted with a bag-mask and oxygen. When the respiratory rate is less than 10 breaths/min or more than 30 breaths/min, minute volume is usually inadequate. The patient will no longer be able to remove carbon dioxide from or deliver supplemental oxygen to the alveoli effectively. (Objective 13)

3. Absence of a radial pulse indicates that peripheral perfusion is poor and that the cardiovascular system is shunting blood from the periphery to the core organs. (Objective 13)

4. Head, chest, abdomen. (Objective 6)

5. The "Golden Hour" is the time period within which a critically injured trauma patient must reach the operating room to have the greatest probability of surviving. EMS has 10 minutes of the Golden Hour to identify a critically injured trauma patient, prepare the patient for transport, and begin moving the patient toward definitive care in the operating room. (Objective 4)

6. Kinetic energy = ½ Mass × Velocity². Because the velocity is squared, it makes a larger contribution to the amount of kinetic energy available to cause damage. (Objective 5)

7. Three. Vehicle versus object, occupant versus vehicle, occupant's organs versus occupant's body wall. (Objective 7)

8. Normal capillary refill time is less than 2 seconds. A prolonged capillary refill time may indicate poor peripheral perfusion. However, capillary refill also can be prolonged by cold environments because cold produces peripheral vasoconstriction. (Objective 13)

9. IV access for critical trauma patients should be obtained en route to the hospital. Attempting to establish IVs on scene delays the patient's reaching definitive care in the operating room. Also, there is no way of knowing whether an IV established in the field will be able to keep up with ongoing blood loss. (Objective 13)

10. The probably locations of injured organs from a gunshot cannot be determined by the locations of entrance and exit wounds for several reasons. First, bullets transmit energy to body tissues through cavitation, which can produce trauma at significant distances from the bullet track. Second, bullets can change their trajectories as they pass through the body, producing a track that is not a straight line. Finally, impacts with bone can produce fragments that become secondary missiles, creating their own wound tracks. (Objective 12)

11. The secondary survey should be performed in the ambulance on the way to the hospital. Performing a detailed history and physical exam on scene delays the patient's receiving definitive care in the operating room. (Objective 13)

12. A "paper bag" pneumothorax results from rupture of the lung that occurs when the chest is compressed while the patient is holding his or her breath. Compression of the chest wall with the glottic opening closed decreases the volume of the chest cavity and raises the pressure in the alveoli. The rise in pressure tears the alveolar walls, allowing air to leak into the pleural space to form a pneumothorax. (Objective 7)

13. The initial efforts should focus on securing an airway, assisting ventilations, and decompressing the possible tension pneumothorax on the left side of the chest. Once the problems with airway and breathing have been corrected, the next priority is support of circulation by controlling external hemorrhage and beginning treatment of hypovolemic shock while en route to the hospital. (Objective 14)

14. The Don Juan syndrome is a pattern of injuries that occurs commonly in patients who land on their feet after a fall. They suffer bilateral fractures of the calcanei (heel bones) from the initial impact and fractures of the lower legs, knees, femurs, and hips. Compression fractures of the thoracic and lumbar spine can occur as the head and torso continue moving downward. (Objective 11)

15. Waddell's triad is a pattern of injuries commonly found in children struck by motor vehicles. Children typically turn to face a vehicle that is about to strike them. This results in an impact by the vehicle's bumper against the legs that results in lower extremity fracture, followed by an impact of the torso against the vehicle's hood that causes thoracic trauma, followed by the child's falling off the vehicle and striking his/her head on the roadway. (Objective 10)

16. This patient has suffered primary blast injuries caused by the blast's pressure wave. (Objective 11)

17. He should be suspected of having other injuries in areas of the body where there is an air-fluid interface such as the lungs or the gastrointestinal tract. (Objective 11)

MULTIPLE CHOICE

1. C. Initiate oxygen therapy, apply a cervical collar, extricate the patient to a long board, assist ventilation, apply MAST, transport, initiate IVs en route. This patient is critically injured and needs to reach the operating room within the Golden Hour. Applying a KED or attempting to establish IVs on the scene will unnecessarily delay transport to definitive care. (Objective 14)

2. B. 2, 3, 4, 1. Highest priority should go to the patient with the compromised airway (Patient 2). The next most critical patient is suffering from an intraabdominal hemorrhage that is producing hypovolemic shock (Patient 3). Patient 4 should be managed next because she has no immediately life-threatening problems with her ABCs but does have a spinal injury that could cause severe disability. Patient 1 has a non–life-threatening extremity injury. (Objective 14)

3. B. The purpose of triage is to ensure that patients with life-threatening conditions receive immediate treatment. (Objective 13)

4. B. EMS has 10 minutes of the "Golden Hour" for on-scene patient assessment and management. This time period has been referred to as the "Platinum 10." (Objectives 4, 13)

5. B. This is an example of indirect violence because the fracture occurred at a location away from the point where the external force was applied to the body. (Objective 7)

6. C. Penetrating or blunt trauma caused by flying debris from an explosion is a secondary blast injury. (Objective 11)
7. D. A level IV trauma center is a medical care facility located in a remote area that stabilizes and prepares trauma patients with moderate or serious injuries for transport to a facility with capabilities for trauma surgery. (Objective 3)
8. A. A level I trauma center is a medical care facility, usually a university teaching center, that commits resources to address all types of specialty trauma 24 hours a day, 7 days a week. (Objective 3)

CASE STUDIES

Case One

1. This patient has cardiac tamponade. The best strategy would be to stop at the level IV trauma center and have the physician perform a pericardiocentesis, and then arrange for transport to the level I trauma center for definitive surgical management of the wound in the patient's heart. Unless the paramedics caring for this patient have been trained to perform pericardiocentesis, attempting to reach the level I center is not a good option, because the patient is unlikely to survive a 20-minute transport. (Objective 3)

Case Two

1. The law of conservation of energy states that energy cannot be created or destroyed, only transformed from one form of energy to another. The law of conservation of energy is relevant to this situation because the kinetic energy that is present when a moving vehicle and its occupants impact a fixed object does not simply disappear. It is transformed into other energy that causes damage to the vehicle and the persons in it. (Objective 5)
2. The first law of motion states that a body in motion will remain in motion unless acted on by an outside force. The first law of motion is relevant in this situation because an unrestrained occupant of a vehicle that suddenly stops moving will continue moving until an outside force applied by an impact with the inside of the vehicle or some other object stops the occupant from moving. (Objective 5)
3. The amount of kinetic energy present is determined primarily by a moving body's velocity: Kinetic energy $= \frac{1}{2}$ Mass $\times$ Velocity^2. Because the velocity is squared, it makes a larger contribution to the amount of kinetic energy available to cause damage. (Objective 5)
4. Vehicle versus object, passengers versus inside of vehicle, passenger's organs versus passenger's body walls. (Objective 5)
5. Sternal or rib fractures, pulmonary contusion, myocardial contusion, pneumothorax, hemothorax, aortic tear, tracheobronchial tree injuries. (Objective 5)

6. The damage suggests the patient's knee impacted the dashboard. (Objective 5)
7. Fracture/dislocation of the patella, dislocation of the knee, femur fracture, hip fracture, hip dislocation, pelvic (acetabulum) fracture. (Objective 5)

Case Three

1. Lower extremity fractures, chest trauma, head trauma. (Objective 10)
2. Waddell's triad. (Objective 10)
3. Children tend to turn toward a vehicle that is about to strike them. The initial impact with the bumper causes lower extremity fractures. The child's chest strikes the hood, causing thoracic trauma. The driver then brakes, and the child falls off the front of the vehicle, striking his/her head on the roadway. (Objective 10)

CHAPTER 44: BLEEDING

MATCHING

1. __A__ Bright red and spurting
   __C__ Dark red and flowing
   __B__ Dark red and oozing
   (Objective 1)

SHORT ANSWER

1. The goal is to stop the bleeding as quickly and completely as possible. Allowing the patient to continue to bleed while attempting ineffective methods of control can lead to poor patient outcome. (Objective 5)
2. Hemorrhage is defined as massive, heavy bleeding. It may be external or internal and may occur acutely or chronically. (Objective 1)
3. Perfusion is the circulation of blood through an organ. Perfusion is critical to the function of cells, tissues, organs, organ systems, and the body as it delivers oxygen and nutrients and removes carbon dioxide and other waste products. (Objective 1)
4. Causes of major blood loss can include solid organ injury, aortic aneurysm, vascular injury, penetrating trauma, gastrointestinal bleeding, ruptured liver or spleen, hemothorax, ruptured ectopic pregnancy, arteriovenous malformation, bleeding esophageal varices, pelvic fractures, femur fractures, bleeding ulcers, placenta previa, abruptio placentae. (Objective 2)
5. Near-complete loss of blood that is not conducive with life. (Objective 2)
6. A loss of 1000 mL in the adult, 500 mL in the child, and 100 t\o 200 mL in the infant is considered serious. (Objective 2)
7. Signs and symptoms of blood loss can include dizziness or light-headedness, pale skin, tachycardia, normal or low blood pressure, narrowed pulse pressure, alterations in mental status. (Objectives 2, 7)

8. Older treatments of elevation and pressure points have been shown to be ineffective in controlling hemorrhage. Normally, direct pressure and pressure bandages will control most bleeding; however, if these do not work a tourniquet should be considered in order to stop the bleeding. Time spent attempting ineffective control measures leads to greater blood loss and greater hypovolemia for the patient. (Objectives 3, 4)

9. The systolic blood pressure should be maintained between 80 and 90 mm Hg unless a head injury is also present, in which case the systolic pressure must be maintained above 90 mm Hg. A systolic blood pressure in this range maintains perfusion to the vital organs without increasing the rate of hemorrhage. (Objectives 4, 8)

10. Direct pressure. (Objective 5)

11. A tourniquet. (Objective 5)

12. A tourniquet controls bleeding by occluding all blood flow to an injured extremity. The resulting ischemic injury can cause loss of the limb. Ischemia from tourniquet application also results in accumulation of lactic acid and potassium in the affected extremity. Sudden release of the tourniquet can result in a release of these substances into the circulation, producing dysrhythmias and depressed myocardial function. Finally, an improperly applied tourniquet can reduce venous return from an extremity without occluding arterial flow, resulting in worsened hemorrhage. (Objective 5)

13. Tissue ischemia results in accumulation of potassium and lactic acid distal to a tourniquet. Sudden release of a tourniquet can lead to "washout" of these substances into the central circulation where they can cause dysrhythmias or depressed myocardial function. Loosening or removing a tourniquet also can cause return of arterial blood flow to an extremity, which can dislodge clots and renew bleeding. (Objective 5)

14. A blood pressure cuff. (Objective 5)

MULTIPLE CHOICE

1. B. The bleeding from the scalp should be controlled first because it is arterial. Because blood flows through arteries under high pressures, arterial hemorrhage can rapidly lead to hypovolemic shock. (Objective 1)

2. C. If a dressing and bandage become soaked with blood you should reinforce the bandage with more gauze and pressure. Removing a bandage can dislodge clots and worsen bleeding. Doing nothing to control obvious bleeding though a bandage can result in more severe hypovolemia. A tourniquet should be applied if direct pressure and a pressure bandage fail to control bleeding. (Objectives 3, 4)

3. B. The first step to control bleeding is application of direct pressure. (Objectives 3, 4)

4. A. Arterial bleeding is bright red and spurting. (Objectives 3, 4)

5. C. The average blood volume is 70 mL/kg. (Objective 2)

6. A. A 10% to 15% loss of blood volume is generally well tolerated by most healthy patients. (Objective 2)

7. D. Warfarin (Coumadin) is an anticoagulant. Patients who are taking these will have an impaired ability to form clots and therefore are more likely to experience severe hemorrhage. (Objective 2)

8. B. High-flow oxygen will be of the most benefit to this patient in order to ensure the blood flowing to the organs is well saturated. (Objective 8)

9. C. Tachycardia, hypotension, and a narrowed pulse pressure are all indicators of hemorrhage, either internal or external. (Objective 8)

10. B. Applying direct pressure is the first step in controlling external hemorrhage. (Objective 5)

CHAPTER 45: SOFT TISSUE TRAUMA

MATCHING

1. __B__ Abrasion
   __D__ Amputation
   __F__ Avulsion
   __A__ Contusion
   __C__ Laceration
   __E__ Puncture
   (Objectives 10, 13)

2. __E__ Collagen synthesis
   __D__ Epithelialization
   __A__ Hemostasis
   __B__ Inflammation
   __C__ Neovascularization
   (Objective 5)

3. __F__ Adherent
   __G__ Nonabsorbent
   __C__ Nonadherent
   __B__ Nonocclusive
   __E__ Occlusive
   __A__ Sterile
   (Objective 21)

SHORT ANSWER

1. Epidermis, dermis, subcutaneous tissue. (Objective 2)

2. Dermis. (Objective 2)

3. Amputated body parts should be placed in a plastic bag. The bag then should be immersed in cold water. (Objective 15)

4. The skin flap should be returned to its normal anatomic position before the injury is bandaged. This reduces the risk of obstructing blood flow to the skin flap when a dressing and bandage are applied. (Objective 15)

5. An impaled object should be left in place unless it compromises the airway. A bulky dressing should be placed around the object to stabilize it. (Objective 15)

6. Bandages should not be removed in the field because of the risk of dislodging clots and restarting bleeding. If a patient bleeds through a bandage, direct pressure over the bandage should be used to control the bleeding; then the bandage should be reinforced with additional material. (Objective 15)

7. Crush syndrome results from prolonged pressure against a body part that results in diminished blood flow into the compressed area. Decreased oxygen delivery results in ischemic injury, tissue necrosis, and accumulation of potentially toxic substances such as lactic acid, potassium, phosphate, and myoglobin. When the pressure on the affected area is removed, these substances are released into the central circulation. (Objective 19)

8. Rhabdomyolysis is breakdown of skeletal muscle. (Objective 18)

9. When rhabdomyolysis results from crush syndrome, myoglobin leaks into the bloodstream. Myoglobin enters the kidney, where it precipitates in the filtering tubules, clogging them. (Objective 18)

10. Rapidly infuse large volumes of normal saline to promote urine output and rapidly push myoglobin through the kidneys. Avoid Ringer's lactate because it contains potassium, which may worsen the hyperkalemia caused by crush syndrome. Consider administration of sodium bicarbonate to alkalinize the urine, decreasing the tendency of myoglobin to precipitate in the filtering tubules. Consider administration of an osmotic diuretic such as mannitol to increase urine output. Avoid loop diuretics such as furosemide because they can worsen electrolyte imbalances and acidify the urine, increasing the risk of myoglobin precipitation. (Objectives 17, 18, 19)

11. Extremity muscles are enclosed in compartments formed by fascia. When a closed injury causes edema within a fascial compartment, the fascia resists the swelling, leading to a rise in pressure within the compartment. When the pressure in the compartment exceeds the pressure in the vessels providing blood to the compartment, ischemia results. (Objective 19)

12. Any fractures should be splinted. The injured part should be elevated and cold packs should be applied to reduce swelling. The patient should be transported rapidly since a fasciotomy to decompress the affected compartment may be necessary. (Objective 19)

MULTIPLE CHOICE

1. B. Control the spurting bleeding from the scalp. Bright red, spurting bleeding is arterial in origin and is an immediate life threat because it can result in hypovolemia and shock. Once the arterial bleeding is controlled, hemorrhage from other sites should be addressed. Assessment of extremity motor/sensory function is not appropriate until all potential life threats have been managed. (Objective 15)

2. D. Avulsed or amputated parts present at a motor vehicle collision should be transported with the patient for possible reattachment. (Objective 15)

3. D. An avulsion is a soft tissue injury in which skin has been torn and is hanging as a flap. (Objective 13)

4. C. A dressing and bandage soaked with blood should be reinforced with more gauze and pressure. (Objective 22)

5. C. The organs should be left exposed and covered with a moist, sterile dressing to protect them, prevent drying, and reduce loss of body heat. (Objective 15)

6. C. Avulsed or amputated body parts should be transported with the patient since it may be possible to reattach them. Although cooling is appropriate, amputated parts should not be packed directly in ice. (Objective 15)

7. C. When an extremity is bandaged, the fingers and toes should be left exposed to permit monitoring of circulation. While the bandage should maintain sufficient pressure over the dressing to help control bleeding, it should not be wrapped so tightly that it occludes circulation to the extremity. Once in place, a bandage and dressing should not be lifted since this action may dislodge clots and restart bleeding. (Objective 21)

8. C. A contusion is a closed soft tissue injury that produces edema and ecchymosis from crushing of skin and subcutaneous tissues. An abrasion results from scraping away of the skin surface. In an avulsion, skin is partially torn away in a flap. A laceration is an open cut in the skin that is longer than it is deep. (Objectives 9, 10, 13)

9. C. A localized collection of blood forming a lump in the tissues is a hematoma. Hematoma means "blood lump." (Objective 11)

10. C. When you are managing a patient with a partial avulsion or amputation, gently straighten and align any skin bridges to promote the best possible circulation through any intact blood vessels. (Objective 15)

11. B. Pain out of proportion to physical findings is the most important indicator that compartment syndrome may be present. Compartment syndrome is most likely to appear 6 to 8 hours after an injury. Pulselessness, paresthesias, and altered motor and sensory function develop late in compartment syndrome and are not dependable findings. (Objective 19)

12. D. Adherent dressings promote clot formation more effectively than nonadherent dressings. However, they are more likely to disturb clots when they are removed. Occlusive dressings block air and fluid movement through themselves. (Objective 21)

CASE STUDY

1. An incision. An incision is a type of laceration in which the wound edges are very smooth. Incisions usually are produced by very sharp objects such as knives, scalpels, razor blades, or pieces of glass. They tend to bleed freely. (Objective 13)

2. The first step in controlling bleeding is to place a dressing over the wound and apply direct pressure. (Objective 15)
3. If direct pressure does not control bleeding, a tourniquet should be used. (Objective 15)
4. The patient is showing signs and symptoms of hypovolemic shock. She should be placed in a supine position with her lower extremities elevated 8 to 12 inches. Oxygen should be administered by nonrebreather mask at 10 to 15 liters per minute. The patient should be covered with a blanket to prevent loss of body heat. She should be transported immediately. An IV of isotonic crystalloid solution should be started en route to the hospital. (Objective 15)
5. Diabetic patients tend to heal slowly and are prone to wound infections. (Objective 6)

CHAPTER 46: BURN INJURY

MATCHING

1. __A__ Burned areas are red and painful. They blanch under pressure. No blisters are present.
   __C__ Burn is gray, white, or charred. Looks thickened and leathery. Pain is absent.
   __B__ Burn is salmon-pink and moist. Severe pain is present. Blisters may be present.
   (Objective 4)
2. __A__ 3% third degree caused by an electrical shock
   __C__ 9% third degree, excluding face, feet, hands, and genitalia
   __B__ 15% first degree caused by exposure to the sun
   __A__ 20% second degree in a patient with a femur fracture
   __A__ 35% second degree, including face and hands
   (Objectives 1, 4)

SHORT ANSWER

1. Epidermis, dermis, subcutaneous tissue. (Objective 2)
2. Dermis. (Objective 2)
3. Loss of body fluid, leading to hypovolemia and shock. Increased loss of body heat, leading to hypothermia. Loss of protective barrier against bacteria, leading to infection. (Objective 3)
4. __9__ Head
   __18__ Anterior trunk
   __18__ Posterior trunk
   __9__ Each upper extremity
   __18__ Each lower extremity
   __1__ Perineum
   (Objective 4)
5. __18__ Head
   __18__ Anterior trunk
   __18__ Posterior trunk
   __9__ Each upper extremity
   __13.5__ Each lower extremity
   __1__ Perineum
   (Objective 4)

6. 1%. (Objective 4)
7. 9% (right arm) + 9% (left arm) = 18%. (Objective 4)
8. 18% (anterior trunk). (Objective 4)
9. In a 3-year-old child, each lower extremity is approximately 16% of the total body surface area. 18% (posterior trunk) + 7.25% (posterior half of right lower extremity) + 7.25% (posterior half of left lower extremity) = 32.5%. To use the rule of nines in children, for each year older than 1 year, subtract from the head and add 0.5% to each lower extremity. (Objective 4)
10. Ringer's lactate. 80 kg × 70% burn × 4 mL/kg/% burn = 22,400 mL (22.4 liters). (Objective 4)
11. 50 kg × 50% burn × 4 mL/kg/% burn = 10,000 mL (10 liters) × ½ = 5000 mL (5 liters). One half of the required fluid volume should be given in the first 8 hours after the patient is burned. The other half should be infused over the next 16 hours. (Objective 4)
12. Ringer's lactate is closer in its composition to normal extracellular fluid than normal saline. In particular, LR contains potassium, while NS does not. Infusion of massive amounts of NS into a burn patient can produce severe hypokalemia, leading to dysrhythmias. (Objective 4)
13. Because fluid loss in burns is the result of a slow leak of fluid from the body, burns do not produce a rapid onset of hypovolemia. Therefore when a burn patient shows a rapid onset of signs of hypovolemic shock, other injuries causing hemorrhage must be present. (Objective 4)
14. Vascular access should be obtained in the upper extremities, even if this necessitates starting an IV through a burn. IVs should never be started in the lower extremities of burn patients. Because patients with large burns frequently are not ambulatory for extended periods of time, IV sites in their lower extremities increase the risk of pulmonary emboli. (Objective 4)
15. With the exception of tetanus prophylaxis (which is given IM), the IV route should be used to administer all medications to burn patients. Burn injuries produce massive peripheral vasoconstriction in response to volume loss and pain. Medications administered by the intramuscular or subcutaneous routes will be absorbed slowly and produce effect unreliably. (Objective 4)
16. Be sure the current is turned off before making contact with the patient. (Objective 20)
17. Taking care to avoid contaminating yourself, you should undress the patient and brush away as much of the powder as possible from any exposed skin surfaces. The small amounts of dry chemical remaining should be washed away with large amounts of water. When a patient is contaminated with large amounts of dry chemical, water should not be used initially because of the risk of causing a chemical reaction that could liberate large amounts of heat. (Objective 12)
18. This patient is at risk of losing her upper airway because of tissue edema caused by the burn. (Objective 4)

19. Place the patient on high-concentration oxygen using a nonrebreather mask. Attach an ECG monitor to detect any dysrhythmias that may result from contact with electrical current. Establish an IV with Ringer's lactate. Give an initial 20 mL/kg fluid bolus followed by additional fluid to maintain adequate perfusion and urine output. Consider administration of sodium bicarbonate (1 mEq/kg) to alkalinize the urine and prevent renal failure secondary to myoglobin precipitation in the kidneys. Consider mannitol (10 g) to promote urine output. Identify and manage any orthopedic injuries that could have resulted from muscle spasms caused by contact with electrical current. Consider the possibility of spinal injury secondary to muscle spasms caused by contact with electrical current. (Objective 20)

20. Low-voltage current tends to follow structures such as muscles, nerves, and blood vessels, which provide low-resistance pathways along which electricity can flow. High-voltage current follows the shortest pathway to ground. (Objectives 14, 15)

21. A patient who has lost consciousness in a smoke-filled environment will no longer hold his or her breath to avoid inhaling products of combustion. Therefore loss of consciousness increases the risk of lower airway injury. (Objective 4)

22. What was burning or what was the toxic substance? Was the smoke or other gas trapped in an enclosed space, increasing its concentration? Was there a loss of consciousness, leading to inability to protect the lower airway by breath-holding? How long was the patient exposed? (Objective 4)

23. Carbon monoxide binds to hemoglobin more efficiently than oxygen, occupying sites that should be used to carry oxygen to the tissues. Therefore carbon monoxide produces tissue hypoxia by reducing the blood's oxygen-carrying capacity. (Objective 4)

24. Carbon monoxide is colorless and odorless. (Objective 4)

25. Children have larger body surface to volume ratios than adults. Therefore for the same percentage of burned body surface area, a child will lose fluid and heat more rapidly than an adult. (Objective 21)

26. Stocking and glove burn patterns in children result from dipping of the hands or feet into hot water. They are signs of intentional injuries resulting from child abuse. (Objective 21)

27. Burn shock occurs as a result of the loss of plasma from the vascular tree. However, unlike true hypovolemic shock, in which the plasma, water, or blood has been lost from the circulation and often the body, in burns the loss is a result of capillary leak. This phenomenon is a result of several factors. First and foremost, capillary integrity is lost because of physical thermal injury to capillaries and larger vessels. Thermal injury causes the destruction of red blood cells, which in large burns (15% to 40% TBSA) contributes to anemia (acute and chronic).

As much as 18% of the red cell mass may be lost in the first 24 hours after a burn.

28. Alpha, beta, and gamma.

MULTIPLE CHOICE

1. D. Flush her eyes with water or saline solution. Although phenol is more soluble in alcohol than in water, no substance other than water or saline should be used to irrigate the eyes. Delaying removal of an acid or alkali from the eyes can result in loss of sight. (Objective 12)

2. A. 8400 mL of Ringer's lactate. Based on the Parkland formula, this patient should receive 70 kg × 60% × 4 mL/kg/% or 16,800 mL of fluid during the first 24 hours following the injury. Half of this amount, 8400 mL, should be given during the first 8 hours. Ringer's lactate should be used because administration of large amounts of normal saline can produce severe hypokalemia. (Objective 4)

3. D. 9% (right arm) + 9% (left arm) + 18% (right lower extremity) + 18% (left lower extremity) = 54%. (Objective 4)

4. B. The material that was burning; the duration of the exposure; whether the fire was located in an enclosed space; whether the patient lost consciousness. The nature of the material that was burning will help identify the toxins present in the smoke. The duration of exposure will help determine the amount of the toxins inhaled. If the fire was in an enclosed space, the toxins will be more concentrated. If the patient lost consciousness, he would have stopped holding his breath to avoid inhaling smoke. (Objective 4)

5. B. 15% (head) + 18% (anterior trunk). To use the rule of nines in children, for each year older than 1 year, subtract 1% from the head and add 0.5% to each lower extremity. A 4-year-old child's head is 15% of the body surface area. (Objective 4)

6. A. Critical. Because this patient has suffered other trauma associated with her burn, the burn should be considered critical, and she should receive care in a burn center. (Objectives 1, 4)

7. B. The burn should be covered with a clean, dry sheet to reduce contamination. Ointments should not be applied to burns during initial management. Blisters should not be ruptured since this increases the area of open wound. Irrigating or applying wet dressings to a large burn increases the risk of hypothermia. (Objective 4)

8. A. An area equal in size to the area of a patient's palm is approximately 1% of the patient's body surface area. The "Rule of Palm" can be used to estimate the size of small or irregularly shaped burns. (Objective 4)

9. C. Children and infants who are burned are more likely to suffer significant fluid loss than adults because their body surface area is larger in proportion to their body volume than in adults. Because they have a higher surface to volume ratio than adults, children will tend to lose fluid and body heat more rapidly through a burn. (Objective 21)

10. B. A 5% third-degree burn excluding the face, feet, hands, and genitalia would be a moderate burn. Any burn including the face, feet, hands, or genitalia is a critical burn. A first-degree burn of the face associated with hoarseness and drooling would be a critical burn. A 20% second-degree burn in a patient with diabetes mellitus would be a critical burn because diabetes slows wound healing and increases the risk of infection. (Objectives 1, 4)

11. B. Brush away as much of the chemical as possible; then wash with water. Applying water to a dry chemical can result in a reaction that generates heat, worsening the patient's injuries. As much of the chemical as possible should be removed by undressing the patient and brushing the chemical from her skin. The remaining chemical can be washed off using large amounts of water from the safety shower. (Objectives 10, 12)

12. A. You should brush away as much of the lime as possible before washing. Addition of water to dry lime generates large amounts of heat, which could worsen the chemical injury already present by causing thermal burns. Although dry lime is a base, you should never attempt to neutralize a base on a patient's skin by adding an acid such as vinegar. Acids react with bases to generate heat, which can worsen the burn. Also, it is difficult to determine how much acid is necessary to achieve neutralization. Adding too much acid could result in acid burns in addition to the alkali burns already present. (Objective 12)

13. C. 18% (head) + 18% (anterior trunk) = 36%. (Objective 4)

14. A. Carbon monoxide poisoning. The patient has been in an environment where carbon monoxide, a product of incomplete combustion of carbon-containing material, could be present. He shows no signs of upper airway injury, pulmonary burns, or hypoperfusion. (Objective 4)

15. B. 90% oxygen via bag-mask. Oxygen by nonrebreather mask would not be adequate because of the patient's slow respiratory rate. A simple facemask or nasal cannula would not deliver the concentrations of oxygen this patient needs. (Objective 4)

16. C. Immediately transport the patient to the hospital. Although the entrance and exit wounds associated with electrical burns frequently are small and do not appear serious, they only mark the starting and ending points of the path electricity followed through the body. Along that path extensive damage not visible from the body's surface can be present. (Objective 20)

17. B. Cardiopulmonary arrest, dysrhythmias, extremity orthopedic injuries, and spinal fractures are all injuries that can be present following contact with a high-voltage electrical current. (Objective 18)

18. B. Second degree (partial thickness). Partial-thickness burns are painful and have a moist, salmon-pink appearance. Partial-thickness burns usually develop a blister, but if blisters are present, the burn is partial thickness. (Objective 4)

19. A. According to the rule of nines an adult's head is 9% of the body surface area and an infant's head is 18%. (Objective 4)

20. A. Get help from trained power company personnel whenever power lines are down. Attempting to remove fallen power lines without proper training and equipment is extremely dangerous. Patients should be told to remain in the vehicle until the electricity has been turned off. (Objective 20)

21. C. Flushing out the eyes with water or saline is the prehospital treatment for a chemical burn of the eyes. Identification of the chemical is unnecessary. Using chemical "antidotes" in the eyes can worsen injury. Delaying removal of the chemical from the eyes can cause loss of sight. (Objective 12)

22. C. Infection by bacteria; extensive fluid loss, leading to hypovolemic shock; inability to regulate body temperature, leading to hypothermia. (Objective 3)

23. C. Commercial gel (and wet) dressings may be applied to burned areas covering no more than 5% of the body surface area. Applying wet dressings to larger areas promotes heat loss and can cause hypothermia. (Objective 4)

24. C. Gamma radiation causes the most damage to human tissues because of its penetration ability. Even brief exposure can cause localized burns and damage to internal organs. (Objective 23)

CASE STUDY

1. This patient's airway should be secured with an endotracheal tube as quickly as possible. Stridor, face and neck burns, and singeing of the eyebrows all indicate the presence of upper airway burns. If an endotracheal tube is not placed immediately, edema from these burns could cause loss of the airway. (Objective 4)

2. A cervical spine fracture may be present. The patient is unresponsive, and the mechanism of injury suggests that an explosion may have thrown him. (Objective 4)

3. No; a diuretic is not indicated in this situation. The wheezes and crackles probably are due to a lower airway burn caused by smoke inhalation. The pulmonary edema that is present is noncardiogenic and does not result from volume overload. Administering a diuretic could worsen the patient's condition by decreasing circulating blood volume. Noncardiogenic pulmonary edema is treated with oxygen, positive-pressure ventilation, and positive end-expiratory pressure. (Objective 4)

4. The patient probably has carbon monoxide poisoning. Carbon monoxide binds to sites on hemoglobin that normally carry oxygen. An oximeter will detect the fact that the patient's hemoglobin is saturated with some other substance, but will not provide information about the nature of the substance that is present. (Objective 4)

223

5. The patient is showing signs of rapidly worsening hypovolemic shock. Since fluid loss from burns does not cause a rapid onset of hypovolemia, the patient probably has other injuries that are causing internal hemorrhage. (Objective 3)

CHAPTER 47: HEAD AND FACE TRAUMA

SHORT ANSWER

1. Cerebrum: center for higher mental functions such as consciousness, learning, reasoning, emotion, and voluntary movement. Cerebellum: Control of posture, balance, equilibrium; fine control of voluntary movements. Brainstem: interconnection of cerebrum, cerebellum, and spinal cord; control of involuntary functions. (Objective 9)
2. Cerebral perfusion pressure = mean arterial pressure (MAP) – intracranial pressure (ICP). (Objectives 13, 15)
3. Increased blood pressure, decreased heart rate, and altered respiratory pattern. Cushing's triad indicates increased intracranial pressure. (Objectives 13, 15)
4. Controlled hyperventilation lowers arterial carbon dioxide levels and produces a mild respiratory alkalosis. In response to these changes, the cerebral blood vessels constrict, decreasing the volume of the cranial cavity's contents and lowering intracranial pressure. (Objective 17)
5. The cerebral vasoconstriction produced by overly aggressive hyperventilation can reduce blood flow and oxygen delivery to the brain. The alkalosis produced by overly aggressive hyperventilation produces a leftward shift of the oxyhemoglobin dissociation curve that can interfere with off-loading of oxygen from the red blood cells to the tissues. Decreased cerebral oxygenation caused by vasoconstriction and alkalosis can worsen cerebral edema and increase intracranial pressure. (Objective 17)
6. An adult cannot lose enough blood into the cranial cavity to produce hypovolemia. Therefore a patient with a closed head injury who shows signs and symptoms of shock must be bleeding elsewhere. (Objective 15)
7. These terms do not have sufficiently specific meanings to allow healthcare professionals to track changes in a patient's mental status precisely over time. If mental status is described in terms of patient responses to specific stimuli, personnel caring for the patient can easily reproduce the stimulus and observe the patient's response to determine whether the patient's mental status is improving or deteriorating. (Objective 16)
8. IV access for patients at risk for increased intracranial pressure should be obtained using an isotonic crystalloid at a keep open rate. Infusion of excessive amounts of fluid or of hypotonic fluids, which rapidly leave the vascular space and enter the tissues, can worsen increasing intracranial pressure. (Objective 17)

9.

	Pulse Rate	Blood Pressure
Head injury	Decrease	Increase
Neurogenic shock	Decrease	Decrease
Hypovolemia	Increase	Decrease

(Objective 15)
10. Periorbital ecchymosis, bruising over the mastoid process (Battle's sign), clear fluid or blood mixed with fluid draining from the nose (CSF rhinorrhea), clear fluid or blood mixed with fluid draining from the ears (CSF otorrhea). (Objective 11)
11. Patients with basilar skull fracture or mid-face trauma are at risk for fracturing of the cribriform plate that separates the roof of the nasal cavity from the cranial cavity. If the cribriform plate is fractured, a tube inserted into the nasal cavity can find its way into the cranial cavity and penetrate the brain. (Objective 12)
12. Involuntary flexion of the upper extremities and extension of the lower extremities that occurs when a brain-injured patient is stimulated. (Objective 16)
13. Involuntary extension of the upper and lower extremities that occurs when a brain-injured patient is stimulated. (Objective 16)
14. Mannitol is an osmotic diuretic that increases urine output. By removing water from the extracellular space, mannitol can cause a shift of edema fluid from the interstitial and intracellular spaces of the brain into the blood vessels, reducing cerebral edema and decreasing intracranial pressure. (Objective 17)
15. Mannitol is a concentrated solution that tends to form crystals. It should be administered through an IV set that contains an in-line filter to avoid introducing solid crystals of mannitol that could act as emboli into the patient's circulatory system. (Objective 17)
16. Pressure against a lacerated eyeball can cause extrusion of the vitreous humor from the eye and cause loss of eyesight. (Objective 4)
17. When one eye moves, the other eye will follow it, a phenomenon called sympathetic movement. If the patient's uninjured eye is not covered, it will continue to move as it follows changes in the environment. As the uninjured eye moves, sympathetic movement will cause the injured eye to move under the bandage, possibly worsening injury. Covering both eyes limits sympathetic movement. (Objective 4)
18. An orbital blow-out fracture. (Objective 3)
19. A hyphema. (Objective 3)

20. A hyphema is significant because the patient can experience repeated episodes of bleeding with increasing severity into the eye's anterior chamber. Since the eye is a closed compartment, the increased pressure from blood accumulation in the anterior chamber can damage the posterior surface of the cornea, causing loss of eyesight. (Objective 3)

21. You should wash the chemicals from the patient's eyes using water or saline solution. Chemical "antidotes" should never be introduced into the eye because of the damage they can cause. (Objective 4)

22. 1. Loss of the airway.
   2. Cervical spine injury.
   3. Concurrent head injury with possible increased intracranial pressure. (Objective 2)

23. The teeth and dental bridge should accompany the patient to the hospital. The dental bridge will be useful in properly realigning the patient's facial bones during reconstructive surgery. The teeth possibly can be reimplanted. Additionally, all teeth that cannot be accounted for must be assumed to have been aspirated, possibly requiring a bronchosopy to locate and remove them. (Objective 2)

24. Air can enter the cardiovascular system through a laceration in the jugular vein and return to the heart. From the heart, the air can be embolized to the lungs. To prevent entry of air, a laceration involving the jugular vein should be sealed with an occlusive dressing. (Objectives 7, 8)

25. Le Fort I—Separation of the maxilla from the rest of the face. Le Fort II—Fractures through the zygomatic arch separate the maxilla and nasal bones from the rest of the face. Le Fort III—Fractures through the zygomatic arch and the orbits of the eye separate the maxilla, zygoma, and nasal bones from the face. (Objective 2)

26. Cornea, aqueous humor, pupil, lens, vitreous humor, retina. (Objective 3)

27. Intraocular foreign body. (Objective 3)

28. Closed head injury with increased intracranial pressure secondary to an intracranial hematoma. (Objective 15)

MULTIPLE CHOICE

1. A. A loose dressing to both eyes. Pressure should be avoided to prevent extrusion of the vitreous humor. Both eyes should be bandaged to limit sympathetic movement of the injured eye as the uninjured eye moves. (Objective 4)

2. D. Open the airway with cervical spine control, intubate the trachea, ventilate with oxygen using a bag-mask at 20 to 24 breaths/min, stabilize the spine, and transport. The patient's unresponsiveness and unequal pupils indicate the presence of an intracranial hematoma. Controlled hyperventilation (20 to 24 breaths/min) can decrease intracranial pressure and buy time to transport the patient to neurosurgical care. Overly aggressive hyperventilation can decrease oxygen delivery to the brain, causing cerebral edema and increasing intracranial pressure. (Objective 17)

3. C. Epidural hematoma. Initial loss of consciousness, followed by a period of awakening, followed by rapid deterioration is a classic sequence of events that characterizes epidural hematoma. Signs and symptoms of subdural hematoma tend to have a slower onset and progression. Patients with concussion may be unresponsive initially, but they do not deteriorate again once they regain consciousness. Patients with cerebral contusions typically do not display the "lucid interval" that characterizes epidural hematoma. (Objective 16)

4. C. Hyphema is blood in the anterior chamber of the eye. In subconjunctival hemorrhage, blood is present under the conjuctiva, making the white of the eye appear red. Patients with blow-out fractures have double vision, paralysis of upward gaze in the affected eye, numbness of the upper lip on the affected side, and nasal discharge. Patients with detached retinas experience loss of vision, bright flashes, and the sensation of a dark object or "curtain" in their visual field. (Objective 4)

5. B. Alterations in consciousness usually are the earliest sign of an expanding intracranial mass lesion. Pupil changes, central neurogenic hyperventilation, and decorticate or decerebrate posturing occur later. (Objective 16)

6. B. The brainstem functions primarily as the regulator of involuntary activity such as respiration and heart rate. The cerebellum is the center for posture, balance, and equilibrium. The vision and speech centers are in the cerebrum. (Objective 9)

7. C. Cervical spine injuries. Injuries to the mandible, teeth, or facial soft tissues may put the patient's airway at risk. However, any procedures performed to control the airway of a patient with maxillofacial injuries must take the possible presence of cervical spine injuries into consideration. (Objective 1)

8. A. Cover the ears with a loose, sterile dressing. The patient is draining cerebrospinal fluid from the ears. Attempting to stop the flow could increase intracranial pressure if cerebral edema or an intracranial hematoma is present. Irrigating the ears could introduce contaminants into the cranial cavity through a basilar skull fracture. Suctioning the fluid possibly could increase the rate of cerebrospinal fluid loss from around the brain and spinal cord. (Objective 12)

9. B. Level of consciousness is the most reliable indication of a head-injured patient's condition. (Objective 16)

10. A. Extension of the lower extremities and extension with external rotation of the upper extremities describe decerebrate posturing. (Objective 16)

11. B. Extension of the lower extremities and flexion of the upper extremities best describe decorticate posturing. (Objective 16)

12. A. Eye opening, motor response, and verbal response are the elements of the Glasgow Coma Scale. (Objective 16)

13. D. Flush her eyes with water or saline solution. Alcohol and baking soda should never be placed in a patient's eyes. Not flushing the phenol from the patient's eyes immediately could result in blindness. (Objective 4)

14. B. The exposed brain tissue should be protected by covering it loosely with a moist sterile dressing. Because the patient received a hard blow to his head, he also could have a cervical spine injury. (Objective 12)

15. B. A concussion is characterized by a brief period of unconsciousness, absence of neurologic deficits, and loss of memory of the events preceding the injury (retrograde amnesia). (Objective 16)

16. C. A large foreign body impaled in the eye should be left in place and protected with a cup. (Objective 4)

17. D. Gently washing the eye with water or saline solution may remove the object. Rubbing the eye, attempting to blow the object from the eye, or bandaging both eyes and transporting could increase the patient's discomfort and worsen the injury. (Objective 4)

18. A. A patient cannot lose enough blood inside his skull to cause shock. A patient with a closed head injury who displays signs and symptoms of hypovolemic shock is bleeding elsewhere. (Objective 13)

19. B. Applying an occlusive dressing to the laceration to prevent possible air embolism. Encircling the neck with a pressure bandage or compressing the carotid artery could reduce blood flow to the patient's brain. Attempting to clamp bleeding vessels can result in inadvertent clamping of nerves, which tend to follow paths that parallel those of blood vessels. (Objective 8)

20. B. Covered with a moist dressing and protected with a loose bandage or cup. (Objective 4)

21. A. Cervical spine injury should be considered first because this will affect the techniques you use to manage the patient's airway. (Objective 2)

22. D. Open and maintain the airway, immobilize the spine, give oxygen by controlled hyperventilation, and transport. The patient's signs and symptoms suggest the presence of an intracranial hematoma with increasing intracranial pressure. Controlled hyperventilation will decrease intracranial pressure and buy time until a neurosurgeon can treat the patient. Because of the mechanism of injury, a cervical spine injury should be suspected. (Objective 17)

23. B. The best indicator of a head-injured patient's condition is always level of consciousness. (Objective 16)

24. A. P—40 beats/min; BP—210/110 mm Hg; R—36 breaths/min deep, irregular. Cushing's triad—a combination of slowing pulse, rising blood pressure, and altered respiratory pattern—indicates the presence of increased intracranial pressure. (Objective 15)

25. A. Basilar skull fracture can produce periorbital ecchymosis ("raccoon eyes"). Intracranial mass lesions do not produce bruising of the face or scalp. (Objective 11)

26. B. The iris regulates the amount of light entering the eye. (Objective 4)

27. C. The covering of the brain located directly against the brain's surface is the pia mater. Moving outward from the surface of the brain, the brain is surrounded by the pia mater, the subarachnoid space, the arachnoid membrane, the subdural space, the dura mater, and the skull. The pia mater, arachnoid membrane, and dura mater collectively are referred to as the meninges. (Objective 9)

28. A. The cerebellum coordinates posture, balance, and equilibrium. (Objective 9)

29. D. An increased blood pressure and a slow pulse would be present in a patient who is bleeding into his cranial cavity but who has no other injuries. (Objective 13)

30. A. Controlled hyperventilation decreases the $PaCO_2$, which will cause cerebral vasoconstriction and decreased intracranial pressure. (Objective 17)

CASE STUDIES

Case One

1. The clinical presentation of a blow to the head that produces unconsciousness, followed by a lucid interval, followed by rapid deterioration of mental status characterizes an epidural hematoma. (Objective 16)

2. Epidural hematoma usually results from injury to an artery. (Objective 16)

3. The middle meningeal artery is located in a grove on the inner surface of the temporal bone. Fractures of the temporal bone can cross the path of the middle meningeal artery, lacerating it and causing an epidural hematoma. (Objective 16)

4. The "lucid interval" is a classic finding in epidural hematoma. However, not all patients with epidural hematoma have a lucid interval as part of their presentation. (Objective 16)

5. As an epidural hematoma expands, it pushes the temporal lobe of the brain on the affected side down onto the third cranial (oculomotor) nerve. As the oculomotor nerve becomes compressed, it stops conducting impulses to the pupil on the affected side, which dilates. (Objective 16)

6. The patient's pulse rate will slow and the blood pressure will rise. (Objective 16)

Case Two

1. The slower onset of symptoms following a blow to the head suggests an acute subdural hematoma. (Objective 16)
2. Subdural hematoma usually results from an injury to a vein. (Objective 16)
3. Because veins are low-pressure blood vessels, blood accumulates more slowly in a subdural hematoma than in an epidural hematoma. (Objective 16)
4. The aging process results in a loss of brain cells that causes the brain to shrink and occupy less space in the cranial cavity. Because the elderly have a smaller brain mass, there is more room in their cranial cavities in which blood can accumulate before signs and symptoms of increased intracranial pressure appear. (Objective 16)
5. The subdural hematoma most likely is on the left side of the brain, because the patient is presenting with weakness on the right side of his body. Motor control for the right side of the body originates in the left side of the brain and vice versa. (Objective 16)

CHAPTER 48: SPINAL TRAUMA

SHORT ANSWER

1. The mechanism of injury is the most important indication a patient may have a spinal injury. Neurologic signs and symptoms such as weakness, paralysis, paresthesias, and loss of sensation result from injury to the spinal cord. A patient with an injury to the spine and its supporting structures who has not yet sustained injury to the spinal cord may present with no neurologic signs and symptoms. The only indicator that a possible spinal injury might be present may be a mechanism that involves forces and movements that could have damaged the spine. (Objective 3)
2. The modified jaw thrust maneuver should be used to open the airway in a patient with a possible cervical spine injury. By pushing anteriorly on the angles of the mandible, the tongue can be lifted from the pharynx without moving the patient's neck. (Objective 12)
3. If the airway cannot be opened using a modified jaw thrust, a head tilt should be performed. Although there is an increased risk of spinal cord injury when a head tilt is performed, the risks associated with not securing an open airway are greater. (Objective 12)
4. The most important action in managing a patient with possible spinal trauma is restricting the movement of the entire spine by securing the patient to a long spine board, including use of a properly sized cervical collar and head immobilization device. (Objective 12)

5. This patient has central cord syndrome. (Objective 14)
6. Central cord syndrome occurs in patients whose necks are forcefully hyperextended. It is most common among older persons who are developing bony extensions of the vertebrae (exostoses) that extend into the spinal canal, narrowing it. When the neck is forcefully hyperextended, the exostoses push against the spinal cord, compressing the cord and causing damage that concentrates near its center. Because the motor tracts that provide output to the upper extremities lie closer to the center of the cord than the tracts that supply the lower extremities, patients with central cord syndrome display greater loss of motor function in the upper extremities than in the lower extremities. (Objective 14)
7. Brown-Sèquard syndrome is a partial cord injury syndrome causes by a penetrating injury that cuts through the cord on one side only (hemitransection). (Objective 14)
8. A patient with Brown-Sèquard syndrome loses motor function and touch sensation on the same side as the injury to the cord. Pain and temperature perception are lost on the opposite side of the body. (Objective 14)
9. Cauda equina syndrome is a partial cord injury syndrome that occurs with injury to the contents of the spinal canal below the level of the second lumbar vertebra. At L2 the spinal cord ends and the spinal canal is filled with a mass of peripheral nerve tracts called the cauda equina because it resembles a horse's tail. Injury to the spine below the level of L1 or L2 can injure these nerve tracts and produce a pattern of patchy motor and sensory deficits in the lower extremities accompanied by dysfunction of the bladder and bowel. (Objective 14)
10. A patient who is in neurogenic shock will have a decreased blood pressure and a decreased heart rate. Injury to the spinal cord can interrupt the output of the sympathetic nervous system, which arises from the thoracolumbar portion of the cord. Loss of sympathetic tone causes the patient to vasodilate, resulting in decreased peripheral vascular resistance, peripheral pooling of blood, decreased venous return to the heart, decreased preload, decreased cardiac output, and a low blood pressure. Because sympathetic output to the heart is interrupted, an excess of vagal stimulation causes the heart rate to slow. (Objective 14)
11. Because neurogenic shock results from the vascular space being larger than the circulating blood volume, the simplest treatment is to infuse an isotonic crystalloid solution to increase the volume of intravascular fluid. If "topping off the tank" is ineffective, a vasopressor that acts primarily on alpha receptors can be used to decrease the size of the vascular space by producing vasoconstriction. (Objective 12)

12. Spinal cord injury can produce peripheral vasodilation secondary to interruption of the sympathetic nervous system's output. Peripheral vasodilation leads to increased heat loss through the skin surface. (Objective 14)

13. Steroids suppress the inflammatory response that develops whenever tissue damage occurs. One of the components of inflammation is edema that develops because of vasodilation and increased capillary permeability in the injured areas. When structures are located in confined spaces such as the cranial cavity or the spinal canal, inflammatory swelling can worsen injury by creating pressure that resists blood flow and produces ischemia. In these situations, limiting inflammatory response by giving a steroid may be beneficial. (Objective 12)

14. Neurogenic shock secondary to spinal cord injury. (Objective 14)

MULTIPLE CHOICE

1. C. T5 and T10. Sensation at the nipple line comes from sensory nerves that enter the spinal cord at T4. Nerves that enter the cord at T10 provide sensation at the umbilicus. Since this patient has sensation at the nipple line but not at the umbilicus, the injury must be between T5 and T10. (Objective 6)

2. C. C6. Because the patient is breathing with her diaphragm but not with her chest wall, she has an injury below C3, but above T1. Injury above C3 would begin to impair function of the diaphragm while injury at the thoracic level of the spine would preserve some chest wall movement. The positioning of the patient's upper extremities isolates the injury to the level of C6. Damage to the spinal cord at this level interrupts motor function in the upper extremity extensors, but spares upper extremity flexor function. This causes the arms to assume a flexed position. (Objective 6)

3. D. Spinal cord injury with neurogenic shock. This patient is showing the decreased heart rate and blood pressure that characterize neurogenic shock. Absence of sweating caused by the impaired sympathetic nervous system also is typical of neurogenic shock. A closed head injury with increased intracranial pressure would be expected to cause a low pulse rate and elevated blood pressure. Ruptured spleen or aortic tear would produce tachycardia and hypotension. (Objectives 6, 10, 14)

4. C. Spinal cord trauma may damage the sympathetic nervous system, cause vasodilation, and result in increased heat loss. (Objective 14)

5. B. Damage to the sympathetic nervous system caused by a spinal fracture can produce peripheral vasodilation, leading to pooling of blood in the vascular system and a fall in blood pressure. Decreased sympathetic tone secondary to spinal cord injury also can produce a bradycardia and hypothermia because of increased heat loss through dilated peripheral vessels. (Objective 14)

6. B. Maintaining the neck in a neutral position and using a jaw thrust or chin lift is the best way to open the airway when a cervical spine injury may be present. (Objective 10)

7. C. The shock that follows spinal cord injury is due to loss of peripheral vascular resistance caused by decreased sympathetic tone. (Objective 14)

8. C. This patient's entire spine should be immobilized. The mechanism of a fall from a significant height onto both feet and the presence of heel pain suggest that the patient may have an injury pattern called Don Juan syndrome, which includes lumbar spine fracture. Because the spinal column is a stack of blocks that easily transmits energy through itself, a patient with an injury at one level of the spine may have injuries at other levels. Also, the only way to effectively restrict motion in one part of the spine is to restrict the motion of the entire spine from skull to pelvis. Therefore spinal immobilization should be an "all or none" decision. (Objective 12)

9. B. P—62 beats/min; BP—70/50 mm Hg; R—26 breaths/min shallow, regular. A decreased heart rate and a decreased blood pressure are most typical of neurogenic shock. (Objective 14)

10. C. The cervical spine should be stabilized through manual control of the head and neck at the same time the airway is being opened and evaluated. (Objectives 10, 12)

11. A. Mechanism of injury is the most important indication that a patient may have a spinal injury. Neurologic deficits result from damage to the spinal cord, not the vertebral column. Back and neck pain may be present in a nondisplaced fracture or may go unnoticed if the patient has other painful injuries. (Objective 3)

12. A. With any spinal injury, the primary treatment is to keep the entire spine immobilized. (Objectives 10, 12)

13. D. The two most common complications to anticipate in a patient who has a spinal cord injury are neurogenic shock and respiratory paralysis or failure. Spinal cord injury causes shock by producing decreased peripheral vascular resistance, not hypovolemia. Vasodilation associated with spinal cord injury can produce a decreased body temperature. (Objective 14)

14. C. A patient with sensation and movement in the upper extremities but none in the lower extremities would most likely have sustained injury to the lumbar or thoracic spinal cord. Neurologic deficits result from spinal cord injury not injury to the vertebral column. Injury to the cervical spinal cord would cause upper and lower extremity neurologic deficits. (Objectives 6, 7)

15. B. The lumbar spine forms the lower back. (Objective 2)

16. B. Manually stabilize the head and neck and apply a rigid cervical collar. If a patient has a suspected

spinal injury, the entire spine from skull to pelvis should be immobilized. Since placement of a spinal immobilization device can cause movement, particularly of the head and neck, the head and neck should be stabilized initially and throughout the application of the device. (Objectives 10, 12)

17. B. The blood vessels below the injury become dilated and there no longer is enough blood to fill them. Although the heart may slow in neurogenic shock, this is caused by decreased sympathetic tone, not by low blood pressure. (Objective 14)

18. B. If an injury to the head or spinal cord is suspected, you should check for pulses, sensation, and movement in all four extremities to identify any neurologic deficits that may be present. Asking a patient with a suspected spinal injury to move her head could worsen the injury. Having the patient sit up also would be dangerous. (Objectives 10, 12)

19. C. When applying a cervical collar, you should continue manual stabilization until the patient's head can be secured to a back board. The cervical collar must be properly sized following the manufacturer's directions for it to be effective. Most of the population does not require a no-neck collar. However, no-neck collars frequently are applied inappropriately because they fit easily on patients with longer necks. (Objectives 10, 12)

20. A. The damage to the vehicle and the presence of neck and back pain strongly suggest the presence of a spinal injury. The patient needs to be moved to a long board using the "standing takedown" technique to minimize movement of his spine. (Objectives 10, 12)

21. D. Because the thickest part of an infant or small child's body is the head, the necks of these patients tend to flex when they are placed in a supine position. To maintain neutral alignment, padding must be placed under the body to align it with the head and neck. Additional padding between the patient and the long board's straps may be necessary to ensure adequate motion restriction. The head must be secured to the board to ensure adequate stabilization of the entire spine. (Objectives 10, 12)

22. D. A helmet worn by an athlete wearing shoulder pads should be left in place unless they interfere with airway assessment and management, allow for excessive head movement, or prevent proper spinal immobilization. (Objective 12)

CASE STUDY

1. The combination of chest wall paralysis, use of the diaphragm to breathe, and flexion of the upper extremities suggests a cervical spinal cord injury. (Objectives 11, 13)

2. The decreased blood pressure and heart rate suggest the presence of neurogenic shock. Spinal cord injury can interrupt the output of the sympathetic nervous system, which arises from the thoracolumbar portions of the spinal cord. Loss of sympathetic tone produces peripheral vasodilation, which results in peripheral pooling of blood and a drop in blood pressure. Unopposed parasympathetic tone acting on the heart causes the heart rate to slow. (Objectives 13, 14)

3. The diaphragm is innervated by the phrenic nerve, which arises from the spinal cord at the level of C3, C4, and C5. The intercostal muscles are innervated by the intercostal nerves, which arise from the thoracic spinal cord. Injury to the spinal cord at the level of C6 would interrupt the movement of nerve impulses to the intercostal muscles. However, the flow of impulses along the phrenic nerve to the diaphragm would remain intact. (Objectives 13, 14)

4. Loss of sympathetic tone caused by a spinal cord injury allows the vagus nerve to act on the heart unopposed. This results in a decrease in the heart rate. (Objectives 13, 14)

5. The sweat glands normally are activated by the sympathetic nervous system. Interruption of sympathetic output by a spinal cord injury will prevent activation of sweat glands below the level of the injury. (Objectives 13, 14)

6. Decreased sympathetic tone leads to peripheral vasodilation and pooling of blood, which cause a decrease in blood pressure. (Objectives 13, 14)

7. An isotonic crystalloid solution should be used. The patient is hypotensive because her blood volume is not large enough to fill her dilated vascular compartment. An isotonic crystalloid solution will tend to stay in the vascular space, increasing the blood volume to match the size of the vascular compartment and restoring an adequate blood pressure. (Objectives 10, 12)

CHAPTER 49: THORACIC TRAUMA

SHORT ANSWER

1. Ribs 1 through 3 are short, thick structures that are well protected by the shoulder girdle and the muscles of the upper chest. Therefore large amounts of force are required to injure them. These forces also can cause severe damage to the trachea, aortic arch, mainstem bronchi, and superior vena cava, which lie nearby. (Objectives 12, 13)

2. The liver. (Objectives 5, 12)

3. The spleen. (Objectives 5, 12)

4. A patient with penetrating trauma below the nipple line should be suspected of having injuries to structures in both the thoracic and abdominal cavities until proven otherwise. The diaphragm is a dome that attaches to the costal arch anteriorly and rises up into the thoracic cavity. During exhalation, the diaphragm can extend up to the level of the fourth rib, which is approximately the nipple line on males. Therefore penetration of the thoracic wall below the level of the fourth rib can result in damage to both thoracic and abdominal structures. (Objectives 5, 12)

229

5. Paradoxical motion means that a segment of the chest wall is moving in a direction opposite from the motion of the rest of chest wall as a patient breathes. (Objectives 13, 16)

6. Flail chest. (Objectives 13, 16)

7. Although some of the ventilatory failure that occurs with a flail chest is caused by interference with the ability of the chest wall to function as a bellows that moves air in and out of the lungs, most of the problem with gas exchange is caused by the presence of a large pulmonary contusion that always underlies a flail segment. (Objectives 13, 15)

8. The two most important treatments in flail chest are early support of oxygenation and ventilation. Splinting the flail segment by placing something over it or placing the patient on the affected side can reduce the patient's ability to oxygenate and ventilate. (Objective 13)

9. A pulmonary contusion is a bruise of the lung. Leakage of blood into the interstitial spaces of the lung from a pulmonary contusion interferes with gas exchange between the alveoli and bloodstream. Pressure from fluid in the interstitial spaces surrounding the alveoli increases the work of breathing. (Objective 23)

10. Pulmonary contusion should be suspected when blunt force has been applied to the chest wall or when a patient has been involved in a sudden deceleration that could have caused the lungs to impact the inner surface of the chest wall. (Objective 23)

11. A patient with a suspected pulmonary contusion who is hemodynamically stable should not be given large volumes of isotonic crystalloid solution. Vessel damage in the area of the contusion can result in leakage of excessive amounts of IV fluid into the injured area of the lung, worsening problems with gas exchange. (Objective 14)

12. A myocardial contusion is a bruise of the heart muscle. (Objective 31)

13. Dysrhythmias are the most common complication of myocardial contusion. A large myocardial contusion also can reduce ventricular contractility and cardiac output, resulting in cardiogenic shock. (Objective 31)

14. A sucking chest wound should be sealed with an occlusive dressing to prevent the wound from competing with the glottic opening as the primary route for air entry into the chest cavity. (Objective 10)

15. If a patient with a sucking chest wound also has a wound on the lung surface, sealing the wound can place the patient at risk for developing a tension pneumothorax. If a patient with a sealed sucking chest wound develops signs and symptoms of a tension pneumothorax, the occlusive dressing should be unsealed long enough to relieve the pressure from air accumulating in the pleural space. (Objective 10)

16. Subcutaneous emphysema is a crackling sensation that can be felt when air has accumulated in the subcutaneous tissues. (Objectives 7, 23)

17. Subcutaneous emphysema on the chest wall suggests the presence of a pneumothorax. (Objectives 7, 22)

18. A patient with a tension pneumothorax would have prolonged capillary refill, a rapid pulse rate, and a low blood pressure. Pressure from air trapped in the pleural space causes a shift of the mediastinum toward the opposite side of the chest. As the mediastinum shifts, the vena cavae become kinked, decreasing venous return to the heart and lowering cardiac output and blood pressure. (Objective 23)

19. The needle should be inserted just above the lower rib. A neurovascular bundle consisting of a nerve, an artery, and a vein follows the lower margin of each rib. Inserting a needle just below a rib can damage the neurovascular bundle and cause bleeding into the pleural space, causing a hemothorax. (Objectives 14, 26)

20. The mediastinal shift caused by air becoming trapped in the pleural space kinks the vena cavae and slows venous return to the heart. Venous blood unable to return to the heart accumulates in the neck veins, distending them. (Objective 23)

21. Beck's triad consists of distended neck veins, hypotension resistant to fluid administration, and muffled heart sounds. Beck's triad is associated with cardiac tamponade. (Objectives 31, 34)

22. In cardiac tamponade, blood accumulates within the pericardial space, compressing the heart. As the ventricles become compressed, the heart cannot fill completely during diastole and venous return slows. Slowing of venous return results in neck vein distention. (Objective 31)

23. Pulsus paradoxus is a drop in systolic blood pressure on inhalation. Clinically, pulsus paradoxus is indicated by disappearance of the distal pulses on inhalation and reappearance on exhalation. In cardiac tamponade, ventricular filling is reduced by blood in the pericardial space compressing the heart. This decreases ventricular preload, cardiac output, and blood pressure. When the patient inhales, the negative pressure in the thoracic cavity slows the return of blood to the heart through the pulmonary veins. Combined with the effect of the cardiac tamponade of ventricular filling, this drop in venous return during inhalation is sufficient to produce a drop in blood pressure detectable by the disappearance of the distal pulses. When the patient exhales, the positive pressure in the thoracic cavity causes an increase in venous return from the lungs, the cardiac preload and output rise, and the distal pulses return. (Objective 31)

24. The aorta is most likely to tear at the ligamentum arteriosum, which attaches the aortic arch to the pulmonary artery. During a sudden deceleration, the aorta obeys Newton's first law of motion and continues forward within the chest cavity. The ligamentum arteriosum resists the tendency of the aortic arch to move, creating a shearing force that can tear the aorta. (Objective 37)
25. Cardiac tamponade. (Objective 31)
26. Tension pneumothorax. (Objective 23)

MULTIPLE CHOICE

1. C. Simple pneumothorax. A tension pneumothorax would produce distended neck veins and weak, rapid distal pulses. A hemothorax would cause hyporesonance over the affected side. A pulmonary contusion would not produce decreased breath sounds on the affected side and would not cause hyperresonance. (Objectives 22, 23)
2. C. Assist the patient's ventilations with a bag-mask and oxygen; establish an IV with Ringer's lactate tko. The patient's ventilations should be assisted to help overcome the problems with gas exchange that can result from a flail chest. Administration of oxygen by mask alone would not correct ventilatory failure. Since the patient is hemodynamically stable, infusion of large amounts of IV fluid should be avoided because it can accumulate in the contused areas of the lung underlying the flail segment. (Objectives 10, 13)
3. D. Traumatic asphyxia. Traumatic asphyxia results from blunt force trauma being applied to the sternum. As the sternum moves posteriorly, it presses against the right side of the heart, forcing blood backwards into the veins of the head, neck, and shoulders. Engorgement of these vessels with blood accounts for the purplish red coloration of the shoulders, neck, and head found in traumatic asphyxia. (Objectives 18, 19)
4. A. Myocardial contusion. The presence of dysrhythmias in a patient who has suffered blunt force trauma to the anterior chest suggests a myocardial contusion. (Objective 32)
5. B. Hemothorax. A patient with a tension pneumothorax would have distended neck veins, hyperresonance on the affected side, and a tracheal shift away from the affected side. A simple pneumothorax would produce hyperresonance on the affected side. A patient with a cardiac tamponade would have equal breath sounds, diminished heart sounds, and distended neck veins. (Objectives 22, 23)
6. A. Cardiac tamponade. The patient has equal breath sounds bilaterally, which rules out the presence of a tension pneumothorax, simple pneumothorax, or hemothorax. The presence of muffled heart sounds, distended neck veins, and hypotension with a narrowing pulse pressure confirms the presence of cardiac tamponade. (Objective 31)
7. C. Leakage of air into the pleural space through a wound that acts as a one-way valve may produce a tension pneumothorax. (Objective 23)
8. D. Rapid, weak pulse; narrowing pulse pressure; and jugular vein distention are signs of cardiac tamponade. Cardiac tamponade does not produce tracheal deviation or hyperresonance to percussion of the chest wall. (Objectives 22, 23, 31)
9. D. Immediately seal the wound with an occlusive dressing; then assist her ventilations as needed. This patient has a sucking chest wound. The wound must be sealed to prevent it from competing with the glottic opening as the primary route for air movement into and out of the thoracic cavity. (Objective 10)
10. C. Temporarily remove the occlusive dressing. The patient has developed a tension pneumothorax from air that has continued to leak into the pleural space through an injury in the lung after the chest wound was sealed. Removing the dressing temporarily will allow this air to escape, relieving the tension pneumothorax. (Objectives 10, 14, 23, 25)
11. A. Give oxygen, apply an occlusive dressing at the base of the knife, stabilize the knife with a bulky bandage, and transport. The knife should be left in place and stabilized. Since air is moving in and out of the chest cavity through the wound, an occlusive dressing should be placed to reduce the risk of air flowing through the wound, competing with the ability of the patient to move air through the trachea. (Objectives 10, 14)
12. A. Assist the patient's ventilations with oxygen flowing to the bag-mask at 12 to 15 L/min. (Objective 10)
13. C. Subcutaneous emphysema is a crackling sensation causes by the presence of air in the soft tissues. (Objectives 7, 22, 23)
14. D. The presence of subcutaneous emphysema in the tissues of the chest wall suggests the patient may have a pneumothorax. (Objectives 7, 16, 22)
15. A. A condition in which two or more ribs are broken in two or more places and the chest wall lying between the fractures becomes a free-floating segment is flail chest. (Objective 13)
16. B. A lacerated liver or a pneumothorax might be suspected in a patient who has penetrating trauma to the right lateral chest below the nipple line. Because the thoracic and abdominal cavities overlap, trauma to the chest below the nipple line should be assumed to involve both thoracic and abdominal organs until proven otherwise. The stomach is located in the left upper quadrant and would be less likely to be damaged than the liver in penetrating trauma to the right side of the body. (Objective 5)
17. B. Paradoxical movement means that a segment of the chest wall moves in the opposite direction from the rest of the chest cage as the patient breathes. (Objective 13)

18. B. Air in the pleural space is called a pneumothorax. (Objective 23)
19. C. Myocardial contusion. A patient with a pneumothorax or hemothorax would have unequal breath sounds. A patient with a cardiac tamponade would have distended neck veins. Since the most common complication of myocardial contusion is dysrhythmias, the presence of an irregular pulse suggests this patient has a myocardial contusion. (Objectives 7, 32)

CASE STUDIES

Case One

1. Traumatic thoracic aortic aneurysm is suggested by the mechanism of injury (sudden deceleration) and the patient's signs and symptoms. (Objectives 36, 37)
2. Traumatic aneurysms most commonly occur in the descending aorta just distal to the left subclavian artery. During a sudden deceleration, the heart continues to move forward within the thoracic cavity while this portion of the aorta remains fixed in place. This applies a shearing force to the aorta that can result in a tear to the aorta's inner lining. The pressure of blood against this weakened point can cause the aortic wall to balloon outward as an aneurysm. (Objectives 36, 37)
3. The aorta arches over the left mainstem bronchus. An aneurysm forming on the aortic arch can compress the left mainstem bronchus and the left lung, interfering with a patient's ability to ventilate. (Objectives 36, 37)
4. The aneurysm is compressing the patient's esophagus. (Objectives 36, 37)
5. The recurrent laryngeal nerves, which supply the vocal cords, travel downward through the neck into the thoracic cavity and then loop around the mainstem bronchi before traveling upward through the neck to reach the vocal cords. As a thoracic aortic aneurysm pushes downward on the left mainstem bronchus, it places tension on the recurrent laryngeal nerve. This interferes with the functioning of the vocal cords and produces hoarseness. (Objectives 36, 37)

Case Two

1. The tibia fracture is at the bottom of the list of priorities in managing this patient. The patient has several injuries that are compromising his breathing and circulation. These problems must be corrected first before non–life-threatening injuries are addressed. (Objective 26)
2. The patient probably has a tension pneumothorax. Breath sounds are absent on the left. The trachea is deviated away from the left side of the chest. The left lung field in hyperresonant to percussion. (Objectives 22, 23)

3. A patient with a tension pneumothorax would be expected to have distended neck veins. However, this patient also appears to have hemorrhaging into his abdominal cavity. His neck veins are flat because he does not have the intravascular volume necessary for the tension pneumothorax to cause distention. (Objective 23)

Case Three

1. Traumatic asphyxia. Use of this term to describe the persistent purplish red color of the head and neck in patients who have suffered blunt trauma to the chest originated with an early description of the condition that likened the appearance of these patients to that of "one who has been hanged." Traumatic asphyxia is not true asphyxiation. (Objective 19)
2. Blunt trauma to the anterior chest forces the sternum against the right side of the heart, driving blood backward into the veins of the neck, head, face, and shoulders. (Objective 18)
3. Patients with traumatic asphyxia are at risk for myocardial contusion, pulmonary contusion, cardiac tamponade, and injuries to the great vessels, trachea, and mainstem bronchi. (Objective 18)
4. Paradoxical motion. (Objective 13)
5. A flail chest. (Objective 13)
6. Flail chest is accompanied by an underlying pulmonary contusion that interferes with adequate oxygenation and ventilation. (Objective 13)
7. Flail chest and the accompanying pulmonary contusion are managed by assisting the patient's ventilations with high-concentration oxygen. Intubation and positive end-expiratory pressure may be added if necessary to support adequate oxygenation and ventilation. (Objectives 10, 13)
8. The patient has a pulmonary contusion caused by the blunt trauma that produced the flail chest. (Objectives 10, 13)
9. Blood from damaged vessels in the contused areas of the lung accumulates in the pulmonary interstitial spaces. This interferes with diffusion of gas between the alveoli and capillary beds and increases the amount of work that must be done to expand the lungs. (Objectives 10, 13, 15)
10. If the patient is hemodynamically stable, administration of large amounts of IV fluid should be avoided. Excessive fluid can accumulate in the contused areas of the lungs, worsening problems with gas exchange and ventilation. (Objectives 10, 13, 15)
11. Myocardial contusion. (Objective 32)
12. A myocardial contusion can cause dysrhythmias. It also can reduce ventricular contractility and cardiac output, producing cardiogenic shock. Leakage of fluid into the pericardial space from a contused area on the myocardial surface can cause cardiac tamponade. (Objective 31)

CHAPTER 50: ABDOMINAL TRAUMA

SHORT ANSWER

1. Hollow — Appendix
    Hollow — Gallbladder
    Solid — Liver
    Solid — Pancreas
    Solid — Right kidney
    Hollow — Sigmoid colon
    Solid — Spleen
    Hollow — Stomach
    (Objective 3)

2. Right lower — Appendix
    Right upper — Gallbladder
    Right upper — Liver
    Left upper and right upper — Pancreas
    Right upper — Right kidney
    Left lower — Sigmoid colon
    Left upper — Spleen
    Left upper — Stomach
    (Objective 3)

3. Hollow organ trauma leads to spillage of the contents of these organs into the abdominal cavity, resulting in peritonitis. (Objectives 6, 17)

4. Solid organ trauma leads to hemorrhage, resulting in hypovolemic shock. (Objectives 6, 21)

5. Cullen's sign is ecchymosis around the umbilicus, which is associated with bleeding into the abdominal cavity, pancreatitis, and ectopic pregnancy. (Objective 7)

6. Grey Turner's sign is ecchymosis of the flanks, which is associated with bleeding into the abdominal cavity and pancreatitis. (Objective 7)

7. Kehr's sign is abdominal pain radiating to the left shoulder. (Objective 7)

8. Kehr's sign suggests injury to the spleen. Bleeding from splenic damage irritates the inferior surface of the diaphragm on the left side, resulting in pain that radiates to the shoulder. Kehr's sign also can occur in ectopic pregnancy. (Objective 7)

9. The pneumatic antishock garment (PASG) is useful in managing patients with intraabdominal bleeding because it applies uniform pressure to the structures within the abdomen. Bleeding occurs because the pressure outside the opening in a blood vessel is lower than the pressure within the vessel. The PASG raises intraabdominal pressure, slowing or stopping hemorrhage from injured blood vessels. (Objectives 14, 15)

10. A diaphragmatic hernia consists of a portion of an abdominal organ that has passed though a tear in the diaphragm into the thoracic cavity. Diaphragmatic hernia usually results from blunt force trauma to the abdomen that drives the abdominal organs against the inferior surface of the diaphragm. (Objective 37)

11. The PASG should not be applied if diaphragmatic hernia is suspected. Pressure against the abdominal wall can displace more of the patient's abdominal contents through the tear in the diaphragm into the thoracic cavity. (Objective 37)

12. Patients with abdominal trauma or disease processes that produce abdominal pain frequently will have diminished bowel activity and an increased risk of vomiting. Placing anything in the GI tract increases the risk of vomiting and aspiration. Also, since these patients frequently must go to the operating room, giving them anything by mouth increases the risk of aspiration during induction of anesthesia. (Objective 14)

13. This patient probably has an injury to his urethra. The urethra passes though the perineum and can be injured when force is applied to this area by a straddling an object. Bleeding from the damaged urethra collects in the scrotum, producing a hematoma, and moves down the medial aspects of both thighs, producing a pattern called a *butterfly bruise*. (Objective 53)

14. Patients in late-term pregnancy should be transported on the left side. In late-term pregnancy, the fundus of the uterus reaches high enough into the abdominal cavity to lie anterior to the inferior vena cava. If a pregnant patient is placed in a supine position, the uterus will move backwards, compressing the inferior vena cava and decreasing venous return to the heart. Placing the patient on her left side displaces the uterus away from the inferior vena cava. (Objective 51)

15. When a PASG is applied to a patient in late-term pregnancy, only the legs of the garment should be inflated. Inflation of the abdominal segment will displace the uterus onto the inferior vena cava, decreasing venous return to the heart and lowering the mother's cardiac output and blood pressure. (Objective 51)

16. Signs of reversal of hypovolemic shock in a woman who is in late-term pregnancy are not an indicator of adequate fluid resuscitation. When a pregnant patient becomes hypovolemic, the first structure to which blood flow is reduced is the placenta. During resuscitation, the placenta is the last structure to which adequate blood flow is restored. Although an injured pregnant woman may be perfusing adequately, the fetus still may not be receiving adequate blood flow. (Objective 51)

17. Management of a pregnant patient should focus on the mother. Supporting adequate maternal oxygenation, ventilation, and perfusion helps ensure that the fetus is adequately oxygenated and perfused. (Objective 51)

MULTIPLE CHOICE

1. B. Trauma to the lower chest wall on the right frequently is associated with injury to the liver, producing hypovolemic shock. (Objectives 21, 22)

2. D. Presence of hematuria associated with signs of a pelvic fracture suggests this patient has an injured urinary bladder. (Objectives 53, 54)

3. A. Rapid, shallow breathing and a rapid pulse (signs of shock) associated with left upper quadrant pain radiating to the left shoulder (Kehr's sign) suggest injury to the spleen. (Objectives 21, 22)

4. A. The patient would be most likely to have a lacerated liver or a pneumothorax. Because the diaphragm is a dome that rises up into the chest cavity during exhalation, any injury to the chest below the level of the fourth intercostal space should suggest both thoracic and abdominal trauma. Since this patient's injuries are on the right, the abdominal organ most likely to be injured is the liver. (Objectives 3, 4, 37)

5. B. The small intestine and urinary bladder are located below the umbilicus. The gallbladder, liver, stomach, and spleen are all located in the upper abdomen and wound be less likely to be injured by a stab would below the umbilicus. (Objectives 3, 4)

6. C. Eviscerated organs should not be replaced into the body. (Objectives 13, 14)

7. C. Normal saline would be the preferred solution to moisten a dressing for an evisceration. Both $D_{50}W$ and sodium bicarbonate are hypertonic solutions that would remove water from the exposed tissues, damaging them. Distilled water is a hypotonic solution, which would move into the cells of the exposed organ, causing it to become edematous. An isotonic solution like normal saline would keep the eviscerated organ moist without causing fluid shifts. (Objectives 13, 14)

8. D. Injury to the left lower chest wall, signs and symptoms of shock, and pain radiating from the left upper quadrant to the left shoulder suggest injury to the spleen. (Objectives 4, 10)

9. C. Pelvic fracture would be most likely to cause this combination of signs and symptoms. An isolated closed head injury will not produce signs and symptoms of shock. A radius/ulna fracture cannot produce enough blood loss to cause hypovolemic shock. A hemothorax would result in absent or diminished breath sounds on the injured side of the chest. (Objectives 4, 10)

CASE STUDY

1. The highest priority lies with the mother. Supporting the mother's oxygenation, ventilation, and perfusion helps ensure that the fetus is adequately oxygenated and perfused. In the prehospital setting, no interventions are available to directly support the fetus. (Objective 51)

2. The abdominal section of the PASG should not be inflated. Inflation of the abdominal section of the PASG could push the uterus onto the inferior vena cava, decreasing venous return to the mother's heart and dropping her cardiac output and blood pressure. Decreasing the mother's blood pressure would harm the fetus by decreasing placental blood flow. (Objective 51)

3. The patient should be placed on her left side. If she is on a spine board, padding should be placed under the right side of the board to tilt the patient toward her left. Placing the patient on her left side displaces the uterus away from the inferior vena cava. (Objective 51)

4. Signs of adequate perfusion in a pregnant patient being treated for hypovolemia do not indicate that she has been sufficiently resuscitated to ensure adequate blood flow to her fetus. The placenta is one of the last structures to regain adequate perfusion following an episode of hypovolemic shock. (Objective 51)

CHAPTER 51: MUSCULOSKELETAL TRAUMA

MATCHING

1. __A__ Bone ends are crushed or broken into more than two pieces
   __C__ Bone ends are driven together at fracture site
   __B__ Bone is only partially broken on one side
   __D__ Fracture line crosses shaft at an angle other than right angle
   __E__ Fracture line coils through bone like a spring
   __F__ Fracture line is at a right angle to the bone's shaft
   (Objectives 5, 6)

SHORT ANSWER

1. Ball and socket. The head of the femur (a ball) articulates with the acetabulum (a cup-shaped socket in the pelvis). (Objective 3)

2. Hinge. The trochlear notch at the head of the ulna articulates with the trochlea, a spool-shaped structure at the distal end of the humerus. The arrangement of the bones allows movement in only one plane, like the hinge of a door. (Objective 3)

3. Hinge. The articulation of the mandible with the skull is a special type of hinge joint called a condylar joint that primarily allows movement in one plane with a small amount of movement in a second plane. This arrangement permits the movements necessary for chewing. (Objective 3)

4. Ligaments attach bone to bone. (Objective 3)

5. Tendons attach muscle to bone. (Objective 3)

6. The outer fibrous covering of a bone is the periosteum. (Objective 3)

7. The origin of a muscle is the point of attachment of the muscle that does not move when the muscle contracts. (Objective 3)

8. The insertion of the muscle is the point of attachment of the muscle that moves when the muscle contracts. (Objective 3)

9. A fracture is any break in the continuity of a bone. (Objective 4)

10. A dislocation is disruption of the continuity of a joint resulting from displacement of the bones from their normal positions. (Objective 4)

11. The fracture site and the joints proximal and distal to the fracture should be immobilized. Because muscles lying adjacent to a bone may originate above the bone's proximal joint or attach below the bone's distal joint, movement at these joints can create forces against the bone that can displace a fracture site. (Objectives 12, 14)

12. The dislocated joint and the bones proximal and distal to the joint. In practice this means that the joints above and below a dislocated joint also must be immobilized. Because tendons connecting muscles to bones cross a joint, movement of these bones can create forces that can further displace a dislocated joint. (Objectives 12, 14, 17)

13. The principal problem associated with any orthopedic injury is the damage the broken or displaced bone ends do to the surrounding soft tissues. (Objective 6)

14. Hemorrhage leading to severe hypovolemic shock. Injury to the blood vessels lying against the pelvis can cause massive loss of blood into the pelvic cavity. (Objectives 6, 8)

15. A fractured femur can cause up to 2000 mL of blood loss into the thigh at the fracture site. (Objectives 6, 8)

16. A pelvic fracture. A femur fracture. Any open fracture with an associated external arterial hemorrhage (Objectives 6, 8)

17. A traction splint. The traction splint stabilizes the bone ends of a femur fracture by overcoming spasms in the large muscles of the thigh. This limits additional soft tissue damage and hemorrhage at the fracture site. (Objective 18)

18. The splint of choice for an ankle or foot fracture is a pillow. A pillow secured with triangular bandages completely surrounds, supports, and cushions an injury to the foot or ankle. (Objectives 12, 14)

19. This patient's orthopedic injuries should be immobilized by securing the patient to a long spine board. A trauma patient who is in respiratory distress and shock must reach the operating room as quickly as possible. Attempting to apply splints in the field to all of a critical trauma patient's orthopedic injuries can unnecessarily delay transport. Securing the patient to a long spine board will temporarily splint every bone and every joint. (Objectives 11, 14, 17)

20. The knee and the ankle. The knee is the joint above the tibia and fibula, and the ankle is the joint below the tibia and fibula. (Objectives 12, 14)

21. By checking skin color, sensation, movement, and capillary refill in the fingers or toes. (Objectives 13, 14)

22. A sprain is an injury to the supporting structures of a joint. A strain is an injury to a musculotendinous unit. In a sprain, forces move a joint beyond its normal range of motion, stretching or tearing the supporting ligaments. After the displacing forces are removed, the bone ends realign, resulting in a joint that is painful and swollen, but not deformed. In a strain, excessive force applied to a musculotendinous unit causes fibers in the muscle or tendon to tear. The classic finding in a strain is pain on active movement but absence of pain when the injured area is moved passively. (Objective 5)

23. Crepitation is the crackling or grinding that can be felt at a fracture site as the broken bone ends grind against each other. Crepitation should not be actively sought as a sign of a fracture because of the risk of causing additional injury. (Objective 9)

24. A Colles' fracture is a fracture of the distal end of the radius. It also frequently is associated with a fracture of the distal end of the ulna. (Objectives 5, 6)

25. The pneumatic antishock garment or another device that provides circumferential pressure such as a pelvic binder or sheet tied around the pelvis is the preferred way to stabilize a pelvic fracture. (Objectives 6, 7, 14, 17)

26. Greenstick fractures and growth plate fractures are unique to children. Growth plates occur only in the bones of children. The pliant bones of children can bend under pressure rather than breaking, resulting in the pattern of compression on one side and splintering on the other that characterizes a greenstick fracture. (Objective 4)

MULTIPLE CHOICE

1. D. Immobilize the leg as found and transport. If a dislocation is interfering with blood flow to an extremity, a single attempt to realign the extremity and restore circulation is appropriate, particularly in situations where transport may be prolonged. However, if resistance is met, the attempt at realignment should be stopped and the extremity should be splinted as found. Continuing to move an injured extremity after resistance is met can result in worsened injury. (Objectives 12, 14, 17)

2. B. Transport the patient with the leg immobilized as it was found. This patient appears to have a fracture through the neck of the femur, commonly referred to as a "hip" fracture. The injury should be immobilized to limit movement during transport. A traction splint could cause further injury by pulling the bone ends of the fractured femoral neck across each other. Attempting to straighten the leg also could cause further injury. (Objectives 12, 14, 17)

3. B. Cool, pale skin and absent pulses distal to a fracture site indicate occlusion of the extremity's arterial supply. (Objectives 9, 10)

4. A. With the fingers slightly flexed as if holding a baseball. Placing an injured hand in the "position of function" midway between full extension and full flexion minimizes stress on the musculoskeletal structures. (Objectives 12, 14)

5. B. Pillow splint. A pillow splint cushions and supports an injured ankle and foot. A short board splint would be difficult to secure to an injured ankle and would be uncomfortable. A traction splint is

235

indicated for femur fractures. An elastic bandage would not provide as much support as a pillow splint and could compromise circulation if the injured part swells. (Objectives 12, 14)

6. C. Blood loss leading to hypovolemia. A femur fracture can produce up to 2000 mL of blood loss into the soft tissues of the thigh, resulting in hypovolemic shock. (Objectives 12, 14, 18)

7. A. Elevate the leg and apply a cold pack to the injury site. Elevating an injured extremity and applying a cold pack help reduce edema at the site of the injury. Placing an injured extremity in a dependent position or applying heat can worsen swelling or bleeding at the injury site. (Objectives 12, 14, 15)

8. B. In a critical patient, orthopedic injuries can be splinted by securing the patient to a long spine board. Most orthopedic injuries are not immediately life threatening and have a low treatment priority. The principal concern in orthopedic trauma is the damage the bone ends cause to the surrounding soft tissues. Attempting to individually splint orthopedic injuries in a multiple systems trauma patient can unnecessarily delay transport to definitive care in the operating room. (Objectives 11, 12)

9. C. A properly applied splint immobilizes the fracture site and the joints above and below the fracture. Failure to immobilize the joints above and below the fracture can result in excessive movement at the fracture site. (Objective 14)

10. D. The most common complication of fractures and dislocations is injuries to the surrounding soft tissues including peripheral nerves and blood vessels. (Objective 6)

11. D. The goal of applying manual traction to a fractured femur is to stabilize the bone fragments and improve alignment of the limb, limiting soft tissue injury and hemorrhage at the fracture site. A traction splint is applied to stabilize the injured limb, not to reduce the fracture or force the limb back into alignment. (Objectives 12, 18)

12. B. A fracture of the pelvis would be most likely to produce hypovolemic shock. (Objectives 6, 8)

13. C. A sprain is a partial dislocation where ligaments are stretched or torn, but the bone ends realign when the stress is removed. A strain is an injury in which the structures of a musculotendinous unit are stretched or torn. (Objectives 5, 6)

14. D. When applied to an injured extremity, a splint should immobilize one joint above and one joint below the injury. (Objectives 12, 14)

15. C. The three types of muscle tissue are skeletal, smooth, and cardiac. Striated muscle is a synonym for skeletal muscle. Smooth muscle also is called involuntary muscle. (Objective 3)

16. A. A fracture is the same as a broken bone. (Objective 5)

17. B. The flat, cordlike bands of connective tissue that connect bone to bone are ligaments. (Objective 3)

18. A. This is an example of direct violence, because the injury occurred at the point of impact. If the fracture had occurred in the shaft of the femur or at the hip, the mechanism would have been indirect violence. (Objective 2)

19. A. A Colles' fracture is a fracture of the distal radius. (Objectives 5, 6)

20. A. A ball and socket joint attaches the femur to the pelvis at the hip. (Objective 3)

21. B. The traction splint is indicated if the patient has a mid-shaft femur fracture. The traction splint is not indicated in hip fracture because it will not pull along the long axis of the injured bone. The traction splint is contraindicated in pelvic injury because the proximal end of the splint will press against the fractured pelvis. Traction splints should not be applied if a partial amputation is present because the pull of the splint could complete the amputation. (Objective 18)

CASE STUDIES

Case One

1. The patient appears to have a dislocated knee with compression of the popliteal artery that has interrupted blood flow to the distal extremity. (Objective 9)

2. One attempt to realign the limb is indicated, particularly if transport times are likely to be lengthy. Early restoration of blood flow will limit damage to structures in the distal extremity. (Objectives 12, 20)

3. If the limb will not realign easily, it should be splinted in the position in which it was found, and the patient should be transported immediately. (Objectives 12, 20)

Case Two

1. The patient probably has fat embolism syndrome. (Objective 5)

2. Fat embolism syndrome is associated with long bone fractures, particularly fractures of the femur. (Objectives 6, 18)

3. Early application of traction to femur fractures has been shown to reduce the incidence of fat embolism syndrome. (Objectives 6, 18)

Case Three

1. This patient's knee was hyperextended, resulting in a temporary dislocation that spontaneously reduced itself. (Objective 6)

2. No; hyperextension of the knee frequently is associated with injury to the popliteal artery, which lies just posterior to the knee joint. Patients with this injury may appear to have intact distal circulation initially, but may later develop a thrombus at the site of injury that can compromise blood flow to the extremity. (Objectives 6, 12)

3. The patient should be transported to a facility that has the diagnostic imaging capabilities necessary to determine whether a popliteal artery injury has occurred. (Objectives 6, 12)

CHAPTER 52: ENVIRONMENTAL CONDITIONS

SHORT ANSWER

1. An environmental emergency is a medical problem that is caused or worsened by the effects of temperature, weather, terrain, or atmospheric pressure. (Objective 1)
2. Age, poor general health, fatigue, predisposing medical conditions, medications. (Objective 3)
3. Homeostasis is the body's ability to maintain a stable internal environment. (Objective 7)
4. Conduction, convection, radiation, evaporation, respiration. (Objectives 10, 12, 13)
5. Temperature regulation is centered in the hypothalamus. (Objectives 10, 12, 13)
6. Sweating and peripheral vasodilation. (Objectives 10, 12, 13)
7. Vasoconstriction, shivering, and voluntary movement of large muscles to create heat. (Objectives 10, 12, 13)
8. The heat-regulating mechanisms of the elderly do not respond as rapidly as those of younger persons. The elderly have fewer sweat glands than younger persons. They are less able to vasoconstrict and vasodilate than younger people because of peripheral vascular disease. They have a diminished thirst drive, so they frequently are mildly dehydrated. They frequently are on fixed incomes and do not adequately cool their dwellings because of concerns about cost. (Objectives 3, 15, 21, 26)
9. Diuretics, beta-blockers, antihistamines, psychotropics. (Objectives 3, 15, 21)
10. Diabetic clients develop autonomic neuropathy, a condition that decreases the ability of the autonomic nervous system to respond to changes in core temperature. (Objectives 3, 15, 21)
11. (A) This patient has classic heat stroke. (Objective 33) (B) Your primary objective in managing this patient is to rapidly lower his body temperature to 102 F. (Objective 33)
12. A patient with an exertional heat stroke will have warm, moist skin rather than warm, dry skin. (Objective 27)
13. If cooling is continued after the body temperature reaches 102 F the patient is at risk for becoming hypothermic. (Objective 33)
14. (A) Heat exhaustion. (Objective 33) (B) Assess airway, breathing, and circulation. Move the patient to a cool environment. Place the patient in a supine position with his lower extremities elevated. Give high-concentration oxygen using a nonrebreather mask. If the patient can drink, administer dilute sports drink to rehydrate him. If he cannot take fluids orally, establish an IV with normal saline. (Objective 33)
15. (A) Heat cramps. (Objective 24) (B) Assess airway, breathing, and circulation. Move the patient to a cool environment. Have the patient consume a dilute sports drink to restore serum sodium to normal levels. The muscles should not be massaged because this can trigger cramping. Heat cramps do not always require transport to the hospital. If the patient is to be released on scene, he should be instructed to avoid the heat and to salt his food more heavily than usual for the next 24 hours. (Objective 24)
16. Giving water without supplemental salt to a patient with heat cramps can lower the sodium concentration in the extracellular fluid and worsen cramping. (Objective 33)
17. Pediatric patients have a large surface-to-volume ratio, which increases the rate at which they lose heat. Children and infants also have less subcutaneous fat to insulate themselves from heat loss. Because children have a smaller muscle mass than adults, they cannot generate as much heat by shivering. (Objective 36)
18. The body temperature regulating mechanisms of the elderly do not respond as rapidly as those of younger persons. They are less able to vasoconstrict and vasodilate than younger people because of peripheral vascular disease. The elderly have lower metabolic rates than younger people and therefore generate less body heat. They may be malnourished, which decreases heat production. They frequently are on fixed incomes and do not adequately cool their dwellings because of concerns about cost. (Objective 36)
19. Alcohol causes peripheral vasodilation, which speeds heat loss. Alcohol also interferes with shivering, decreasing the ability to produce heat. By decreasing the level of consciousness, alcohol interferes with the ability of the patient to self-rescue by moving to shelter. (Objective 36)
20. (A) The patient is hypothermic. (Objective 43) (B) The patient's ventilations should be assisted with a bag-mask and oxygen, if possible using warm, humidified oxygen. The patient should be moved to a warm environment. His wet clothing should be removed, and he should be wrapped in blankets to prevent further heat loss. The ECG should be monitored. An IV should be established with normal saline. If a gag reflex is absent, an endotracheal tube should be placed to secure the airway. (Objective 43) (C) Hypothermic patients who are unresponsive or not responding appropriately should not be actively rewarmed. Cold exposure causes peripheral vasoconstriction that produces tissue ischemia and anaerobic metabolism. Active rewarming of the periphery can cause a return of lactic acid and potassium from the periphery to the body core, triggering cardiac dysrhythmias and depressing myocardial function. As blood flows into the cold

peripheral tissue, it will cool. When this blood returns to the central circulation, it can cause a drop in core temperature. (Objective 43)

21. Patients who become hypothermic before experiencing cardiac arrest have an increased probability of surviving. CPR should be performed using standard rates and ratios. If ventricular fibrillation is present, an initial shock may be given. Further shocks and medication administration should be delayed until the patient is rewarmed to a body temperature above 86° F. The patient may be intubated and ventilated with warmed, humidified oxygen. When the body temperature exceeds 86° F, ACLS medications may be administered; however, dosing intervals should be increased to compensate for slower metabolism of drugs. (Objective 42)

22. Frostbitten body parts should not be rubbed. Ice crystals form in frostbitten tissue. Rubbing a frostbitten area will move the ice crystals in the tissues, causing mechanical trauma and worsening the injury. (Objectives 50, 51)

23. 102° to 104° F. (Objectives 50, 51)

24. The patient should be transported to the hospital for observation. Aspiration of freshwater can damage the alveolar-capillary membrane and remove surfactant from the alveoli. These effects can lead to delayed pulmonary edema and ventilatory failure in patients who initially survive a near-drowning. Additionally, aspiration of large amounts of freshwater can cause hemolysis, electrolyte disturbances, cardiac dysrhythmias, and renal failure. (Objectives 58, 59, 60)

25. In addition to hypoxia, acidosis, and aspiration of water, the patient also may have a head injury, a neck injury, and hypothermia. (Objectives 58, 59, 60)

26. The patient probably has an arterial gas embolism. (Objectives 66, 67, 69, 71, 73)

27. When air is breathed under pressure using SCUBA apparatus, nitrogen becomes dissolved in the blood plasma and other body fluids. If the diver surfaces too rapidly, nitrogen comes out of solution and forms bubbles. Bubbles in the joint spaces and in the capillary beds of the large muscles cause musculoskeletal pain known as "the bends." Nitrogen bubbles in the capillary beds of the brain can cause strokelike signs and symptoms. Nitrogen bubbles in the spinal cord can cause paraplegia or quadriplegia. Rapid bubbling of nitrogen in the bloodstream can clog the pulmonary circulation, resulting in respiratory failure ("the chokes"). (Objectives 63, 64, 65)

28. Nitrogen narcosis is a state of altered mental status and impaired judgment that results from breathing nitrogen gas under pressure during deep SCUBA dives. (Objectives 67, 68)

29. Headache, nausea, vomiting, altered mental status, ataxia, and occasionally focal neurologic signs. (Objectives 81, 83)

30. Dry cough, mild shortness of breath on exertion, slight pulmonary crackles. Can progress to severe dyspnea, cough productive of frothy sputum, coma, death. (Objectives 80, 83)

MULTIPLE CHOICE

1. B. Heat loss by the movement of air over the surface of the body is called convection. (Objectives 10, 11)

2. B. Frostbitten tissue should not be thawed if there is a risk of refreezing. Dry, sterile dressings should be used to cover frostbitten areas. If a decision is made to rewarm frostbitten tissue, rewarming should take place rapidly using warm water. (Objectives 50, 51)

3. A. Heat is generated within the body by cellular metabolism and physical activity. (Objectives 10, 11)

4. D. The most effective means of cooling patients with heat exhaustion is to place them in an air-conditioned environment. Patients suffering from heat exhaustion can still sweat, so covering them with a wet sheet is unnecessary. (Objective 32)

5. C. The temperature control center of the body is located in the hypothalamus. (Objectives 10, 12, 13)

6. A. Medications should be given to hypothermic patients at longer intervals because they will be metabolized more slowly. (Objective 42)

7. B. The person at greatest risk for classic heat stroke, assuming the environment's temperature and humidity are high, would be a 65-year-old male with a history of type 1 diabetes who is taking a walk outside. (Objective 21)

8. C. Mild alterations of mental status are most likely to occur in a patient who has heat exhaustion. (Objectives 24, 25)

9. A. The patient probably is suffering from classic heat stroke. Classic heat stroke tends to occur in patients with chronic health problems that interfere with the body's ability to remove heat. Classic heat stroke is characterized by altered mental status and hot, dry skin. (Objective 27)

10. B. The most important action in treating a patient with heat stroke would be to begin cooling the patient immediately. (Objectives 32, 33)

11. D. You should begin CPR immediately and transport. Following submersion in cold water, the effects of hypothermia and the mammalian diving reflex can increase the time during which a patient may be successfully resuscitated. Patients who are severely hypothermic must be rewarmed slowly from the body's core outward. (Objectives 42, 43)

12. B. Because of the transport time to a hospital, rewarming the patient's frostbitten hands would be appropriate. Rewarming should take place rapidly. Once frostbitten tissues are thawed, they should never be allowed to refreeze. (Objectives 50, 51)

13. C. *Active* external rewarming techniques are indicated for hypothermia patients who are responding appropriately. (Objectives 38, 43)

14. A. *Passive* external rewarming techniques are indicated for hypothermia patients who either are not responding appropriately or are unconscious. Actively rewarming a patient who is severely hypothermic can promote the return of cold, acidotic blood from the periphery to the body's core, lowering core temperature and depressing myocardial function. (Objectives 38, 43)

15. A. Carotid pulse assessment should be performed for as long as 30 to 45 seconds. If a pulse is felt during that time, chest compressions should not be performed. (Objective 42)

16. B. Deep cold injury (frostbite) should be covered with dry dressings. If jewelry is present, it should be removed. Hot packs should not be applied to frostbitten tissue. Frostbitten tissue should not be rubbed. (Objectives 46, 50, 51)

CASE STUDIES

Case One

1. The patient is suffering from heat exhaustion. (Objective 24)

2. The patient's skin is cool and pale because his sympathetic nervous system has been activated in response to inadequate perfusion. Increased sympathetic tone is producing peripheral vasoconstriction. (Objective 24)

3. A patient develops heat exhaustion because the combination of volume loss from sweating and vasodilation in an attempt to radiate away excess heat creates a situation in which the blood volume is inadequate to fill the vascular space. The tachycardia is an attempt to circulate the remaining blood volume more rapidly to maintain adequate perfusion. (Objective 24)

4. Patients with heat exhaustion are usually hypotensive. This patient has a systolic blood pressure above 90 mm Hg. However, she has a history of hypertension. A systolic blood pressure of 100 mm Hg probably is significantly below normal for her. (Objective 24)

5. Heat exhaustion is caused by a combination of vasodilation and volume loss from sweating that results in hypoperfusion. (Objective 24)

6. A patient suffering from heat exhaustion will have a body temperature that is normal or possibly slightly below normal. (Objective 24)

7. Patients with hypertension are at increased risk of developing heat exhaustion because they frequently take diuretics and vasodilators that potentiate the effects of heat exposure on the body. (Objective 21)

8. Assess the patient's airway, breathing, and circulation. Move her to a cool environment. Place her in a supine position with her lower extremities elevated. Give high-concentration oxygen by nonrebreather mask. If the patient can drink, give her diluted sports drink to replace lost fluid volume. If she cannot drink because of nausea or altered mental status, establish an IV. Monitor ECG. Transport to the hospital. (Objective 33)

Case Two

1. The patient is suffering from heat cramps. (Objective 24)

2. Patients with heat cramps do not have altered mental status. Patients with heat exhaustion do. (Objective 24)

3. Heat cramps are caused by excessive loss of sodium from the body in sweat. Heat exhaustion is caused by loss of intravascular fluid volume and vasodilation. (Objective 24)

4. The muscle spasms in heat cramps are caused by hyponatremia (low serum sodium concentration). (Objective 24)

5. The patient should be moved to a cool environment. He should be given diluted sports drink to replace lost sodium. The muscles should not be massaged because this can trigger cramping. Heat cramps do not always require transport to the hospital. If the patient is to be released on scene, he should be instructed to avoid the heat and to salt his food more heavily than usual for the next 24 hours. (Objective 24)

6. Drinking large amounts of pure water would worsen this patient's muscle cramps by further decreasing the concentration of sodium in the extracellular fluid. (Objectives 24, 31)

Case Three

1. This patient is suffering from frostbite. (Objectives 44, 46, 49)

2. Exposure to subfreezing temperatures causes peripheral vasoconstriction, which decreases delivery of heat from the body core to the most distal portions of the circulation. As the peripheral tissues cool, ice crystals form in the interstitial spaces, drawing water out of the cells. The ice crystals expand, damaging tissue. Drawing of water from the cells increases intracellular electrolyte concentrations, further damaging the cells. (Objectives 44, 51)

3. The affected area should not be thawed if there is any possibility of refreezing. After administering analgesia, immerse the frostbitten areas in water warmed to 102° to 104° F. Warm water will have to be added frequently during the thawing process. The thawed parts should be covered with a loosely applied dry, sterile dressing. The affected area should be kept elevated to reduce edema. Blisters should not be punctured or drained. (Objectives 50, 51)

4. If transport times are short, the affected areas should be bandaged with dry, sterile dressings, and the patient should be transported to the hospital for rewarming under controlled conditions. (Objectives 50, 51)

5. The patient should not rub or slap his hands together. Rubbing or massaging frostbitten tissue moves the ice crystals about in the interstitial spaces, worsening tissue damage. (Objectives 50, 51)

Case Four

1. The patient has an arterial gas embolism. (Objective 67)
2. When a patient is using SCUBA, she is breathing air that is at the same pressure as the surrounding water. If the patient holds her breath while surfacing, expansion of the pressurized air in the alveoli can tear the alveolar walls, allowing air to enter the pulmonary circulation. The air returns to the left side of the heart where it is pumped into the systemic circulation. If air bubbles enter the circulation of the patient's brain, they can block the capillary beds and cause a stroke. (Objectives 63, 66)
3. Assess the patient's ABCs. Administer high-concentration oxygen using a nonrebreather mask. Keep the patient in a supine position to help ensure adequate cerebral blood flow. Establish a keep open IV. Check the blood glucose level. Monitor the ECG. Consult with medical control about possible administration of steroids to reduce cerebral edema. If the patient deteriorates rapidly and shows signs of increasing intracranial pressure (ICP), controlled hyperventilation can be used to decrease ICP. The patient should be transported to a hyperbaric chamber for recompression to drive the air bubbles clogging her cerebral circulation into solution so they can pass through the capillary beds. (Objective 73)

Case Five

1. The patient has decompression sickness. (Objectives 64, 65)
2. When a patient uses SCUBA, nitrogen gas dissolves under pressure in the blood and other body fluids. If the patient does not surface slowly to give the dissolved nitrogen an opportunity to escape through the lungs, nitrogen bubbles will form in the interstitial spaces and bloodstream. (Objective 63)
3. In an arterial gas embolism, air bubbles enter the bloodstream from tears in the alveolar walls caused by rapid expansion of pressurized gas. In decompression sickness, nitrogen dissolved under pressure in the extracellular fluid forms bubbles as the diver ascends. To be at risk of decompression sickness, a diver must descend to a depth of greater than 33 feet, the equivalent of 1 additional atmosphere of water pressure. An arterial gas embolism can occur if a diver holds his/her breath while surfacing from any depth of water. (Objective 63)
4. The Navy Dive Tables used by SCUBA divers to time their ascent from dives to allow adequate decompression are based on the assumption that the diver will remain near sea level for at least 24 hours following the last dive. Divers who fly shortly after

their last dive may develop decompression sickness even though they followed the Dive Table recommendations precisely. (Objective 63)
5. Assess the patient's airway, breathing, and circulation. Keep the patient in a supine position. Administer high-concentration oxygen using a nonrebreather mask. Establish a keep open IV with an isotonic crystalloid. Consult with medical control about administration of steroids to decrease the inflammation in the central nervous system triggered by nitrogen bubbles in the tissues. Transport the patient to a hyperbaric chamber for recompression. (Objective 73)

Case Six

1. The patient has high-altitude cerebral edema (HACE). (Objectives 81, 82, 84)
2. At high altitudes, unacclimatized persons increase their respiratory rates to compensate for the decreased partial pressure of oxygen in the inspired air. The increased respiratory rate causes increased carbon dioxide removal from the body, resulting in metabolic alkalosis. Metabolic alkalosis causes a leftward shift in the oxyhemoglobin dissociation curve, which results in inadequate tissue oxygenation. Hypocarbia also results in periodic episodes of respiratory arrest while the patient sleeps, producing hypoxia. Hypoxia produces cerebral vasodilation, resulting in increased intracranial pressure. Hypoxia also damages the capillary walls causing fluid to leak into the interstitial spaces of the brain, producing cerebral edema. (Objectives 76, 81, 82, 86)
3. The patient should be given high-concentration oxygen and moved to a lower altitude immediately. Administration of steroids should be considered to reduce cerebral edema. (Objectives 76, 81, 82, 86)

Case Seven

1. The patient has high-altitude pulmonary edema (HAPE). (Objectives 80, 82, 84)
2. The patient should be given high-concentration oxygen and moved to a lower altitude. If her respiratory function deteriorates, CPAP or intubation with PEEP can be used to maintain adequate oxygenation. (Objectives 76, 80, 82, 86)
3. Morphine and Lasix are not indicated in the management of HAPE. (Objective 85)
4. HAPE is a noncardiogenic pulmonary edema caused by increased capillary permeability. Morphine and Lasix are useful in managing pressure pulmonary edema associated with volume overload and decreased left ventricular function. Giving morphine to a patient with HAPE can worsen his/her condition by depressing the respiratory drive and worsening hypoxia. Administration of Lasix can cause hypovolemia, worsening the dehydration that tends to occur at high altitude. (Objective 85)

SHORT ANSWER

1. Farmers typically are independent individuals who rely on their own resources and those of their neighbors before requesting outside help. Also, they frequently will transport themselves or have a relative drive them rather than waiting for an ambulance. This combination of factors means that when EMS is called the situation typically is a severe one that has not been managed successfully with the resources immediately available to the farm family, and that a significant amount of time already has passed before outside help was summoned. (Objective 1)

2. Tractors and other machinery. (Objective 1)

3. When a large tissue mass is compressed, blood flow and oxygen delivery decreases. Anaerobic metabolism in the tissues results in production of lactic acid. As acidosis worsens, potassium moves from the intracellular space to the extracellular space, producing hyperkalemia. As muscle tissue begins to die, myoglobin leaks into the bloodstream and begins to be filtered into the urine by the kidney. When myoglobin enters the acidic environment of the kidney's filtering tubules, it precipitates and clogs the tubules, causing renal failure. As long as tissues are compressed, release of lactic acid, potassium, and myoglobin into the circulation is slowed. Sudden restoration of circulation by removing a crushing force can rapidly introduce these toxic substances into the circulation, resulting in myocardial failure, dysrhythmias, shock, and renal failure. (Objective 2)

4. Normal saline solution is preferred because it can be used to replace extracellular fluid volume without adding potassium, which would worsen the hyperkalemia already present in crush syndrome. (Objective 2)

5. Correction of lactic acidosis. Creation of a mild alkalosis that displaces potassium back into the intracellular space, correcting hyperkalemia. Alkalinization of the urine, which decreases the tendency of myoglobin to precipitate in the tubules of the kidney. (Objective 2)

6. The ECG may show widening of the QRS complex and increased amplitude of the T wave. Both of these abnormalities are produced by hyperkalemia. (Objective 2)

7. Muscles are surrounded by layers of fascial tissue that form compartments. If a muscle is injured and swells, the pressure inside the fascial compartment can exceed the pressure in the vessels supplying the compartment's contents with blood. Oxygenated blood cannot enter the fascial compartment and waste products cannot exit. Damage occurs to the muscle and the blood vessels and nerves within the affected compartment. (Objective 3)

8. Application of a cold pack and elevation of the affected extremity can help lower pressure within the affected fascial compartment. Surgery frequently is required to relieve the pressure. (Objective 3)

9. Physical distention of tissues, which compresses blood vessels and causes ischemic necrosis. Chemical irritation, which leads to inflammatory edema and further vascular compromise. Secondary bacterial infection, which leads to inflammatory edema and further vascular compromise. (Objective 4)

10. Skin absorption. (Objective 5)

11. Organophosphates inhibit the action of acetylcholinesterase, which normally breaks down the neurotransmitter acetylcholine. Inhibition of acetylcholinesterase results in a buildup of acetylcholine in the synapses of the parasympathetic nervous system and at the neuromuscular junction. Excessive stimulation of muscarinic receptor sites by acetylcholine causes the classic SLUDGE syndrome of cholinergic crisis (*s*alivation, *l*acrimation, *u*rination, *d*efecation, *g*astrointestinal cramping, and *e*mesis) as well as bradycardia and constricted pupils. Buildup of acetylcholine at the neuromuscular junction causes muscle twitching followed by weakness and paralysis. (Objective 5)

12. Atropine blocks the effects of excess acetylcholine at the muscarinic receptor sites and reverses the SLUDGE syndrome as well as increasing the heart rate. (Objective 5)

13. The definitive antidote for organophosphate toxicity is 2-PAM (pralidoxime), which reactivates acetylcholinesterase by uncoupling the organophosphate molecule from it; however, atropine is considered the mainstay therapy, particularly in the prehospital setting. (Objective 5)

14. Carbamates also are acetylcholinesterase inhibitors, and they produce a clinical picture similar to that of organophosphate toxicity. However, carbamates spontaneously uncouple themselves from acetylcholinesterase over time. Therefore carbamate toxicity is managed by giving atropine and waiting for the patient's acetylcholinesterase to reactivate. 2-PAM is not administered in carbamate poisoning. (Objective 5)

15. Oxygen should not be given to patients who have been poisoned by Paraquat. Paraquat tends to concentrate in the lung cells that produce surfactant. Administration of oxygen accelerates Paraquat's toxic effects on these cells. (Objective 5)

16. Silo gas is a reddish brown gas consisting of nitrogen dioxide and nitrogen tetroxide that accumulates as a result of fermentation of plant material in silos. (Objective 6)

17. Silo gas is most likely to be present if the material in the silo has been fermenting for a period of 3 weeks or less. (Objective 6)

18. At moderate concentrations, silo gas does not cause sufficient acute discomfort to cause workers to leave environments where it is present or to hold their breath. As the gas is inhaled into the lower airway, it reacts with water to form nitric acid, which causes a chemical burn to the airway walls and the alveoli. This can result in severe pulmonary edema 6 to 12 hours after exposure. (Objective 6)

19. Anhydrous ammonia reacts with water on the mucous membranes of the airway, the surface of the eye, and the skin to form ammonium hydroxide, which causes alkali burns to the tissue. The high affinity of anhydrous ammonia for water also causes water to be pulled from the tissues, resulting in cell death and tissue necrosis. Exposure to anhydrous ammonia can cause blindness (from necrosis of the eyeball), burning of the upper airway (which results in edema and obstruction), bronchospasm, and chemical burns of the lower airway (which cause pulmonary edema). (Objective 6)

20. After taking appropriate steps to avoid exposing themselves, the rescuers should undress the patient and decontaminate the skin using large amounts of water. The eyes also should be irrigated with large amounts of water or saline solution. If signs of impending upper airway obstruction (stridor, hoarseness, drooling) are present, an endotracheal tube should be placed. Albuterol should be administered if bronchospasm is present. Assisted ventilation with positive end-expiratory pressure may be necessary if pulmonary edema occurs. The pulmonary edema present following exposure to anhydrous ammonia is noncardiogenic in origin and should not be treated with nitroglycerin, morphine, or furosemide. (Objective 6)

21. Hydrogen sulfide is most likely to be present in pits under barns and feed lots that are used to collect manure for use as fertilizer. The hydrogen sulfide present in this environment is referred to as "manure gas." Hydrogen sulfide sometimes also is referred to as "rotten egg gas" because of its distinctive odor. (Objective 6)

MULTIPLE CHOICE

1. D. Most serious injuries and deaths on farms are caused by tractors and other machinery. (Objective 1)
2. D. Crush syndrome should be suspected if a patient has had a large muscle mass compressed for longer than 60 minutes; the syndrome is considered to exist if the patient has been entrapped for 4 to 6 hours. (Objective 2)
3. D. Sodium bicarbonate should be given to correct acidosis and to decrease the risk of renal failure. Normal saline is the preferred IV fluid in crush syndrome because it does not contain potassium and will not worsen hyperkalemia. IVs should be started on patients suffering from partial crush syndrome and adequate extracellular fluid volume should be restored before the patient is freed from entrapment. (Objective 2)
4. C. Swelling from hydraulic injection injury typically begins 1 to 3 hours post injury. Typically there is little or no pain at the time the injury occurs. Injection can occur at distances of several inches from the hydraulic fluid leak because of the extremely high pressures involved. Surgery typically is required to correct the problem. (Objective 4)
5. D. The patient is displaying SLUDGE syndrome, which indicates exposure to an organophosphate. (Objective 5)
6. C. The excess salivation, incontinence, and pupillary constriction are due to increased parasympathetic tone caused by an excess of the neurotransmitter acetylcholine. (Objective 5)
7. A. The patient should be given atropine to block the effects of acetylcholine and reverse the SLUDGE syndrome and bradycardia. The pinpoint pupils and slow respirations are a result organophosphate poisoning, not a narcotic overdose, so the patient will not respond to Narcan. The crackles and rhonchi are due to overproduction of pulmonary secretions caused by increased parasympathetic tone, not to volume overload from heart failure. Therefore furosemide is not indicated. Flumazenil antagonizes the effects of benzodiazepines and could be dangerous in this case since patients suffering from organophosphate poisoning are at risk of having seizures. (Objective 5)
8. B. 2-PAM (pralidoxime) is the definitive antidote for organophosphate poisoning. (Objective 5)
9. A. Death in Paraquat poisoning usually results from respiratory failure caused by destruction of the surfactant-forming cells in the lungs. Paraquat poisoning typically takes place by ingestion rather than absorption. Cases of poisoning by absorption usually involve either exposure to large amounts or contact with broken skin. Oxygen administration will worsen the effects of Paraquat poisoning by accelerating the damage to the surfactant-producing cells. Paraquat ingestion can result in significant gastrointestinal fluid losses and electrolyte imbalances that should be corrected with IV fluids. (Objective 5)
10. B. Because most farms are exempt from OSHA inspection, farmers often do not follow OSHA-mandated confined space entry procedures. However, EMS personnel and other rescuers are not exempted from following all applicable safety standards during confined space rescues on farms. (Objective 6)
11. B. Breathing moderate concentrations of silo gas will produce few immediate symptoms followed by inflammation of the lower airway and pulmonary edema 6 to 12 hours later. (Objective 6)
12. B. Hydrogen sulfide or "manure gas" is characterized by an odor like rotten eggs. (Objective 6)

242

Answer Keys

CASE STUDY

1. Because of the prolonged transport time, a helicopter should be called. In cooperation with the fire department officer-in-command, a decision should be made about requesting additional heavy-duty rescue equipment as needed to lift the tractor. (Objective 2)

2. Movement of personnel and equipment through the muddy field will be difficult. Four-wheel-drive vehicles available on the farm could be used to move personnel and equipment to and from the site of the tractor overturn. (Objectives 1, 2)

3. The tractor needs to be shut off and stabilized. Any leaks of fuel or other fluids from the tractor should be secured. If the tractor was applying any chemicals to the field, they should be identified and appropriate steps should be taken prevent or manage spills. (Objective 2)

4. Because of the nature and length of entrapment, the patient probably is suffering from crush syndrome. Before any attempts are made to move the tractor, IVs should be established with normal saline and fluid should be infused to replace any volume losses and ensure adequate urine output. Sodium bicarbonate should be administered to correct acidosis and hyperkalemia and minimize the risk of myoglobin precipitating in the filtering system of the kidney. The patient's body temperature should be assessed because he is at risk for hyperthermia, and appropriate steps should be taken to keep him cool. Because the patient may have suffered pelvic and lower extremity fractures, arrangements should be made to stabilize these structures with a spine board and appropriate splinting devices (pelvic binder, pneumatic anti-shock garment) when the tractor is removed. (Objective 2)

5. All personnel will have to be monitored closely for heat stress and volume depletion. Steps will have to be taken to ensure stable footing around the patient and tractor. Spine boards or pieces of plywood could be used to prevent personnel from sinking or tripping in the mud. (Objectives 1, 2)

6. Because of the remote location of the incident, a helicopter should be requested. Extrication of the patient should be coordinated with the arrival of the helicopter so that time between removal of the tractor and initiation of transport is minimized. (Objectives 1, 2)

CHAPTER 54: WILDERNESS EMS

SHORT ANSWER

1. Wilderness medicine is medical management of situations where care and prevention are limited by environmental considerations, prolonged extrication, or resource availability. (Objective 1)

2. A wilderness EMS system is a formally structured organization, integrated into or part of the standard EMS system, configured to provide care in austere environments. (Objective 2)

3. Prolonged patient care, austere or hostile environments, minimal resources, delays in comprehensive care. (Objective 3)

4. The practice environment of wilderness EMS differs from that of traditional EMS in the following ways:
   - Increased environmental hazards for patients and caregivers
   - Increased complexity in accessing and removing patients
   - Decreased availability of resources
   - Increased duration of care
   - Longer transport times
   - Increased demands for high-level operational and medical decision making

   (Objective 3)

5. EMS personnel providing care in wilderness areas must have offline protocols that allow them to provide an expanded range of interventions needed to care for patients in extreme environments for extended periods of time. These offline protocols must be combined with access to online medical control for support during unanticipated or complex, dynamic situations. Specific areas not considered in traditional EMS protocols that must be addressed in protocols for wilderness EMS include:
   - More liberal criteria for clearing spinal injuries
   - Packaging to prevent pressure ulcers during prolonged transport
   - Patient waste elimination
   - Patient protection against extremes of heat and cold during prolonged extrication and transport
   - Hydration and nutrition for patients during prolonged extrication and transport
   - Management of intravenous therapy (fluid and electrolyte balance) over extended time periods
   - Wound cleaning and closure
   - Antibiotic therapy
   - Reduction of dislocations
   - Removal of impaled objects
   - Management of analgesia over extended time periods
   - Criteria for termination of resuscitation and pronouncement of death

   (Objective 4)

6. Personnel who provide wilderness EMS must be trained to provide a broader range of care necessary to manage patients over extended time periods in settings where resources are limited. Additionally, they must be prepared to protect themselves and their patients from the effects of extreme environments. However, there is no national standard curriculum that defines the knowledge and skill necessary for providing wilderness EMS and only two states provide formal certification for EMS personnel who practice in wilderness areas. Multiple private organizations provide training and certifications relevant to EMS practice in wilderness environments. EMS personnel must evaluate the quality and reputation of sponsoring organizations carefully. (Objective 5)

7. Wilderness EMS is provided in austere environments where equipment must be carried to the patient over long distances and then carried out along with the patient. These factors limit the amount of equipment available to EMS personnel and require equipment to be smaller, lighter, and, when possible, usable for multiple purposes. Much of the equipment required to provide wilderness EMS involves vehicles and gear needed to access the patient, including all-terrain vehicles, helicopters, boats, high-angle and swift water rescue equipment, and hiking equipment such as packs and footwear. (Objective 7)

8. Wilderness EMS generally is characterized by reduced availability of resources. While wilderness EMS personnel may have increased access to aircraft, rescue gear, and extended care equipment, problems with access and egress may limit the usefulness of these resources. A patient often can be reached and removed only on foot, significantly increasing the number of personnel required for wilderness EMS operations. (Objective 8)

9. Wilderness EMS personnel must interface with a larger number of other providers during the course of patient care. Increased interaction creates more opportunities for conflict, miscommunication, and errors and demands more sophisticated systems for command and coordination. (Objective 9)

10. The National Park Service, Department of the Interior; the Department of Defense; the National Disaster Medical System, Department of Health and Human Services; Urban Search and Rescue Task Forces, Federal Emergency Management Agency, Department of Homeland Security. (Objective 10)

11. National Ski Patrol, Mountain Rescue Association, National Cave Rescue Commission, Diver Alert Network, National Association for Search and Rescue. (Objective 10)

12. Absence of a coordinating or certifying body at the national level and in most states. Philosophical and political disputes over whether a society has a responsibility to rescue and care for persons who voluntarily enter wilderness areas. Philosophical and political disputes over responsibility for the costs of rescuing and caring for persons injured in wilderness areas. Shortages of paramedics and park rangers. Increasing interest in outdoor and wilderness activities as a form of recreation. A heavy dependence on volunteers and the impact of this dependence on system sustainability. (Objective 11)

MULTIPLE CHOICE

1. B. Including a physician or other healthcare provider within a group that is going into a wilderness area for an extended time is an example of expedition wilderness medicine. (Objective 1)

2. C. Professional wilderness medicine involves individuals or groups that preplan to provide care in austere environments and then are called on to perform this duty when needed. The term *professional* includes both volunteer groups and groups that are compensated for their services. (Objective 1)

3. D. The paramedic providing care to the injured hiker is an example of the recreational model of wilderness medicine. (Objective 1)

4. B. Maine and Maryland currently provide formal certification in wilderness medicine. (Objective 1)

5. B. The National Disaster Medical System includes Disaster Medical Assistance Teams, Disaster Veterinary Assistance Teams, and Disaster Mortuary Response Teams. Urban Search and Rescue Task Forces are not part of the National Disaster Medical System. (Objective 10)

CHAPTER 55: ASSESSMENT-BASED MANAGEMENT

SHORT ANSWER

1. Assessment-based management is delivery of patient care based on the information obtained from evaluation of the scene and from the history and physical examination rather than simply applying a protocol to the patient's chief complaint. At times, assessment-based management requires deviating from or modifying a protocol. In essence, assessment-based management is treating the patient rather than the protocol. (Objective 1)

2. Protocols must be based on the assumption that a patient has only a single disease process producing his/her chief complaint and has no other factors that would complicate or contraindicate the treatments prescribed in the protocol. Unfortunately, patients frequently suffer from multiple disease processes and take a variety of medications that could make strict application of the treatment outlined in a protocol ineffective or dangerous. (Objective 1)

3. Pattern recognition is use of combinations of signs and symptoms that typically accompany a disease process to rapidly identify a patient's problem. (Objective 1)

4. Pattern recognition allows a paramedic to rapidly identify the problem(s) producing a patient's chief complaint by matching the patient's clinical presentation to the pattern of signs and symptoms associated with specific disease processes. (Objective 1)

5. Sources of information to support practice of assessment-based management include the patient's history and physical exam findings, any diagnostic studies available in the field, family members, bystanders, and the environment. (Objective 1)

6. Pattern response is the specific set of therapies that should be performed to provide care to a patient who presents a particular clinical picture. For example, a patient with squeezing substernal chest pain associated with nausea, diaphoresis, and shortness of breath generally should be managed with high-concentration oxygen, ECG monitor, an IV, aspirin, a 12-lead ECG, nitroglycerin, and morphine. A patient complaining of shortness of breath that awakened her as well as crackles in both lung bases and pedal edema generally should be managed with high-concentration oxygen, assisted ventilations, ECG monitor, an IV, a 12-lead ECG, nitroglycerin, furosemide, and morphine. (Objective 9)

7. Effective assessment-based management involves matching a pattern of signs and symptoms indicating a particular disease process with a pattern of therapies that are appropriate for that disease process. A practitioner who is skilled in assessment-based management is like a master chess player who sees the pattern of pieces on the board (the clinical picture) rather than analyzing the positions of individual pieces (a list of signs and symptoms). (Objective 9)

8. Because assessment-based management is based on recognition of patterns and clinical pictures, a paramedic must be able to present patient information in a way that allows other practitioners to see the same clinical picture as the paramedic. Effective presentation ensures that all personnel responsible for the patient's care are working from the same impression of the patient's problem(s). Since assessment-based management sometimes involves deviating from or modifying protocols, a paramedic must have excellent presentation skills to justify changes in standard patient care procedures to an online medical control physician. (Objectives 8, 13)

9. Tunnel vision is an error in clinical reasoning that involves making a diagnosis prematurely and then refusing to acknowledge assessment findings that contradict that diagnosis. (Objectives 3, 5)

10. Tunnel vision interferes with effective assessment-based management because it prevents the practitioner from seeing elements of the clinical picture that are essential to identifying and correcting the patient's true problem. (Objectives 3, 5)

11. The inverted pyramid approach to clinical reasoning involves using a patient's chief complaint to generate a list of possible problems that could be producing that complaint (a differential diagnosis) and then using the results of the history and physical exam to eliminate problems from the list until one problem (the working or "field" diagnosis) remains. (Objective 1)

12. The inverted pyramid approach helps prevent tunnel vision by forcing a practitioner to consider a wide range of possible field diagnoses that could produce the patient's chief complaint rather than quickly focusing on one problem. (Objectives 1, 5)

13. Personal attitudes, uncooperative patients, lack of patient compliance, distracting injuries, environmental distractions, personnel distractions. (Objectives 3, 4)

14. Assessment by committee is the practice of having multiple personnel asking the patient questions and performing physical examination procedures simultaneously. Assessment by committee is not an effective practice because it fragments the clinical picture necessary for pattern recognition and assessment-based management. (Objective 8)

15. I. Scene size-up
II. Primary survey (initial assessment)
 a. General impression
 b. Level of consciousness (AVPU)
 c. Airway
 d. Breathing
 e. Circulation
 f. Disability (brief neurologic examination)
 g. Expose and examine
III. Secondary survey
 a. History (focused or detailed)
 b. Physical examination (focused or head-to-toe)
IV. Reassessment (ongoing assessment)
(Objective 12)

16. Patient contact, history, physical exam, presents patient, handles documentation, EMS command. (Objective 9)

17. Scene cover, scene information, talks with bystanders, vital signs, performs interventions, triage officer. (Objective 9)

18. Every 15 minutes. (Objective 12)

19. Every 5 minutes. (Objective 12)

CASE STUDIES

Part One

1. A focused assessment of the injured hand should be performed. The patient is a stable trauma patient with an isolated injury.

2. A more detailed assessment should be performed. Although this trauma patient appears to be stable, the mechanism of injury suggests she may have more extensive injuries than are immediately obvious.

3. A focused assessment of the cardiovascular system should be performed. This is a conscious medical patient who is able to provide a chief complaint and history that suggest a cardiovascular problem.

4. A more detailed assessment should be performed. This appears to be an unresponsive medical patient, although trauma cannot be completely ruled out. Because the patient cannot provide a chief complaint to focus the exam, a detailed exam is necessary to obtain the information needed to develop a field diagnosis. (Objective 12)

Part Two

1. Congestive heart failure with pulmonary edema.
2. Acute myocardial infarction.

3. Cerebrovascular accident with increased intracranial pressure secondary to a subarachnoid hemorrhage.
4. Cardiac tamponade.
5. Preeclampsia.
6. Tension pneumothorax.
7. Hypovolemic shock.
8. Neurogenic shock secondary to spinal cord injury.
9. Chronic obstructive pulmonary disease (emphysema) with a spontaneous pneumothorax.
10. Pulmonary embolism. (Objective 2)

Part Three

1. Administration of nitroglycerin should be deferred because of recent use of an erectile dysfunction drug. Administration of nitrates to a patient who has recently taken an erectile dysfunction drug can produce severe hypotension. Because the patient has signs of right-sided heart failure and ECG findings suggesting a right ventricular infarction, his preload should be augmented by infusion of an isotonic crystalloid before giving morphine or any other vasodilating drug. Administration of a vasodilator to a patient with right ventricular failure can produce hypotension. Expansion of intravascular volume to augment preload can counteract this effect. Because of the history of asthma and the presence of wheezing, administration of metoprolol should be deferred, or the dose should be reduced and titrated to the minimum needed to decrease the heart rate. Concurrent administration of an inhaled $beta_2$ agonist should be considered. Although metoprolol is $beta_1$ selective, it still has the potential to worsen bronchospasm in patients with asthma and chronic obstructive pulmonary disease. (Objectives 2, 8)

CHAPTER 56: CLINICAL DECISION MAKING

SHORT ANSWER

1. Paramedics carry out the same tasks as other clinicians in uncontrolled and unpredictable environments under circumstances that do not exist in other clinical settings and without information gathered from laboratory results or diagnostic images. (Objective 1)
2. Patient acuity is the severity of a patient's condition. (Objective 2)
3. Critically life-threatening, potentially life-threatening, non–life-threatening. (Objective 2)
4. Protocols, standing orders, and patient care algorithms provide precompiled, standardized approaches to patient care that reduce the need to process large amounts of data and recall critical information in stressful situations. (Objective 3)
5. Protocols, standing orders, and patient care algorithms address only "classic patients." They must be based on the assumption that a patient has only one problem and does not have other disease processes or is not taking medications that would

complicate or contraindicate the steps directed by the protocol. (Objective 3)
6. The hormones released during the fight-or-flight response can improve reflexes and increase concentration and focus on the situation. (Objective 5)
7. The hormones released during the fight-or-flight response can interfere with the ability to analyze large amounts of data from multiple sources and to think critically about a situation. The stress hormones predispose the brain to tunnel vision. (Objective 5)
8. A reflective thinking style involves taking the time to thoughtfully, analytically, and deliberately work through a situation to the best solution. (Objective 4)
9. Reflective thinking is most appropriate in complex situations where a patient is stable and in no acute distress. (Objective 4)
10. An impulsive thinking style means reacting instinctively to a situation without stopping to reflect. (Objective 4)
11. Impulsive thinking is most appropriate in life-threatening situations where immediate action is required. (Objective 4)
12. A paramedic with an anticipatory thinking style approaches patient management by assuming that the patient is always going to progress to the next step in the evolution of his/her disease process and that the treatment being performed is not going to correct the problem. A paramedic with an anticipatory style is like a chess player who is always thinking at least one move ahead. (Objective 4)
13. Stress tends to narrow focus and interfere with critical thinking skills. Practicing technical skills until they can be performed at a pseudo-instinctive level without thinking, frees additional thinking capacity that can be called on during a crisis to help reason through a complex situation to an appropriate solution. (Objective 4)
14. Gather data and form a concept about the patient, scene, and situation. Interpret the data to develop a field diagnosis. Apply your protocols and the principles of medicine to devise a management plan. Evaluate the effectiveness of your plan. Reflect on your field diagnosis and patient management plan as a way to improve management of future cases. (Objectives 4, 6)
15. *R*ead the scene, *r*ead the patient, *r*eact by determining the nature of the problem, and treating accordingly, *r*eevaluate, *r*evise the management plan, *r*eview your performance. (Objectives 4, 6)

MULTIPLE CHOICE

1. D. A positive effect of the sympathetic nervous system response on clinical decision making is that this response narrows the paramedic's focus of attention, improving concentration on the decision-making task. However, this effect also can predispose paramedics to tunnel vision in complex, high-stress situations. (Objective 5)

2. B. In medicine, the term *acuity* refers to the severity of the patient's condition. (Objective 2)
3. D. A clinical policy that allows giving nitroglycerin to a patient with cardiac chest pain without contacting online medical control is an example of a standing order. (Objective 3)
4. C. A 20-year-old male involved in a motor vehicle crash with a heart rate of 100 beats/min would have the lowest acuity. The other patients display an alteration of mental status, respiratory function, or cardiovascular function that could indicate a life-threatening problem. (Objectives 2, 6)

CASE STUDIES

Case One

1. In spite of her low heart rate the patient appears to be perfusing well; therefore her low heart rate probably is not a source for immediate concern. It would be helpful to determine the type of track or field event in which she competes. If she is a long distance runner or another type of endurance athlete, her low heart rate definitely can be attributed to good conditioning and ignored in favor of dealing with her injured ankle as the primary problem. (Objectives 2, 4, 6)

Case Two

1. The patient has altered mental status, cool skin, and prolonged capillary refill. All of these signs indicate poor perfusion. He also has abdominal pain in the left upper quadrant and pain referred to an uninjured left shoulder. Along with the mechanism of a lateral impact to the driver's side of the vehicle, these findings suggest an injury to the spleen. However, the patient does not have the tachycardia that normally would be present with internal bleeding. He also has a blood pressure in the normal range. It would be helpful to determine if this patient is being treated for hypertension using beta-blockers. Patients with hypertension become dependent on their elevated blood pressure to maintain adequate tissue perfusion. They can be severely hypoperfused at what appear to be "normal" blood pressures. Because beta-blockers antagonize the effects of epinephrine and norepinephrine on the heart, a patient receiving beta-blocker therapy will not develop a tachycardia, even with severe volume loss. (Objectives 2, 4, 6)

CHAPTER 57: GROUND AND AIR TRANSPORT OF CRITICAL PATIENTS

MATCHING

1. __A__ At a constant temperature, the volume of a gas is directly proportional to its pressure.
   __B__ At a constant pressure, the volume of a gas is inversely proportional to its temperature.
   __D__ The amount of gas dissolved in a liquid is proportional to the partial pressure of the gas.
   __C__ The total pressure of a gas mixture is the sum of the partial pressures of the gases making up the mixture.

SHORT ANSWER

1. Rapid transport in situations in which time required for ground transport poses a threat to the patient's survival. Access to remote areas. Access to specialty units such as neonatal intensive care units and burn centers. Access to personnel with specialized skills. Access to specialty supplies and equipment. (Objective 5)
2. Weather and environmental restrictions to flight. Limitations on patient weight. Limitations on number of patients that can be transported. High cost. Difficulties delivering patient care because of limited access, limits on amounts of equipment and supplies, and restrictions on lighting. (Objective 5)
3. Decreased partial pressure of oxygen. Atmospheric pressure changes. Thermal changes. Decreased humidity. Noise. Vibration. Fatigue. (Objective 7)
4. Early hypoxia will produce confusion, restlessness, and anxiety. (Objective 7)
5. The areas of the body affected most by pressure changes as an aircraft changes altitude are the gastrointestinal tract, lungs, sinuses, and ears. (Objective 7)
6. Barosinusitis, also called sinus block, occurs when persons with acute or chronic inflammation of one or more of the paranasal sinuses experience a change in atmospheric pressure. Inflammation of the passage-ways connecting the sinuses to the nasal cavity prevents the air in the sinuses from equalizing its pressure with the atmosphere during pressure changes, resulting in severe pain. The pain typically occurs during descent. (Objective 7)
7. The aircraft should reascend until pressure between the sinuses equalizes with that of the atmosphere followed by a more gradual descent. Inhaled vasoconstrictors such as phenylephrine can be used to open the inflamed sinus passageways. (Objective 7)
8. A patient who is only 6 hours status post bowel resection is unlikely to have normal peristalsis in the gastrointestinal tract. The patient should have a nasogastric tube in place that is vented to ambient air or low intermittent suction. The nasogastric tube will help prevent expansion of any gases present in the patient's inactive bowel. The colostomy bag should be emptied and adequately vented before flight to prevent rupture of the bag by expanding gases trapped in it. (Objective 8)
9. During flight, patients can be given earplugs to limit the effects of noise. However, the earplugs must be removed before the aircraft descends or negative pressure can pull the earplugs toward the tympanic membrane. (Objective 8)

10. Vibration transfers mechanical energy to the patient's tissues, where it is degraded into heat. This can produce an increase in body temperature, metabolic rate, and carbon dioxide production. (Objective 8)

11. A flare or a vehicle with its headlights on low beam should be used to mark each corner of the landing zone with a fifth marker placed on the upwind side. At night a light should never be directed toward a helicopter because of the risk of temporarily blinding the pilot. (Objective 8)

12. Describe your position relative to the helicopter—for example, "Air 1, we are at your nine o'clock position." This will tell the pilot you are to his left near the midline of the aircraft. Describing positions relative to your location are not useful because the pilot does not know where you are in relationship to his or her aircraft. (Objective 8)

13. A helicopter should be approached from the front. This allows the pilot to keep you in sight. (Objective 8)

14. The area of greatest danger is at the rear of the aircraft where the tail rotor is located. A spinning tail rotor is almost invisible. Except during operations involving helicopters that load from the rear, personnel should never go beyond the aircraft's three o'clock to nine o'clock line and should never cross under the ship's tail boom. (Objective 8)

15. Having the fire department apply a light water fog to the landing zone to wet the dirt can reduce the size of the dust cloud created by the rotor wash. (Objective 8)

MULTIPLE CHOICE

1. D. A landing zone for a helicopter should be 100 by 100 feet (Objective 8)
2. C. The landing zone should be 100 to 200 feet downwind from the patient care area. (Objective 8)
3. C. Any bystanders, livestock, or motor vehicles should be a minimum of 200 feet from the landing zone. (Objective 8)
4. A. The slope of the surface of a helicopter landing zone should not exceed 5 degrees. (Objective 8)
5. A. As air cools it holds less moisture; therefore as altitude increases, humidity decreases. (Objective 7)
6. C. Civilian use of helicopters for medical transport grew out of benefits demonstrated by the military during the Korean War. (Objective 1)
7. C. Fixed-wing aircraft generally used for patient transport when transport distances exceed 100 miles. (Objective 5)
8. B. The first step taken to manage a patient who develops signs and symptoms of hypoxia during flight should be to administer high-concentration oxygen. (Objective 7)

CHAPTER 58: EMS DEPLOYMENT AND SYSTEM STATUS MANAGEMENT

SHORT ANSWER

1. System status management is the art and science of matching the production capacity of an emergency medical services system to the changing patterns of demand placed on that system. (Objective 1)

2. Fixed station (static) deployment and full (flexible) deployment are the two primary ambulance deployment strategies. Some EMS systems use a mixed deployment strategy that combines features of static and flexible deployment. (Objective 3)

3. Fixed station or static deployment places ambulances and personnel at stations within designated service areas. All stations typically are staffed 24 hours a day, 7 days a week. Staffing levels remain constant, with the same number of ambulances and personnel available at the same locations at the same times. (Objective 3)

4. Demand for emergency medical services can fluctuate dramatically according to day of week and time of day (temporal demand) as well as location within the EMS system's service area (geospatial demand). As call volume fluctuates through the day, there are times when the system is underutilized and times when it may be overwhelmed. As people change locations throughout the day, changes in population density produce changes in call locations. If ambulances continue to respond from fixed locations, prolonged response times to some requests for service may result. (Objective 4)

5. Full or flexible deployment uses computer-aided dispatch to shift ambulances throughout the system's service area, following changing temporal and geospatial demand. Rather than being dispatched from fixed stations, ambulances respond from "posts" that move throughout the service area based on requests for service. Fluid deployment frequently is combined with peak-load staffing, which varies the number of ambulances and personnel available based on predicted call volume for the time of day and day of week. (Objective 3)

6. By placing more ambulances closer to locations where requests for service are likely to be generated, flexible deployment shortens response times. Combined with peak-load staffing, which keeps available only the number of ambulances and personnel needed to meet projected demand for service, flexible deployment decreases system costs and improves efficiency. (Objective 4)

7. Because systems using flexible deployment operate ambulances from posts rather than stations and shift post locations based on projected demand, personnel in these systems can spend significant amounts of time sitting in their vehicles or driving throughout their service areas. This can lead to decreased morale and productivity. (Objective 4)

8. A unit hour consists of a fully equipped and staffed vehicle available or on assignment for 1 hour. (Objective 5)

9. Unit hour utilization (UhU) is a measure of ambulance service productivity and staff workload calculated by dividing the number of unit hours available during a period of time by the number of responses or number of transports during the same period of time. (Objective 5)

10. Flexible deployment tends to decrease response times at the expense of crews being in their units moving throughout their service areas for longer periods of time. Combining flexible deployment with peak-load staffing, which increases the number of ambulances and personnel available to respond during periods when demand is higher, can decrease stress on crews. This strategy decreases the number of responses and post moves by crews during peak-load periods. Some systems have established a maximum number of calls to which a crew is expected to respond during a shift. Other systems provide amenities such as CD players and televisions for crews that must spend extended time periods "on post." (Objective 5)

MULTIPLE CHOICE

1. A. This system is using a fixed deployment strategy because it is operating units from stations rather than from posts that change locations based on demand. In a system with flexible or full deployment, units shift position throughout the service area based on projected demand rather than responding from stations. Mixed deployment strategies combine fixed and flexible deployment. (Objective 3)

2. C. The system 120 unit hours available during a 24-hour shift. 24 hours × 5 units = 120 unit hours. (Objective 5)

3. A. The unit hour utilization-transport (UhU-T) during a 24-hour shift for the EMS system described in the previous question is 0.3. 36 transports/120 unit hours = 0.3 transports/unit hour. (Objective 5)

4. D. The unit hour utilization-response (UhU-R) during a 24-hour shift for the EMS system described in the previous question is 0.5. 60 calls/120 unit hours = 0.5 calls/unit hour. (Objective 5)

5. B. The UhU-T for this crew is 0.25. 3 transports/12 unit hours = 0.25 transports/unit hour. (Objective 5)

6. C. The UhU-R for the crew in the previous question is 0.33. 4 calls/12 unit hours = 0.33 calls/unit hour. (Objective 5)

7. D. The unit hour utilization-time deployed (UhU-TD) for the crew in the previous question is 0.66. 4 calls + 4 post changes/12 unit hours = 8/12 = 0.66. (Objective 5)

CHAPTER 59: CRIME SCENE AWARENESS

SHORT ANSWER

1. You do not upset the family by attracting unnecessary attention to their situation. You avoid attracting a crowd, which can lead to a less stable and less safe environment. You avoid warning persons on the scene of your impending arrival and disturbing the scene. (Objective 3)

2. Request that the communications center place a call back to the number to determine if anyone will answer. Request an immediate response by the police. Do not approach the house. (Objective 3)

3. Park at least 15 feet back from the vehicle with the ambulance angled to the left 10 degrees and the front wheels turned all the way to the left. This position places the cover provided by the ambulance's engine block and wheels between you and the vehicle. It also creates a safe zone along the driver's side of the vehicle where the ambulance shields you from traffic moving on the roadway. (Objective 3)

4. Concealment is something that can hide you from view, but that will not stop bullets. (Objective 6)

5. Cover is something that will stop bullets. (Objective 6)

6. The engine block and the wheel rims. (Objective 6)

7. Stand on the doorknob side of the door in line with the door's frame. You are in less danger if someone decides to shoot through the door. Anyone opening the door must lean out to make contact with you. (Objective 3)

8. Knock on the door; then quickly retreat several feet until someone answers. (Objective 3)

9. The contact provider knocks on the door and makes the initial contact with the occupants. The cover provider stays back several feet in a position where he/she can scan the scene for hazards, and, if necessary, escape to obtain help. (Objective 6)

10. Ask them to lead you to the patient. This avoids the danger associated with strangers (you and your partner) surprising the patient in his bedroom. (Objective 3)

11. Domestic disputes are dangerous because the parties involved in the dispute may both turn on EMS personnel or law enforcement officers who attempt to intervene in their dispute. (Objective 5)

12. Law enforcement. The primary role of EMS is to provide care to any persons injured during the dispute. (Objective 5)

13. Ask them to please remain where you can see them. If they refuse and leave your sight, immediately leave the scene. There is a high risk they may return with a weapon. Following them is not a good idea since you may be out of contact with your partner and unable to warn him/her or escape from a dangerous situation. (Objective 5)

14. Tell your patient it is time to go to the hospital, and immediately leave the scene. (Objective 5)

15. Leave the scene anyway. Request a response by the police. Thoroughly document the fact that you attempted to get the patient to accompany you but that you left the scene because you feared for your personal safety. (Objective 5)

16. Arrange to meet with the responding police officers to brief them on the situation before they enter. (Objective 5)

17. Evidence is anything that can be used to connect a suspect to a victim, a victim to a suspect, or a suspect to the scene of a crime. (Objective 7)

18. It is impossible to go anywhere without leaving evidence that you were there and without taking evidence with you. (Objective 7)

19. A crime scene is a location where any part of a criminal act took place and all routes for entering and leaving that location. Since EMS personnel must access locations where criminal acts took place to provide patient care, they are passing through the crime scene long before they reach the patient. As they move through the crime scene, they may disturb or destroy evidence. (Objective 7)

20. Cut around, rather than through, bullet or knife holes. Avoid shaking the clothing or turning the clothing inside out. Place it in a paper or cloth bag. Avoid letting it come into contact with clothing removed from other victims. Turn it over to a law enforcement officer as quickly as possible. (Objective 7)

21. Cover the patient's hands with paper bags or loose gauze bandages to protect any skin or blood under the fingernails. (Objective 7)

22. Airtight containers promote growth of molds and bacteria that can destroy evidence. (Objective 7)

23. If at all possible, they should avoid washing or using the toilet until they can be examined at the hospital. An exam at the hospital may be able to recover evidence that can identify the assailant. (Objective 7)

24. Because first statements are made in an excited state without consideration of their consequences, they may represent events more accurately than statements made at a later time. (Objective 7)

25. Debris left on a crime scene by EMS personnel can be interpreted by law enforcement officers as evidence and disrupt the progress of an investigation. (Objective 7)

26. Because a drug laboratory is a hazardous materials hot zone, you should not risk spreading contamination by returning to your ambulance. Leave the lab with your patient and call for the fire department hazardous materials team and the police. Wait on the scene until you and your patient can be decontaminated. (Objective 5)

27. Transport the patient immediately. Advise the hospital you are en route with a contaminated patient. The patient, your ambulance, you, and your partner will need be decontaminated on arrival at the hospital. (Objective 5)

28. Medical monitoring of fire department and law enforcement personnel working in the hot zone. (Objective 5)

MULTIPLE CHOICE

1. C. Cover will stop bullets; concealment will hide the rescuer, but not stop bullets; the box of the ambulance provides concealment; the ambulance engine block provides cover. (Objective 6)

2. D. When you knock on the door of a residence or apartment, the best position to be in is to the side of the door, opposite the hinges (the doorknob side). In this position, you are in less danger if someone shoots through the door. When the door is opened, the occupant will have to lean out of the door to see you if you stand on the doorknob side. (Objectives 3, 6)

3. C. Your best response to this situation should be to leave the scene immediately whether or not the patient is willing to go with you. Following an angry individual is not a good idea since you may find yourself alone with a person who now has a weapon. Physical restraint is not appropriate because you or your partner is not being attacked. Attempting to restrain one party in a domestic dispute can trigger an attack by the other party. If you fear for your personal safety, you are not obligated to remain with a patient who refuses to leave the scene with you. (Objective 5)

4. B. At this point the best course of action would be to move both patients to a safe distance from the structure but not to the ambulance, call for a fire department hazardous materials' team response, and remain on the scene until the HAZMAT team arrives. You have been called to a clandestine drug lab, which means you and your partner now have been inside what must be considered a hazardous materials' hot zone. Returning to your ambulance would place the ambulance inside the hot zone. Because the male patient has minor injuries, you can wait for the HAZMAT team to decontaminate you, your partner, and both patients. (Objective 5)

5. D. An appropriate strategy for managing this situation would be to show respect to the bystanders and acknowledge their concern for the patient. Openly disrespecting gang members will result in retaliation against you and other members of your organization. Move the patient to the ambulance immediately, transport, and assess and treat the patient en route to the hospital. Attempting to treat a gang member in the open is very dangerous. Remaining on scene in the ambulance also is dangerous because his fellow gang members may decide to "encourage" you to transport. You should avoid cutting the patient's shirt or bandana if at all possible because his "colors" are a mark of his membership in the gang. Damaging "colors" shows disrespect to the gang and invites retaliation. (Objective 5)

CHAPTER 60: DISPATCH ACTIVITIES

SHORT ANSWER

1. The communications center serves as the first point of contact in the continuum of patient care. It controls the triage, initial response, and initial treatment for most cases the system handles. (Objective 1)

2. 9-1-1 and emergency call receiving
   Incident address verification
   Patient assessment and call triage
   Identification of scene hazards
   Responder case assignment and unit alerting
   Prearrival instructions
   Incident communication and coordination
   Response time measurement
   Unit status tracking
   Critical staff notifications
   Posting and deploying available units
   Scheduling interfacility and nonemergency transports
   (Objective 2)

3. A primary 9-1-1 center receives all initial requests from the public for police, fire, and emergency medical services. The primary 9-1-1 center may then transfer calls to secondary 9-1-1 centers that manage only police, fire, or EMS-related requests. (Objective 3)

4. ANI/ALI is a type of detailed caller identification system used to help communications center personnel determine the origin of calls. The Automated Number Identification (ANI) provides the communications center with the telephone number from which the call is originating. The Automated Location Identification (ALI) provides the address of the call. (Objective 4)

5. Mobile telephone service and Internet service using Voice Over Internet Protocol (VOIP) are the principal technologic challenges to ANI/ALI systems. (Objective 4)

6. 1. Use of medical dispatch protocols
   2. Provision of prearrival instructions
   3. Emergency medical dispatcher training
   4. Emergency medical dispatcher certification
   5. Quality control and improvement processes
   (Objective 5)

7. Accreditation is a proven method for attaining significantly improved service quality. The accreditation process gives agencies the standards and incentives to implement protocols, policies, and procedures consistent with industry best practices. Accreditation also provides opportunities for centers to benchmark by comparing their policies, procedures, protocols, and performance to one another. (Objectives 6, 10)

8. To match the EMS resource used with the patient's clinical need. To limit the use of lights and siren responses to only the most critical cases. (Objective 13)

9. Dispatchers understand policy, protocol, and practice.
   Dispatchers comply with policy, protocol, and practice.
   Compliance deficiencies are corrected.
   Policies, protocol, and practices are updated regularly. (Objective 16)

10. Correct chief complaint identification
    Compliance to basic case information protocols
    Correct final call typing
    Compliance to interrogation protocol for all cardiac arrest cases
    Compliance to prearrival instruction protocol for all cardiac arrest cases
    Compliance to prearrival instruction protocol for all near arrests and cases of respiratory failure
    (Objective 21)

11. Call received at EMS communications center
    Call answered by emergency medical dispatcher
    Address and phone number verification
    Dispatcher evaluation of patient and scene conditions
    Case queued for dispatch
    Unit selected/EMS crew notified (Objective 25)

12. In a performance-based response system, the local government sets specific time requirements for emergency and nonemergency calls. The EMS provider provides monthly response time reports that are subject to audit. EMS managers must develop unit deployment plans that match EMS responder resources to call demand to meet the response requirements set in the performance-based contract. (Objective 28)

13. Because callers to EMS communications centers sometimes report symptoms consistent with contagious, potentially pandemic diseases, emergency medical dispatchers equipped with appropriate surveillance software can identify patterns in numbers and types of requests for service that should trigger an increased level of alert for public health officials on a local, state, or national basis. (Objective 31)

MULTIPLE CHOICE

1. B. A protocol is a predictable, reproducible process for addressing a medical problem; a guideline is a less-structured, more subjective process. (Objective 8)

2. C. Sudden cardiac arrest would trigger the highest priority response. (Objective 12)

3. D. Unknown problem would trigger an intermediate-priority response. (Objective 12)

4. B. Minor trauma with injured ankle would trigger a low-priority response. (Objective 12)

5. D. Engine, ALS ambulance, quick response ALS unit, and defibrillator-equipped police all responding with lights and siren would be appropriate for a high-priority call. (Objective 12)

6. A. ALS ambulance responding with lights and siren would be appropriate for an intermediate-priority call. (Objective 12)
7. B. BLS ambulance responding without lights and siren would be appropriate for a low-priority call. (Objective 12)
8. B. The National Institutes of Health recommends auditing 7% to 10%. (Objective 20)
9. A. Call processing time is the elapsed time from the moment an emergency call is received at the 9-1-1 center until the closest available responders have been notified with all information necessary to respond. (Objective 22)
10. D. Proper use of dispatch protocols is under the control of the EMS communications center. (Objective 23)

CHAPTER 61: EMERGENCY VEHICLE OPERATIONS

MATCHING
1. __B__ Type I
   __A__ Type II
   __C__ Type III
   (Objective 3)

SHORT ANSWER
1. (1) Exceed the posted speed limit. (2) Pass through a stop sign or red traffic signal. (3) Disregard restrictions on turning and direction of travel. (4) Stop, park, or stand the vehicle where otherwise prohibited. (Objectives 5, 11)
2. The emergency vehicle operator must make use of appropriate visual and audible warning devices and must exercise the privileges with due regard to the safety of the lives and property of others. (Objectives 5, 11)
3. (1) Am I responding like other crews would in the same situation? (2) Am I using my warning devices appropriately to give other motorists and pedestrians time to respond? (3) Am I driving safely based on traffic, road, and weather conditions? (Objectives 5, 11)
4. Intersections. (Objectives 5, 11)
5. Other drivers' "timing" lights. Emergency vehicles following each other. Multiple emergency vehicles converging on same location. Motorists going around stopped traffic. Vision of pedestrians in crosswalk obstructed by other vehicles. (Objectives 5, 11)
6. Slow down at intersections. Ensure other drivers have seen you and stopped before you proceed. (Objectives 5, 11)
7. Because police vehicles accelerate more rapidly than ambulances, a large gap frequently will open between the police unit and the ambulance it is escorting. A driver of a vehicle waiting at an intersection may hear the police vehicle's siren, wait

for the police vehicle to pass, and then pull into the intersection, colliding with the ambulance. (Objectives 5, 11)
8. Defibrillator, glucometer, cardiac monitor, oxygen system, automated transport ventilator, pulse oximeter, suction unit, laryngoscope batteries and lights, lighted stylets, flashlights, penlights, and other battery-operated equipment (Objectives 4, 6)
9. A tiered response system is an EMS system that operates units with several different levels of patient care and transport capability. Typically a tiered system includes a larger number of units with basic life support capability than with advanced life support capability. When a request for service is received, the dispatcher uses a protocol to determine which types of units to send. Frequently, both a BLS unit and an ALS unit will respond to the same call. If the patient needs care by a paramedic, the ALS unit will transport. If the patient requires only basic care, the BLS unit will transport, and the ALS unit will return to service. (Objective 7)
10. Location of facilities to house ambulances. Location of hospitals. Anticipated volume of calls. Local geographic and traffic considerations (Objective 7)

MULTIPLE CHOICE
1. B. Intersections are the most common location where ambulances are involved in collisions. (Objective 10)
2. C. Ambulances usually are not authorized to pass school buses that are loading and unloading children. You should stop, but leave your warning lights operating as a signal to the bus driver that you are responding to an emergency and need to pass as quickly as possible. After the driver secures the children on the bus, he or she will signal you on. (Objectives 9, 10)
3. A. When operating with lights and sirens, an ambulance may disregard regulations governing direction of travel if proper caution is used. (Objectives 9, 10)
4. A. Multiple vehicle responses are extremely hazardous and extreme care should be used when proceeding through an intersection in which another emergency vehicle has already passed. (Objective 10)
5. C. The federal agency that establishes guidelines for ambulance equipment and design that are related to infection control is the Occupational Safety and Health Administration. (Objective 4)
6. B. Use of a siren is unlikely to save a significant amount of time during most emergency responses. Motorists are more likely to yield if the siren tone is changed intermittently. Use of the siren can cause the driver to increase driving speed by 10 to 15 miles per hour. Use of the siren can increase the anxiety of sick or injured patients. (Objective 10)
7. B. The General Services Administration issues the federal guidelines that specify ambulance design. (Objectives 1, 2)

8. B. If no fire or escaping liquids or fumes are present, the ambulance should be parked a minimum of 50 feet from the site of a motor vehicle crash. (Objective 10)
9. B. If a fire is present, the ambulance should be parked a minimum of 100 feet from the site of a motor vehicle crash. (Objective 10)

CASE STUDIES

Case One

1. Position the ambulance so it protects the collision site from traffic. (Objective 10)

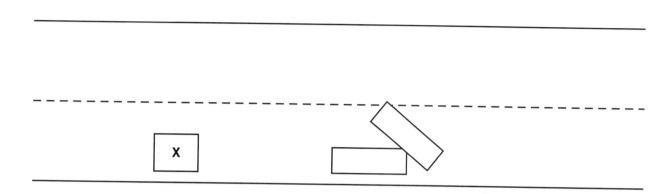

Case Two

1. Position the ambulance beyond the collision site so the wreckage and the police vehicle protect it from traffic. In this position, the ambulance's warning lights also alert oncoming traffic to the presence of danger. (Objective 10)

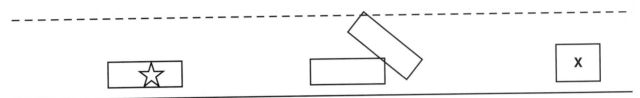

CHAPTER 62: EMS OPERATIONS COMMAND AND CONTROL

SHORT ANSWER

1. A multiple-casualty incident is any incident that depletes the available on-scene resources at any given time. The specific number of patients necessary to create an MCI depends on the resources available to the EMS system. (Objective 3)

2. Mitigation. Preparedness. Response. Recovery. (Objective 5)

3. (1) Mitigation is preventing or limiting the impact of emergencies. Examples of mitigation activities include zoning ordinances, building codes, and safety inspections. (2) Preparedness consists of activities that take place before an emergency that are intended to ensure an efficient, effective response. Preparedness includes development of evacuation and emergency response plans, training, exercises, and stockpiling of essential equipment and supplies. (3) Response consists of activities following an incident that are intended to save lives and property and stabilize the situation that is producing the emergency. (4) Recovery involves restoring the responding agencies and the community to normal. Activities taken during the recovery phase can also be used to mitigate the impact of future incidents. (Objective 5)

4. Life safety. Incident stability (open or closed). Property conservation (Objective 16)

5. A closed incident, also known as a stable or contained incident, is not likely to generate further patients. An open incident, also known as an unstable or uncontained incident, has the potential to generate additional patients. (Objective 16)

6. Command: responsible for coordinating all activities and making all decisions on an emergency scene.
   Finance-administration: responsible for maintaining personnel and time records. Finance also estimates costs, pays claims, and handles procurement of items required at an incident.
   Logistics: coordinates distribution of equipment and supplies needed at an incident. Logistics also ensures adequate food, water, restrooms, lighting, power, and other support resources are available.

Operations: does the actual work necessary to manage the incident.
Planning: provides past, present, and future information about an incident and helps operations and command develop the incident action plan. (Objective 6)

7. Information: collects data about the incident and releases it to the media as directed by Command.
   Safety: monitors on-scene actions and ensures they do not create any potentially harmful situations.
   Liaison: coordinates all incident operations that involve outside agencies not participating in the unified command structure. (Objective 6)

8. In a single command, one individual representing a single agency is responsible for coordinating the response to an incident. In a unified command, personnel representing several agencies are responsible for coordinating the response to an incident and share responsibility for command. Single command is best suited for incidents that involve primarily a single agency from one jurisdiction and that are unlikely to evolve over time. Unified command is preferred in situations that involve multiple agencies or multiple jurisdictions or that are likely to evolve over time. (Objective 12)

9. One member of the first arriving EMS crew must assume command of EMS operations and coordinate EMS activities with those of other responding agencies. Another member of the first arriving EMS crew must assume responsibility for initial triage of any patients. (Objective 11)

10. Staging manages the staging area, a location to which resources respond initially to wait for assignments from Command. Staging is responsible for maintaining an inventory of units that have responded and their capabilities. Staging also is responsible for assigning units as directed by Command.
    Extrication/rescue is responsible for locating and rescuing any patients.
    Triage is responsible for initially assessing patients within the area impacted by the incident and assigning priorities for their movement to the treatment area(s).

Treatment is responsible for coordinating on-scene management of patients in the treatment area(s).

Transport is responsible for coordinating transport of patients from the scene to appropriate medical facilities, including maintenance of records that can be used to track patient movement.

Rehabilitation is responsible for providing food, water, rest, and medical monitoring for personnel responding to the incident.

Morgue is responsible for maintaining an area where the bodies of persons killed in an incident can be collected; morgue is also responsible for coordinating with the medical examiner, coroner, law enforcement, and other appropriate agencies. (Objective 18)

11. A command post is a location near the site of an incident where representatives of responding agencies can meet to coordinate their activities. During small incidents of short duration, the command post provides both strategic and operational/tactical direction. During large incidents, the command post focuses on operational/tactical control and coordination of strategy shifts to the emergency operations center. (Objective 14)

12. The emergency operations center is a fixed facility that serves as a location for strategic decision making and control during large-scale or long-term incidents. The EOC also serves as a site for interaction between high-level officials from local, state, and federal governments. During large incidents the EOC determines who, what, when, and where. The field command posts determine how. (Objective 14)

13. Physicians can be used to make difficult triage decisions, to perform advanced treatment in the treatment area, to perform emergency surgery to extricate patients, and to provide on-site medical direction in the treatment area. (Objective 19)

14. Primary triage takes place in the area impacted by the incident where patients are first found. Secondary triage takes place after patients are moved to the treatment area. (Objective 25)

15. Primary triage takes place at the locations where patients are found initially. Secondary triage takes place at the treatment areas. (Objective 26)

16. (Objective 27)

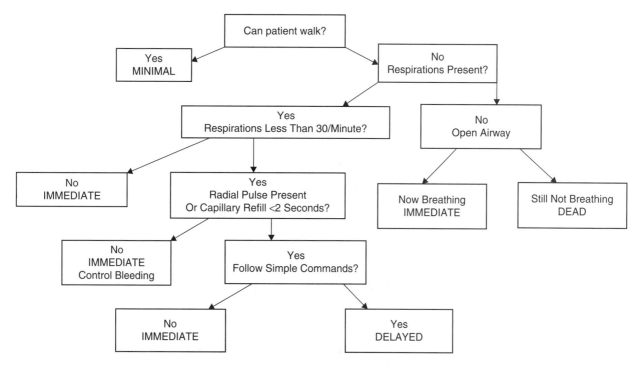

17. Divisions are responsible for a specific geographical area of an incident. Groups are responsible for a function that needs to be performed anywhere within the area impacted by the incident. (Objective 13)

18. Red indicates IMMEDATE.
    Yellow indicates DELAYED.
    Green indicates MINIMAL.
    Black indicates DEAD or DYING. (Objective 28)

19. Early in the incident, the communications center should contact area hospitals and request information on the number of patients they can accept. This information should be communicated to the transport unit supervisor. Patients should be sent to facilities capable of managing their injuries. Attempts should be made to avoid exceeding the rate at which facilities can receive and manage patients. (Objective 21)

20. A destination log should be maintained by the transport supervisor that includes each patient's triage tag number, triage priority, age, gender, major injuries, transporting unit, destination, and departure time. As the transport unit supervisor advises the communications center or command hospital that patients are being transported, the communications center or command hospital should maintain a duplicate log of transport destinations and triage priorities. Maintaining duplicate logs allows the number and destinations of patients to be accounted for more reliably following an incident. (Objective 21)
21. Radio traffic should be kept to an absolute minimum to avoid overloading available channels. Use of codes and signals should be avoided. Transporting units should not make radio reports to receiving facilities. Information about inbound patients should be provided by the transport unit supervisor by relaying it through the communications center or a designated command hospital. Communications to supervisory personnel should be addressed to the position they occupy in the incident management system rather than to their unit number. (For example, "Staging to Command," not "744 to 720.") (Objective 17)
22. (Objective 6)

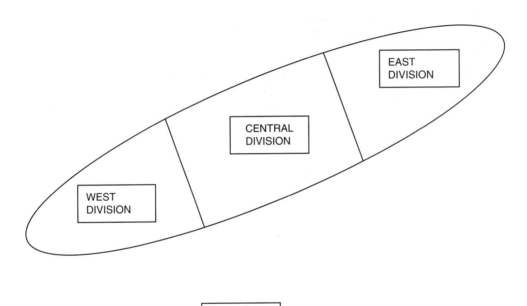

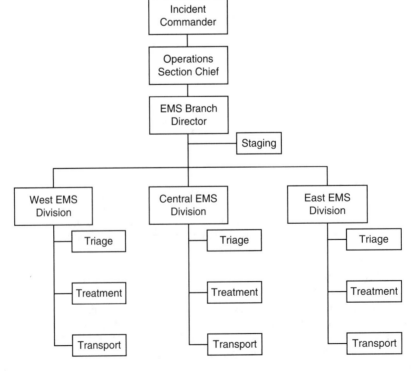

23. (Objective 6)

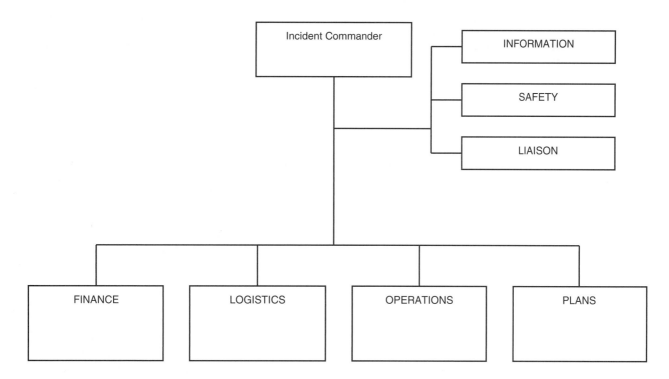

MULTIPLE CHOICE

1. A. Under the START triage system, the first distinction is based on patient's ability to walk. (Objective 27)
2. D. During triage, the best way to assess perfusion quickly and accurately is radial pulse. Capillary refill can be slowed by environmental factors such as exposure to cold. (Objective 27)
3. C. The optimum number of subordinates that one supervisor can manage effectively during an incident is 5. (Objective 13)
4. B. The safety officer has the authority to bypass the chain of command and issue direct orders if necessary to correct an unsafe situation. (Objectives 6, 18)
5. C. Under the incident management system (IMS), the person responsible for EMS on the scene usually will report to the operations section chief. (Objective 6)
6. B. Under the incident management system, the principal distinction between the roles of the incident commander and the operations section chief is that the incident commander deals with strategic goals and objectives while the focus of the operations chief is on operational and tactical concerns. (Objectives 6, 11)
7. D. In the incident management system, the information officer is responsible for interacting with the news media and disseminating public information. All information released to the media must be approved by and coordinated with the incident commander. (Objective 6)

8. C. A staging area is a location where resources are held until given an assignment. All personnel responding to an incident who have not been given another specific assignment should report to the staging area. (Objective 18)

CASE STUDIES

Case One

1. No; the incident commander's optimum span of control has not been exceeded. The optimum span of control is five. There are currently four units on-scene. Because the incident commander will be communicating only with the officer in charge of each of these units, the optimum span of control has not been exceeded. (Objective 13)
2. Because the incident involves hazardous materials and the need to perform rescues, the incident commander should immediately establish a safety officer position. (Objective 18)
3. Wind direction should be monitored continuously throughout the incident. Early in the incident, information should be obtained from the National Weather Service or another reliable source about possible shifts in wind direction during the time period over which the incident is likely to continue. (Objectives 14, 16)
4. The district chief should report to the command post and receive a briefing from the incident commander.

Only after the district chief has been briefed should he accept command of the incident. The communications center and all units operating on the incident should be advised of the change in command by an announcement over the radio net. (Objective 15)

5. Because this incident involves multiple agencies and is likely to evolve over time, a unified command structure should be used. (Objective 12)

Case Two

1. A. Red, because of absent radial pulses.
   B. Green, because of ability to walk.
   C. Black, because respirations were absent initially and after repositioning the airway.
   D. Yellow, because the patient cannot walk but has acceptable breathing, circulation, and neurologic status.
   E. Red, because the patient's respirations are >30 breaths/minute.
   F. Black, because respirations were absent initially and after repositioning the airway.
   G. Red, because respirations were absent initially but were present after the airway was repositioned. (Objective 24)

CHAPTER 63: VEHICLE RESCUE AND RESCUE AWARENESS OPERATIONS

SHORT ANSWER

1. Rescue is the process of extricating or disentangling victims who will become your patients. (Objective 1)
2. Paramedics should be trained and equipped to recognize situations requiring specialized rescue capabilities, to request these resources, to establish incident command when first on the scene, to recognize hazards and either correct them or call for appropriate assistance, to access patients so appropriate initial assessment and stabilization can be performed, and to provide appropriate medical balance to the technical skills of the rescue team. (Objective 3)
3. 1. Arrival and size-up
   2. Hazard control
   3. Patient access
   4. Medical treatment
   5. Disentanglement
   6. Patient packaging
   7. Removal and transport
   (Objective 6)
4. Helmets. Eye protection. Hearing protection. Respiratory protection. Gloves. Foot protection. Flame/flash protection. Personal flotation devices. Lighting. Hazardous materials suits and self-contained breathing apparatus. Extended, remote, and wilderness protection including protective equipment for inclement weather, provisions for drinking water, snacks, temporary shelter, a butane lighter, and redundant light sources. (Objective 8)

5. The purpose of the "patient access" phase of the rescue operation is to enable a medically-trained rescuer to reach the patient to perform an initial assessment and begin providing stabilizing care. (Objective 6)
6. An incident management system should be in place with a designated safety officer. Access should be based on plan approved by the incident commander and safety officer. All personnel should understand plan before it is implemented. (Objective 6)
7. Every rescue operation requires a safety officer. (Objective 5)
8. Apparatus placement: Apparatus should be placed so it protects the scene while causing minimal reduction in traffic flow. The ambulance loading area should NOT be exposed to traffic. Ideally, law enforcement vehicles or fire apparatus vehicles are placed to protect the scene while the ambulance is parked beyond the wreck in the direction of traffic flow, so the other emergency services vehicles and the wreck protect the ambulance loading area.
   Headlights and emergency vehicle lighting: A minimum of warning lights should be used to alert traffic of a hazard and define the size of the ambulance. Too many lights can confuse or blind drivers. Headlights should be turned off with amber parking lights used to indicate the location of vehicles.
   Cones, flares: Traffic cones or flares should be placed early in the incident. Flares should not be placed near spilled fuel or brush. Lighted flares should NOT be picked up in an attempt to extinguish them. Allow flares to burn out.
   Reflective and high visibility clothing: Turnout coats or vests with reflective tape should be worn to highlight rescuers. (Objective 13)
9. Airbag/supplemental restraint devices: Airbags can deploy suddenly, striking and injuring rescuers. Airbags should be deactivated before the rescue begins. If the airbags cannot be deactivated, rescuers should avoid placing themselves into the area where the bag will deploy. Rescuers should remember that an increasing number of vehicles include side airbags.
   Conventional fuel systems: Conventional fuel systems can spill gasoline or diesel fuel, increasing the risk of a fire.
   Alternate fuel systems: High-pressure tanks filled with natural gas create a risk of fire or explosion. Hybrid vehicles contain high-voltage batteries that create electrical shock hazards or ignite spilled fuels. (Objective 10)
10. The A post supports the roof at the windshield. The next post, immediately behind the front seat doors, is the B post. The third post in sedans and station wagons is the C post. Station wagons have a fourth roof support near the rear of the vehicle, the D post. (Objective 16)

11. Down power lines, underground electrical feeds for streetlights, transformer pads. (Objective 14)

12. Tempered glass in the side and rear windows of a vehicle will shatter easily into small, rounded fragments when it is struck forcefully near the window's corner. Safety glass in the windshield is designed not to break. Windshields must be removed intact by cutting around their edges and lifting them out of their frames. (Objective 10)

13. Immersion hypothermia can produce incapacitation and the ability to self-rescue as well as interfere with the victim's ability to grasp a line or flotation device or to follow rescuer instruction. Inability to self-rescue or follow rescuer instructions significantly increases the risk of drowning. (Objective 21)

14. Hypothermia decreases tissue oxygen demand. Immersion of the face in cold water can trigger the mammalian diving reflex, which shunts blood from the body's periphery to the core and slows the heart rate, circulating blood very slowly. These effects can increase the length of time following submersion when the victim may be successfully resuscitated. (Objective 22)

15. Low-head dams and other large uniform obstructions to water flow can cause recirculating currents to form. (Objective 20)

16. A recirculating current, also known as a *drowning machine*, is a current moving against a river's flow that forms where water flows over a large uniform object. Recirculating currents can trap victims against the objects that create the currents. (Objective 20)

17. A strainer is an object such as a downed tree, grating, or wire mesh that will allow water to flow through it but will trap other objects, including people. (Objective 20)

18. If you are unable to talk the patient into self-rescue, reach with a pole. If this is not effective, try throwing a flotation device. If the patient is too far out to reach with either a pole or a thrown floation device, use a boat to go after them. As a last resort, enter the water to rescue the patient. (Objective 26)

19. Water entry is the last resort because it significantly increases the rescuer's risk of becoming a victim. Boat and water entry rescues should never be attempted without proper specialized training. (Objective 25)

20. Float on your back with your feet pointing downstream. Steer with your feet and point your head toward the nearest shore at a 45-degree angle, so the water will push you toward it. (Objective 27)

21. HELP is a technique that can be used to decrease the speed at which immersion hypothermia develops. Keep your head above water and pull your arms and legs into a fetal position. (Objective 23)

22. Keeping the head out of water slows heat loss from this very vascular area. Pulling the arms and legs into a fetal position decreases surface to volume ratio and slows heat loss. (Objective 23)

23. Oxygen-deficient atmospheres. Toxic or explosive chemicals. Engulfment in materials stored in the confined space such as grain, coal, or sand. Machinery entrapment. Electricity. Structural concerns such as protruding supports, unusual shapes, inadequate light levels. (Objectives 29, 30)

24. Hydrogen sulfide, carbon dioxide, carbon monoxide, methane, chlorine, ammonia, nitrogen dioxide, nitrogen tetroxide. (Objective 30)

25. Only personnel with appropriate equipment and training should attempt confined space rescues. O_2 levels will have to be monitored before entry. Depending on the nature of the space, levels of other gases may have to be monitored. Ventilation systems may have to be set up to improve air exchange. All power to space must be shut off. All stored charge must be dissipated. All switches and breakers must be locked out and tagged out. SCBA may have to be used. Personnel may have to resort to air lines because of shape and size of space. Full-body harnesses may be needed in case emergency retrieval is necessary. (Objective 31)

26. Secure scene, perimeter. Establish command. Call for trench rescue team. Interview on-site supervisor, witnesses. Number of patients? Extent of entrapment/burial? Unnecessary personnel, equipment away from trench edges. Trench properly shored before rescue begins. Personnel in trench wear helmets, protective clothing. Use hand tools, not heavy equipment. Determine location of all underground utility lines on site. Priority—uncover patient's face, chest; begin oxygen administration. Keep weight away from patient's chest. Lie flat, stand on planks to spread weight, avoid compressing patient's chest. Do not pull on patient at any time. Consider crush syndrome during prolonged rescues. (Objective 33)

27. Low angle: A slope on which rescuers primarily support themselves with their feet. Ropes may be used for stability or pulling the rescue litter up the hill, but they are not required. A fall on this terrain would not be fatal.

    High angle: A cliff or the side of a building upon which the rescuer cannot walk or support themselves with their feet. A rope system is used for safety purposes and falls result in serious injury or death.

    Belay: Safeguarding a climber's progress by controlling a rope attached to an anchor.

    Rappel: To descend by sliding down a fixed double rope.

    Scrambling: Walking on a low-angle slope using the hands and arms for support.

    Hasty rope slide: Use of a rope anchored to a fixed object to steady personnel moving on a low-angle slope. (Objective 33)

28. Nonpharmacologic pain control includes using proper splinting, distracting the patient by talking and asking questions, scratching or creating other sensory stimuli when doing painful procedures. Pharmacologic pain control includes use of narcotic (morphine, fentanyl) or non-narcotic agents (ketorolac, ketamine) for pain control. Risks associated with use of pharmacologic pain control include alteration of mental status, depressed respirations, hypotension, and removal of pain responses that could warn rescuers that a maneuver they are attempting is harming the patient. (Objective 32)

29. Patients entrapped for extended periods of time are at risk for developing either hypothermia or hyperthermia, depending on the ambient temperature. In cold environments, patients should be covered with blankets to prevent heat loss. Large trash bag liners can be used as an additional vapor barrier to prevent heat loss in cold environments. Properly wrapped chemical hot packs can be used to keep the patient warm. In hot environments, a sheet soaked with water can be placed over the patient to promote evaporative heat loss and cooling. (Objective 32)

30. Crush syndrome occurs when a portion of the body with significant soft tissue mass is compressed with a force large enough to obstruct blood flow. Because the tissues in the compressed area do not receive adequate oxygen, anaerobic metabolism occurs, producing lactic acid and causing a shift of potassium from the intracellular to the extracellular space. Damage occurs to the cell membrane, resulting in loss of extracellular fluid into the intracellular space and leakage of myoglobin from muscle cells into the bloodstream. If perfusion to the compressed area is restored suddenly, lactic acid and potassium can return to the central circulation, depressing myocardial function and producing dysrhythmias. Shifting of fluid into the intracellular space can lead to hypovolemia. Myoglobin entering the bloodstream from damaged muscle cells can precipitate in the filtering tubules of the kidney, causing renal failure. If the mechanism of injury suggests the possibility of crush syndrome, an IV should be established with normal saline and volume resuscitation should begin. Fluid should be infused at a rate that ensures adequate urine output, to help avoid renal failure from myoglobin precipitation in the kidneys. Administration of bicarbonate can help correct acidosis and hyperkalemia and prevent myoglobin precipitation in the kidneys. An osmotic diuretic such as mannitol can be used to promote urine production. Loop diuretics such as furosemide should be avoided because they acidify the urine and can enhance precipitation of myoglobin. (Objective 32)

MULTIPLE CHOICE

1. D. Your ambulance is the first unit to arrive at a report of a person trapped by the collapse of a ditch at a construction site. Your initial action should be to secure the perimeter and request a specialized trench rescue team. Entry into the trench should not be made until a trained rescue team properly shores the walls of the trench. (Objective 32)
2. A. As your first priority, you should ensure that the vehicle is stable. (Objective 15)
3. A. You should gain access to the patient by breaking the side window. The goal of gaining access is to place a medically trained rescuer with the patients as quickly as possible. Attempting to pry a door or cut through the roof could delay patient care. Windshields are made of safety glass and will not break easily. (Objective 15)
4. A. If you fall into swift water, you should float on your back with your feet pointed downstream. (Objective 27)
5. A. During a water rescue, anyone whose responsibilities require them to work in, on, or near the water should wear a personal flotation device. (Objective 8)
6. A. The most common hazard associated with rescue in confined spaces is oxygen deficiency. (Objective 29)
7. A. In newer model vehicles the safest method for displacing a steering column may be to push the A-post and the dash forward. Pulling on the steering column of a front-wheel drive vehicle can cause it to break at the firewall and strike the patient. Cutting a unibody construction vehicle's roof significantly decreases the structural integrity of the rest of the vehicle. Glass in an automobile's windshield is safety glass, which resists breaking. (Objective 17)
8. B. You should start CPR immediately and transport. The combination of hypothermia, the mammalian diving response, and the patient's age significantly increases her probability of surviving. Patients with severe hypothermia must be warmed from the body core outward. Attempting to warm these patients peripherally can produce "rewarming shock," a failure of the circulatory system caused by release of lactic acid and potassium from ischemic peripheral tissues. (Objective 22)
9. A. The primary function of paramedics during the disentanglement phase of extrication is assessing and monitoring the condition of the patient. (Objective 3)

CASE STUDY

1. A specialized trench rescue team should be requested. (Objective 32)
2. Personnel in the trench must wear helmets, protective clothing. Because soil is dry, use of dust masks and eye protection should be considered. The patient also should have a helmet, eye protection, and respiratory protection placed as quickly as possible. Because of

the high heat and humidity, the safety officer should be prepared to have to repeatedly enforce the wearing of proper protective clothing by personnel in the trench. (Objective 8)

3. The scene and its perimeter should be secured as quickly as possible. Unnecessary personnel and equipment must be kept away from trench edges. The backhoe, semi-truck, and other heavy equipment on site must not move. The location of all underground utility lines should be established before rescue attempts begin. (Objectives 5, 32)

4. The trench walls must be shored before rescue begins. The priority should be to remove pressure from the chest of the partially buried worker and begin oxygen administration. Weight should be kept away from his chest by rescuers lying flat or working on spine boards or planks to spread their weight. All digging should be done with hand tools. No attempts should be made to remove the patient by pulling on him. (Objective 32)

5. The patient and rescuers should be observed carefully for signs of hyperthermia or volume depletion because of the high heat and humidity. Because of the mechanism of entrapment, the possibility of crush syndrome should be considered. (Objectives 5, 32)

6. Because of the location of the incident and the time of day, the possibility of prolonged ground transport times exists. Possible use of air transport should be considered. (Objective 6)

CHAPTER 64: RESPONSE TO HAZARDOUS MATERIALS INCIDENTS

SHORT ANSWER

1. Understanding what hazardous substances are and the risks associated with them. Understanding potential outcomes associated with an emergency created when hazardous substances are present. Ability to recognize the presence of hazardous substances. Ability to identify hazardous substances if possible. Understanding first-responder awareness responsibilities including site security and control and the Emergency Response Guidebook. Ability to recognize need for additional resources and make appropriate notifications to the communications center. (Objective 1)

2. Primary contamination is contamination that results from direct contact with a spilled or released hazardous material. (Objective 14)

3. Secondary contamination is contamination that results from contact with a person or thing that has suffered primary contamination. (Objective 14)

4. Acute toxicity is an effect of a hazardous substance that manifests itself immediately or shortly after exposure.

Delayed toxicity is an effect of a hazardous substance that manifests itself from hours to years after exposure.

Route of exposure is the way a hazardous substance enters a patient's body. The routes of exposure are inhalation, absorption, injection (which includes entry through open wounds), and ingestion.

Local effects are effects of a substance involving the immediate area around the point where the substance came into contact with the patient (for example, burns caused by hydrofluoric acid).

Systemic effects are effects that occur throughout the body following contact with a substance (for example, hypocalcemia and dysrhythmias following absorption of hydrofluoric acid into the bloodstream).

Dose response is the toxicologic concept that a larger dose of a toxin will produce more significant effects. Because of dose response effects, patients exposed to a hazardous material should be decontaminated as quickly as possible.

Synergistic effects are effects produced by interaction of two chemicals that neither chemical can produce on its own. Synergistic effects are important in management of patients who have been exposed to hazardous materials because they can result in unexpected responses to drugs given by EMS personnel. (Objective 6)

5. Threshold limit value/time-weighted average (TLV/TWA): The maximum concentration of a substance in air that a person can be exposed to for 8 hours a day, 40 hours per week, without suffering adverse health effects.

Threshold limit value/short-term exposure limit (TLV/STEL): The maximum concentration of a substance that a person can be exposed to for 15 minutes not more than four times a day with 60 minutes of rest between each exposure.

Threshold limit value/ceiling level (TLV/CL): The maximum concentration of a substance that should never be exceeded.

50% lethal concentration (LC50): The concentration of a substance in air that results in the death of 50% of exposed test subjects.

50% lethal dose (LD50): The concentration of a substance that results in the death of 50% of exposed test subjects when injected, ingested, or absorbed.

Parts per million (ppm): The number of units of a substance per 1 million units of air or solution in which it is dissolved.

Parts per billion (ppb): The number of units of a substance per 1 billion units of air or solution in which it is dissolved.

Immediately dangerous to life and health (IDLH): The concentration of a substance that causes an immediate threat to life. (Objective 6)

6. Triage and decontamination at a hazardous materials incident have two goals: minimizing exposure time of contaminated persons and prevention of secondary contamination. Thoroughness of decontamination must always be balanced against the risks of delaying transport of patients to definitive care. When patients have self-extricated from the hot zone, when critically injured patients also are contaminated, or when the substance is known or suspected to be highly toxic, it may be necessary to perform an emergency decontamination that may not be as thorough as the decontamination that can be obtained through setup of a complete decontamination line. (Objective 15)

7. Corrosives (acids/alkalis) cause skin burns, respiratory burns, and airway/pulmonary edema. Some corrosives also have systemic effects. Dry particles should be brushed from the skin followed by washing with large amounts of water. Liquids should be washed away with large amounts of water. Vomiting should not be induced in corrosive ingestions. It may be necessary to secure the airway by endotracheal intubation, to administer nebulized bronchodilators for bronchospasm, and to provide PEEP to support oxygenation and ventilation if noncardiogenic pulmonary edema is present.

Pulmonary irritants produce burning of the mucosa of the upper and lower airways. They also can cause burns of the skin and damage to the eyes. The patient should be undressed to remove any contaminants on or trapped in the clothing. The eyes and any exposed skin should be flushed with large amounts of water. Intubation may be necessary to protect the airway. Nebulized bronchodilators may be given for bronchospasm. PEEP may be needed to support oxygenation and ventilation if noncardiogenic pulmonary edema is present.

Pesticides (carbamates/organophosphates) bind to and inactivate acetylcholinesterase, the enzyme that removes acetylcholine from the synapses. This effect causes excess acetylcholine to accumulate. Effects of excess acetylcholine in the parasympathetic synapses include salivation, lacrimation, urination, defecation, gastrointestinal distress, and emesis. Pinpoint pupils and a slow heart rate also may be present. Excess acetylcholine at the neuromuscular junction causes muscle weakness and paralysis. The patient should be undressed and washed with large amounts of water. The airway and breathing should be supported. Atropine should be given in a dose necessary to eliminate the excess secretions. In organophosphate poisoning, pralidoxime should be given to reactivate acetylcholinesterase. Pralidoxime is not indicated in carbamate poisoning.

Chemical asphyxiants (cyanide/carbon monoxide) interfere with the body's use of oxygen for aerobic metabolism. Carbon monoxide interferes with oxygen transport to the tissues by binding to hemoglobin. Cyanide inhibits the use of oxygen by the electron transport chain by binding to cytochrome oxidase. Chemical asphyxiants produce signs of severe tissue hypoxia in the presence of bright red venous blood and high oxygen saturation readings. Management involves removal from exposure, support of airway and breathing, administration of high concentrations of oxygen. Hyperbaric oxygen therapy may be useful in severe cases of carbon monoxide poisoning. Use of nitrite and thiosulfate therapy is indicated in cyanide toxicity.

Hydrocarbon solvents (xylene, methylene chloride) damage the alveolar capillary membrane in the lungs, causing pulmonary edema. They also can cause dysrhythmias by sensitizing the myocardium to catecholamine effects, hypoglycemia by damaging the liver, and seizures from injury to the central nervous system. If skin contaminants are present, the patient should be washed with warm water and soap. Vomiting should not be induced. Endotracheal intubation and PEEP may be necessary to support adequate oxygenation and ventilation. Diazepam can be used to stop seizures. Intravenous glucose should be given to correct hypoglycemia. Caution should be used in administering catecholamines because they may produce increased myocardial irritability. (Objective 15)

8. Boiling point is the temperature at which the vapor pressure of a liquid equals atmospheric pressure and the liquid becomes a gas.

Flash point is the temperature at which a liquid will give off enough vapors to ignite.

Upper and lower flammable limits are the highest and lowest concentrations of a vapor in air at which ignition will result in combustion. Above the upper flammable limit there is not enough oxygen to support combustion. Below the lower flammable limit there is insufficient fuel to support combustion.

Ignition temperature is the lowest temperature at which a liquid will give off enough vapors to support combustion. Ignition temperature is slightly higher than flash point.

Specific gravity is the ratio of the weight of a volume of liquid to the weight of an equal volume of water. If the specific gravity is less than 1, the liquid will float on water. If the specific gravity is greater than 1, it will sink in water.

Vapor density is the ratio of the weight of a volume of a gas to the weight of an equal volume of air. A gas with a vapor density of less than 1 will rise. A gas with a vapor density of greater than 1 will sink.

Vapor pressure is the pressure of a vapor against the walls of a container. As temperature increases, vapor pressure increases. The vapor pressure of a liquid is a measure of the liquid's tendency to evaporate. At a given temperature, a liquid with a higher vapor pressure will evaporate more quickly.

Water solubility is a measure of the tendency of a substance to dissolve in water.

Alpha, beta, gamma radiation are the three types of ionizing radiation. Alpha particles consist of two protons and two neutrons (a helium nucleus) released from the nucleus of a radioactive substance. Alpha particles are stopped by paper, clothing, or intact skin. Beta particles are electrons released by the nucleus of a radioactive substance. They will penetrate a few millimeters of skin. Gamma radiation consists of high-energy photons released from the nucleus of a radioactive substance. Gamma radiation will penetrate several feet of lead and is the most dangerous form of ionizing radiation. (Objectives 4, 5)

9. (Objective 9)

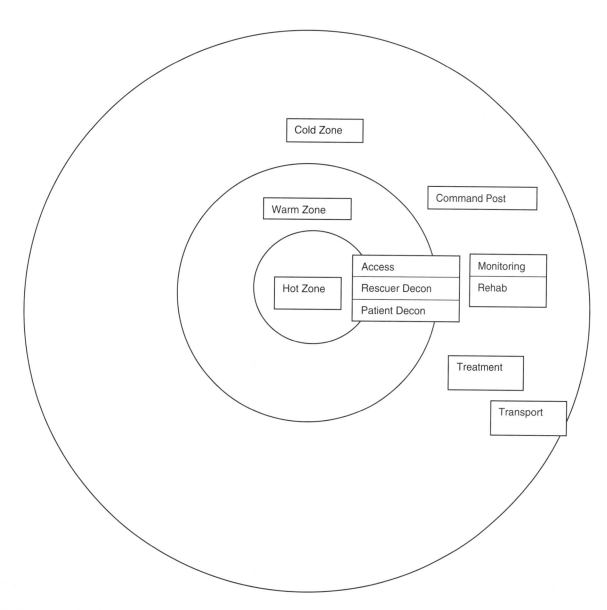

10. Remove and isolate clothing, jewelry, shoes. Brush off solid or particulate contaminants as completely as possible. Blot visible liquid contaminants from the body with absorbent material. Rinse the patient with large amounts of warm water using low pressure, avoid splashing or overspray. Using mild liquid soap and soft brushes wash the patient beginning with the head/face followed by areas of tissue damage or gross contamination. Pay special attention to hair, nailbeds, and skin folds. Perform a final rinse with large amounts of water. (Objective 14)

11. Before entry HAZMAT team members should have the following baseline parameters measured and documented: blood pressure, pulse, respiratory rate, temperature, body weight, ECG, and mental status. Abnormal findings should exclude a team member from entering. Entry team members should prehydrate with 8 to 16 ounces of water or dilute

sports drink. On exit, team members should have the same parameters evaluated as were measured before entry. Team members should not be allowed to reenter the hot zone until they are alert, non-tachycardic, normotensive, normothermic, and within a reasonable percentage of their normal body weight. (Objective 12)

12. A level A suit prevents cooling from evaporation, conduction, convection, and radiation. Factors determining the amount of heat stress this will produce include environmental temperature and humidity, prehydration, duration and degree of activity, and the team member's overall physical fitness. (Objective 12)

13. A flow sheet should be available to record team members' blood pressures, pulses, respiratory rates, temperatures, ECG findings, body weights, and mental status. Personnel performing medical monitoring should work from a set of physician-approved guidelines to determine whether a team member is fit for entry. (Objective 12)

MULTIPLE CHOICE

1. B. A product with a high vapor pressure will evaporate more rapidly than one with a low vapor pressure. (Objective 4)
2. C. The product probably will be emitting enough vapors to ignite since the ambient temperature exceeds the flash point. (Objective 5)
3. D. A product that has a vapor density of 1.5 would sink and accumulate in low-lying areas around the site of release. Depending on the topography of the site, the product could spread over an extensive area. (Objective 4)
4. A. Based on this information, you can determine that the product is a nonflammable gas that must be identified more specifically before any action is taken. Products placarded as nonflammable gases include oxygen and anhydrous ammonia. (Objective 3)
5. A. A product that has a specific gravity of 0.8 will tend to float on water. (Objective 4)
6. B. Immediate decontamination of casualties is part of their emergency medical care because it limits the dose of the hazardous substance to which they are exposed. (Objective 14)
7. C. Shipments of certain classes of material must be placarded regardless of the quantity of material being shipped. Placards for each hazard are not required. Placards indicate only the principal hazard of a material. Shipments of some types or amounts of materials are not required to be placarded. The DANGEROUS placard can indicate a mixed load, a respiratory irritant, or a shipment of some types of low-level explosives. (Objective 3)

8. C. In a HAZMAT situation, the most common route of exposure is respiratory inhalation. (Objective 6)
9. D. Structural firefighting equipment provides level D of HAZMAT protection. (Objective 11)
10. B. At this point, a call to CHEMTREC will be unable to provide you with information from the CHEMTREC communicator on the probable nature and properties of the products of reactions between the spilled chemicals. The CHEMTREC communicators are not chemists and are trained only to provide information about individual substances contained in their databases. Information about interactions between spilled products will have to come from a professional chemist. (Objective 7)
11. B. The transportation warning placard for a flammable gas will have a red color, a flame symbol, and a hazard class "2" number. (Objective 3)
12. D. The most hazardous type of radiation is gamma radiation. (Objective 5)

CHAPTER 65: TACTICAL EMS

MATCHING

1. __C__ Cold zone
   __A__ Hot zone
   __B__ Warm zone
   (Objective 9)
2. __B__ First line
   __D__ Fourth line
   __A__ Second line
   __C__ Third line
   (Objective 11)

SHORT ANSWER

1. Tactical emergency medical services is the comprehensive out-of-hospital medical support for law enforcement's tactical teams during training and special operations. (Objective 2)
2. Barricaded suspects. Hostage situations. Felony warrants. Tactical searches and rescues. Officers/casualties down in line of fire. Dignitary protection. Mobile field force (riot control). Mass-casualty shootings with one or more active shooters. Weapons of mass destruction/terrorism incidents. (Objective 1)
3. Casualty care in the inner perimeter of tactical missions and during high-risk training. Medical intelligence and treat assessment before missions. General assessment and health maintenance of team members during extended training or missions. Remote assessment of casualties in the line of fire. Medical assessment and clearing of suspects before incarceration. Medical training of tactical operators. Physical readiness qualification at the tactical operator level. (Objective 3)

4. Field medicine, tactical skills, personal fitness. (Objective 4)
5. Exsanguination from extremity wounds, tension pneumothorax, airway obstruction. (Objective 7)
6. A set of guidelines encompassing all appropriate field care rendered to casualties from the point they are injured until they are out of the combat zone and delivered to the closest appropriate facility. (Objective 6)
7. Priority one: Fire superiority
   Priority two: Prevent further casualties
   Priority three: Triage
   Priority four: Treat according to Tactical Combat Casualty Care guidelines
   (Objective 8)
8. Concealment is anything that will prevent you from being seen by an adversary, but that will not stop bullets. (Objective 5)
9. Cover is anything that will stop bullets. (Objective 5)
10. Armed tactical medics are able to defend themselves and their patients, eliminating the need for an armed tactical officer to accompany them at all times. Armed tactical medics provide additional firepower available to the team during extreme scenarios such as large-scale ambushes in which multiple team members are wounded simultaneously. (Objective 12)
11. Arming the tactical medics creates a responsibility to ensure they remain proficient in use of firearms as well as their medical and other tactical skills. Presence of an armed medic on the team creates a temptation for the team leader to use the medic as an operational asset instead of holding him/her in reserve to provide patient care as needed. Armed tactical medics may experience an increase in role conflict that interferes with their ability to care for injured suspects, particularly in situations where the medic is responsible for the suspect being wounded. (Objective 12)

MULTIPLE CHOICE

1. B. The most common cause of preventable death in combat situations is exsanguination from extremity wounds. (Objective 7)
2. A. When treatment is provided according to Tactical Combat Casualty Care guidelines, the highest patient care priority is controlling hemorrhage from extremity wounds. (Objective 8)
3. B. Once fire superiority has been established, appropriate treatment in the hot zone would include applying a tourniquet to control extremity hemorrhage. Application of dressings, decompression of a tension pneumothorax, or insertion of a dual-lumen airway should take place in the warm zone in a position of cover and concealment. (Objective 9)
4. A. The sequence of priorities in Tactical Combat Casualty Care is (1) achieve fire superiority, (2) prevent

further casualties, (3) triage, and (4) treat according to TCCC guidelines. (Objective 8)
5. D. Equipment that should be readily accessible in pockets of the tactical medic's vest or body armor includes tactical tourniquet, tactical battle dressing, roller gauze, chest seals, chest decompression needles, dual-lumen airway, and trauma shears. An epinephrine autoinjector, SAM splints, and flex cuff restraints should be carried in the tactical medic's backpack. (Objective 11)
6. D. Cover provides protection from enemy fire and can be provided by a vehicle's engine block. Concealment prevents an enemy from seeing you. Bullets can penetrate walls of most structures. (Objective 5)
7. A. Medical equipment every member of the tactical team should carry and be trained to use includes one tactical tourniquet and one tactical battle dressing. (Objective 11)
8. C. The problem most commonly managed by tactical medics is minor injuries or illnesses during training evolutions or extended missions. (Objective 2)
9. B. When critical injuries occur during a tactical operation, the first medical priority is to immediately assess any injured tactical officer, regardless of potential injuries that may have occurred to suspects. A tactical officer is less of a potential threat to the medic than a suspect. Additionally, tactical officers frequently are unaware of their own physical condition when involved in a critical mission and may compensate up to their last moment of consciousness. (Objective 8)

CHAPTER 66: DISASTER RESPONSE AND DOMESTIC PREPAREDNESS

MATCHING

1. __E__ Collects and evaluates information about incident and response
   __A__ Directs, orders, and controls all resources used to manage an incident
   __C__ Locates and organizes facilities, services, and materials needed to manage incident
   __D__ Manages all tactical operations at an incident
   __B__ Tracks incident costs
   (Objective 4)
2. __A__ Chlorine, anhydrous ammonia, phosgene
   __C__ CS, CNB
   __D__ Cyanide, cyanogens chloride
   __B__ Sulfur mustard
   __E__ Tabun, sarin, soman, VXE
   (Objectives 7, 8)
3. __B__ Trauma from flying debris
   __C__ Trauma from patient being thrown by blast
   __A__ Trauma from pressure wave
   (Objective 13)

SHORT ANSWER

1. Disaster responses must be preplanned because they involve events that are infrequent but that produce high demands for service from public safety agencies, stress the logistics infrastructures of responding agencies, require large amounts of resources to resolve, and require cooperation among agencies and levels of government that frequently do not work together on a daily basis, including agencies that normally do not have emergency response as a primary mission. (Objective 1)

2. The purpose of the National Response Plan is to provide structure and processes to join the efforts and resources of federal, state, local, tribal, private sector, and nongovernmental organizations in a coordinated approach to management of and recovery from natural and man-made disasters and other emergencies. (Objective 2)

3. ESFs are activities that must take place during the response to a disaster or other emergency. ESFs provide a way to logically group government agencies and private organizations that respond to or support responses to disasters and other emergencies to help them plan and coordinate their activities more effectively. (Objective 2)

4. The Department of Health and Human Services coordinates the Public Health and Medical Services function under the National Response Plan. (Objective 3)

5. The Department of Health and Human Services administers and coordinates the National Disaster Medical System. (From 2003 to 2007, the NDMS was coordinated by the Department of Homeland Security.) (Objective 3)

6. DMATs are field-deployable hospital teams that include physicians, nurses, EMS personnel, and other medical and nonmedical support personnel. (Objective 3)

7. NMRT-WMDs are quick-response specialty groups trained and equipped to provide mass-casualty decontamination and patient care after release of a chemical, biologic, or radiologic agent. (Objective 3)

8. DMORTs are teams made up of forensic and mortuary professionals trained to deal with human remains after disaster situations. (Objective 3)

9. Greater case loads of the disease than normally expected. More severe cases than normally expected or unusual routes of transmission. A disease that is unusual for the geographic area or the time of year, or that is occurring in the absence of its normal vector for transmission. Multiple, simultaneous epidemics of different diseases. An outbreak of the same disease simultaneously among animals and humans. Unusual strains, variants, or antimicrobial resistance patterns. Higher incidence among persons in specific environments or locations. Intelligence that a terrorist group has access to a particular agent. Claims by a

terrorist group to have released a biologic agent. Equipment, munitions, or other direct evidence of intentional release. (Objective 9)

10. Electromagnetic pulse is an intense burst of electromagnetic radiation from a high-altitude nuclear weapon detonation. EMP will disable electronic equipment within the affected area. (Objective 11)

11. Because they are easy to acquire or build, easy to conceal, and highly effective. Chemical, biologic, and radiologic weapons require a higher level of skill to build and use. (Objective 12)

MULTIPLE CHOICE

1. D. The staging area manager. All units arriving at a scene where the incident management system is in effect should report to the staging area and standby there until given a specific assignment. (Objective 4)

2. A. Five. The number of subordinates that one supervisor should manage during an incident is three to seven with the optimum number being five. (Objective 4)

3. B. The safety officer has authority to bypass the chain of command to prevent unsafe acts. The liaison officer interacts with outside agency representatives. The public information officer disseminates information to the media. Activation of the emergency operations center usually is a decision made at the level of the incident commander or higher. (Objective 4)

4. C. Operations section chief. Although some EMS personnel may be assigned to assist with the planning or logistics functions, the primary role of EMS during most disasters is caring for casualties of the incident. Since this is a tactical function, the supervisor in charge of EMS activities typically will report to the operations section chief. (Objective 4)

5. B. The incident commander deals with strategic goals and objectives while the focus of the operations chief is operational and tactical concerns. (Objective 4)

6. D. The information officer is responsible for interfacing with the news media and disseminating public information. (Objective 4)

7. C. A staging area is a location where resources are held until given an assignment. (Objective 4)

8. D. Public information. The information officer fills a special staff position under the incident management system. Logistics, finance and administration, and planning and intelligence are primary functional areas under the incident management system and are supervised by chiefs who are general staff officers. (Objective 4)

9. A. The position of incident commander always is established at every incident. Because the incident management system builds from the top down, there

must always be an incident commander, who then determines the other IMS positions that should be filled. (Objective 4)

10. A. Cyanide has a faint odor of bitter almonds. However, some people cannot smell this odor. (Objective 8)

11. C. Phosgene smells like freshly cut grass or hay. Cyanide has an odor like bitter almonds. Chlorine smells like bleach. Anhydrous ammonia has an odor like that of window cleaner. (Objective 8)

12. D. Cyanide binds to the iron ion in cytochrome a_3, interfering with the transfer of electrons to oxygen. This blocks the process of electron transport, shutting down the cell's ability to make ATP. (Objective 8)

13. A. Amyl nitrite, sodium nitrite, and sodium thiosulfate are the antidotes for cyanide toxicity. (Objective 8)

14. C. A patient who is exposed to phosgene will develop pulmonary edema 2 to 24 hours after exposure. Although phosgene may cause some discomfort in the upper airway and produce a mild cough during initial exposure, it is a nonirritating gas that can be inhaled into the lower airway. In the bronchioles and alveoli it reacts with water to form hydrochloric acid, which causes chemical injury leading to pulmonary edema. (Objective 8)

15. B. Nerve agents are toxic because they inhibit the action of the enzyme that breaks down acetylcholine. This causes buildup of acetylcholine in the synapses of the parasympathetic nervous system and at the neuromuscular junction. Excess stimulation of muscarinic acetylcholine receptors causes the classic SLUDGE toxidrome of cholinergic crisis. Excess acetylcholine at the neuromuscular junction prevents skeletal muscles from repolarizing, resulting in weakness and respiratory failure. (Objective 8)

16. D. Weakness or paralysis of respiratory muscles causes must deaths from nerve agent toxicity. (Objective 8)

17. C. Encephalitis is classified as a category B pathogen by the Centers for Disease Control and Prevention. Anthrax, botulism, and tularemia are category A pathogens. (Objective 10)

18. D. The lesions of smallpox occur primarily on the face, arms, and legs, including the palms and soles, and tend to all look alike as the disease progresses. Chickenpox lesions tend to occur primarily on the trunk and do not appear on the palms and soles. As the disease process progresses, chickenpox lesions include a mixture of vesicles, pustules, and scabs. (Objective 10)

19. A. All three forms of plague present initially with fever, chills, and myalgia. Bubonic plague is the most common, but least severe form of the disease.

Pneumonic plague is less common but is more severe. Septicemic plague develops when bacteria spread to the bloodstream from untreated bubonic plague lesions. (Objective 10)

20. B. Tularemia can progress to a pulmonary syndrome that includes sore throat, nonproductive cough, and bronchitis. Exposure to as few as 10 bacteria can cause a case of tularemia. The disease is not easily transmitted from person to person, so no protective measures beyond standard precautions are necessary. (Objective 10)

21. A. Simple radiologic devices typically are gamma emitters. While they can expose patients to dangerously high radiation levels, simple radiologic devices do not cause secondary contamination or make exposed persons or things radioactive. (Objective 11)

22. A. A dirty bomb is a combination of a radioactive source and a conventional explosive designed to spread large amounts of radioactive contaminants. One of the features of dirty bombs that make them an attractive tool for terrorism is that their construction does not require sophisticated knowledge or skill in nuclear technology. (Objective 11)

23. A. Radiation exposure tends to have its greatest effects on cells in the bone marrow and gastrointestinal tract because they are rapidly dividing. Death of these cells produces nausea, vomiting, diarrhea, anemia, and immunocompromise. (Objective 11)

24. A. This patient has a primary blast injury, specifically a pneumothorax caused by the blast's pressure wave rupturing alveoli and allowing air to leak into the pleural space. (Objective 13)

25. C. Explosives are the preferred secondary devices because they are easy to acquire, build, and hide. (Objective 13)

CASE STUDIES

Case One (Objectives 7, 8)

1. A nerve agent.
2. Nerve agents inhibit the action of acetylcholinesterase, the enzyme that breaks down the neurotransmitter acetylcholine. This action causes a build up of acetylcholine in the synapses of the parasympathetic nervous system and at the neuromuscular junction.
3. Atropine can be used to block the stimulation of muscarinic receptor sites by excess acetylcholine and reverse the SLUDGE syndrome associated with nerve agent poisoning.
4. 2-PAM (pralidoxime) is the definitive antidote for nerve agent toxicity. 2-PAM detaches the nerve agent from acetylcholinesterase, reactivating the enzyme so it can remove the excess acetylcholine.

Case Two (Objectives 7, 8)

1. Cyanide.
2. Cyanide interferes with use of oxygen in cellular respiration by blocking the action of cytochrome a_3.
3. Because cyanide has shut down the electron transport chain, the process of cellular respiration no longer is consuming oxygen. Oxygen is remaining on the hemoglobin in the red cells, producing bright red venous blood and high oxygen saturations.
4. Amyl nitrite, sodium nitrite and sodium thiosulfate are the antidotes include in the Taylor or Lilly antidote kits.
5. The nitrites oxidize the iron in hemoglobin from the 2+ state to the 3+ state, inducing a condition called methemoglobinemia. Since cyanide has a high affinity for 3+ iron, it detaches from cytochrome a_3 and binds to the methemoglobin in the red blood cells. This reactivates electron transport. Sodium thiosulfate provides rhodonese, a naturally occurring enzyme, with the sulfide it needs to convert cyanide to thiocyanate, a less toxic compound that is excreted through the kidneys.
6. Cyanide is a nonpersistent agent that enters the body through inhalation. Therefore the patients do not need to be decontaminated.

Glossary

800 MHz A type of radio signal in the ultra-high-frequency range that allows splitting a frequency into individual talk groups used as communication links with other system users.

9-1-1/E9-1-1 A set of three numbers that automatically sends the call to the emergency dispatch center. E9-1-1 is enhanced 9-1-1, which gives the dispatcher the ability to determine the caller's location by routing the call through several CAD systems.

Abandonment Terminating care when it is still needed and desired by the patient and without ensuring that appropriate care continues to be provided by another qualified health care professional.

Abbreviation A shorter way of writing something.

Abdominal compartment syndrome Syndrome caused by diffuse intestinal edema, a result of fluid accumulation in the bowel wall. It may be caused by overresuscitation with crystalloids and results in shock and renal failure.

Abdominal evisceration An injury in which a severe laceration or incision of the abdomen breaches through all layers of muscle to allow abdominal contents, most often the intestines, to protrude above the surface of the skin.

Aberrant Abnormal.

Abortion The ending of a pregnancy for any reason before 20 weeks' gestation; the lay term miscarriage is referred to as a *spontaneous abortion.*

Abruptio placentae Separation of the placenta from the uterine wall after the twentieth week of gestation.

Abscess A collection of pus.

Absence seizure A generalized seizure characterized by a blank stare and an alteration of consciousness.

Absolute refractory period Corresponds with the onset of the QRS complex to approximately the peak of the T wave; cardiac cells cannot be stimulated to conduct an electrical impulse. no matter how strong the stimulus.

Absorption Movement of small organic molecules, electrolytes, vitamins, and water across the digestive tract and into the circulatory system. Also the movement of a drug from the site of input into the circulation.

Abuse Use of a substance for other than its approved, accepted purpose or in a greater amount than prescribed.

Acalculus cholecystitis Inflammation of the gallbladder in the absence of gallstones.

Acceptance A grief stage in which the individual has come to terms with the reality of his or her (or a loved one's) imminent death.

Accessory muscles Muscles of the neck, chest, and abdomen that become active during labored breathing.

Accessory pathway An extra bundle of working myocardial tissue that forms a connection between the atria and ventricles outside the normal conduction system.

Accreditation Recognition given to an EMD center by an independent auditing agency for achieving a consistently high level of performance based on industry best practice standards.

Acetylation A mechanism in which a drug is processed by enzymes.

Acetylcholinesterase A body chemical that stops the action of acetylcholine (a neurotransmitter involved in the stimulation of nerves).

Acid Fluid produced in the stomach; breaks down the food material within the stomach into chyme.

Acid-base balance Delicate balance between the body's acidity and alkalinity.

Acidic pH less than 7.0.

Acids Materials that have a pH value less than 7.0 (e.g., hydrochloric acid, sulfuric acid).

Acquired immunity Specific immunity directed at a particular pathogen that develops after the body has been exposed to it once (e.g., immunity to chickenpox after first exposure).

Acquired immunodeficiency syndrome (AIDS) An acquired immunodeficiency disease that can develop after infection with HIV.

Acrocyanosis A condition in which the core of a newborn is pink and the extremities are cyanotic.

Action potential A five-phase cycle that reflects the difference in the concentration of charged particles across the cell membrane at any given time.

Activated charcoal An adsorbent made from charred wood that effectively binds many poisons in the stomach; most effective when administered within 1 hour of intake.

Activation phase In phases of immunity, the stage at which a single lymphocyte activates many other lymphocytes and significantly expands the scope of immune response in a process known as amplification.

Active immunity Induced immunity in which the body can continue to mount specific immune response when exposed to the agent (e.g., vaccination).

Active listening Listening to the words that the patient is saying as well as paying attention to the significance of those words to the patient.

Active range of motion The degree of movement at a joint as determined by the patient's own voluntary movements.

Active transport A process used to move substances against the concentration gradient or toward the side that has a higher concentration; requires the use of energy by the cell but is faster than diffusion.

Acute arterial occlusion A sudden blockage of arterial blood flow that occurs because of a thrombus, embolus, tumor, direct trauma to an artery, or an unknown cause.

Acute care Short-term medical treatment usually provided in a hospital for patients who have an illness or injury or who are recovering from surgery.

Acute coronary syndrome (ACS) A term used to refer to patients presenting with ischemic chest discomfort. Acute coronary syndromes consist of three major syndromes: unstable angina, non–ST-segment elevation myocardial infarction and ST-segment elevation myocardial infarction.

Acute exposure An exposure that occurs over a short timeframe (less than 24 hours); usually occurs at a spill or release.

Acute renal failure (ARF) When the kidneys suddenly stop functioning, either partially or completely, but eventually recover full or nearly full functioning over time.

Acute respiratory distress syndrome (ARDS) Collection of fluid in the alveoli of the lung, usually as a result of trauma or serious illness.

Addiction The involvement in a repetitive behavior (gambling, substance abuse, etc.). In physical addiction the individual has become dependent on an external substance and develops physical withdrawal symptoms if the substance is unavailable.

Addictive behavior The involvement in repetitive behavior such as gambling or substance abuse.

Additive effect The combined effect of two drugs given at the same time that have similar effects.

Adenosine triphosphate (ATP) Formed from metabolism of nutrients in the cell; serves as an energy source throughout the body.

Adipocyte A fat cell; a connective tissue cell that has differentiated and become specialized in the synthesis (manufacture) and storage of fat.

Adipose (fat) connective tissue Tissue that stores lipids; acts as an insulator and protector of the organs of the body.

Administrative law A branch of law that deals with rules, regulations, orders, and decisions created by governmental agencies.

Adrenergic Having the characteristics of the sympathetic division of the autonomic nervous system.

Adrenocortical steroids Hormones released by the adrenal cortex essential for life; assist in the regulation of blood glucose levels, promote peripheral use of lipids, stimulate the kidneys to reabsorb sodium, and have antiinflammatory effects.

Adsorb To gather or stick to a surface in a condensed layer.

Acute respiratory distress syndrome (ARDS) A life-threatening condition that causes lung swelling and fluid buildup in the air sacs.

Advance directive A document in which a competent person gives instructions to be followed regarding his or her health care in the event the person later becomes incapacitated and unable to make or communicate those decisions to others.

Advanced emergency medical technician (AEMT) An EMS professional who provides basic and limited advanced skills to patients who access the EMS system.

Adverse effect (reaction) An unintentional, undesirable, and often unpredictable effect of a drug used at therapeutic doses to prevent, diagnose, or treat disease.

Advocate A person who assists another person in carrying out desired wishes; a paramedic should function as a patient's advocate in all aspects of prehospital care.

Aerosol A collection of particles dispersed in a gas.

Affect Description of the patient's visible emotional state.

Afferent division Nerve fibers that send impulses from the periphery to the central nervous system.

Affinity The intensity or strength of the attraction between a drug and its receptor.

Afterload Pressure or resistance against which the ventricles must pump to eject blood.

Ageism Stereotypical and often negative bias against older adults.

Agonal respirations Slow, shallow, irregular respirations resulting from anoxic brain injury.

Agonist A drug that causes a physiologic response in the receptor to which it binds.

Agonist-antagonist A drug that blocks a receptor. It may provide a partial agonist activity, but it also prevents an agonist from exerting its full effects.

Agoraphobia Consistent anxiety and avoidance of places and situations where escape during a panic attack would be difficult or embarrassing.

Air emboli Bubble of air that has entered the vasculature. Emboli can result in damage similar to a clot in the vasculature, typically resulting in brain injury or pulmonary emboli when neck vessels are damaged.

Air embolism Introduction of air into venous circulation, which can ultimately enter the right ventricle, closing off circulation to the pulmonary artery and leading to death.

Air trapping A respiratory pattern associated with an obstruction in the pulmonary tree; the breathing rate increases to overcome resistance in getting air out, the respiratory effort becomes more shallow, the volume of trapped air increases, and the lungs inflate.

Airbag identification The various shapes, sizes, colors, and styles of visual identification labels indicating that an airbag is present.

Airbags Inflatable nylon bags designed to supplement the protection of occupants during crashes; one of the most common new technology items confronting responders at crash scenes; also known as *supplemental restraint systems.*

Air-reactive materials Materials that react with atmospheric moisture and rapidly decompose.

Alarm reaction The body's autonomic, sympathetic nervous system response to stimuli designed to prepare the individual to fight or flee.

Alcoholic ketoacidosis (AKA) Condition found in patients who chronically abuse alcohol accompanied by vomiting, a built-up of ketones in the blood, and little or no food intake.

Alcoholism Addiction and dependence on ethanol; often develops over many years.

Aldosterone A hormone responsible for the reabsorption of sodium and water from the kidney tubules.

Alkali A substance with a pH above 7.0; also known as a *base* or *caustic*.

Alkaline pH greater than 7.0.

Alkaloids A group of plant-based substances containing nitrogen and found in nature.

Allergen A substance that can provoke an allergic reaction.

Allergic reaction An abnormal immune response, mediated by immunoglobulin E antibodies, to an allergen that should not cause such a response and to which the patient has already been exposed; usually involves excessive release of immune agents, especially histamines.

All-hazards emergency preparedness A cross-cutting approach in which all forms of emergencies, including manmade and natural disasters, epidemics, and physical or biologic terrorism, are managed from a common template that uses consistent language and structure.

Allografting Transplanting organs or tissues from genetically nonidentical members of the same species.

All-terrain vehicle (ATV) Any of a number of models of small open motorized vehicles designed for off-road and wilderness use; three-wheeled (all-terrain cycles) and four-wheeled (quads) versions are most often used for personnel insertion; six- and eight-wheeled models exist for specialized applications.

Alpha particle A positively charged particle emitted by certain radioactive materials.

Altered mental status Disruption of a person's emotional and intellectual functioning.

Altitude illness A syndrome associated with the relatively low partial pressure of oxygen in the atmosphere at altitudes encountered during mountain climbing or travel in unpressurized aircraft.

Alveolar air volume In contrast to dead air space, alveolar volume is the amount of air that does reach the alveoli for gas exchange (approximately 350 mL in the adult male). It is the difference between tidal volume and dead-space volume.

Alveoli Functional units of the respiratory system; area in the lungs where the majority of gas exchange takes place; singular form is *alveolus.*

Alzheimer's disease Progressive dementia seen mostly in the elderly and marked by decline of memory and cognitive function.

Amniotic sac (bag of waters) The fluid-filled protective sac that surrounds the fetus inside the uterus.

Amplitude Height (voltage) of a waveform on the ECG.

Ampule A sealed sterile container that holds a single dose of liquid or powdered medication.

Amygdala Almond-shaped structure at the end of each hippocampus that attaches emotional significance to incoming stimuli; has a large role in the fear response; plural form is *amygdale.*

Amylase Enzyme in pancreatic juice.

Amyotrophic lateral sclerosis (ALS) Autoimmune disorder affecting the motor roots of the spinal nerves, causing progressive muscle weakness and eventually paralysis.

Anal canal Area between the rectum and the anus.

Analgesia A state in which pain is controlled or not perceived.

Anaphylactic reaction An unusual or exaggerated allergic reaction to a foreign substance.

Anaphylactoid reaction Reaction that clinically mimics an allergic reaction but is not mediated by immunoglobulin E antibodies, so not a true allergic reaction.

Anaphylaxis Life-threatening allergic reaction.

Anasarca Massive generalized body edema.

Anatomic plane The relation of internal body structures to the surface of the body; imaginary straight line divisions of the body.

Anatomic position The position of a person standing erect with his or her feet and palms facing the examiner.

Anatomy Study of the body's structure and organization.

Anchor point A single secure connection for an anchor.

Anchors The means of securing the ropes and other elements of the high-angle system.

Anemia Deficiency in red blood cells or hemoglobin; most common form is iron-deficiency anemia.

Anesthesia A process in which pain is prevented during a procedure.

Aneurysm Localized dilation or bulging of a blood vessel wall or wall of a heart chamber.

Anger A stage in the grieving process in which the individual is upset by the stated future loss of life.

Angina pectoris Chest discomfort or other related symptoms of sudden onset that may occur because the increased oxygen demand of the heart temporarily exceeds the blood supply.

Anginal equivalents Symptoms of myocardial ischemia other than chest pain or discomfort.

Angioedema Swelling of the tissues, including the dermal layer; often found in and around the mouth, tongue, and lips.

Angle of Louis An angulation of the sternum that indicates the point where the second rib joins the sternum; also called the *manubriosternal junction.*

Anhedonia Lack of enjoyment in activities one used to find pleasurable.

Anion A negatively charged ion.

Anorexia nervosa Eating disorder characterized by a preoccupation that one is obese; drastic, intentional weight loss; and bizarre attitudes and rituals associated with food and exercise.

Anoxia A total lack of oxygen availability to the tissues.

Antagonist A drug that does not cause a physiologic response when it binds with a receptor.

Antegrade amnesia The inability to remember short-term memory information after an event during which the head was struck.

Antepartum The period before childbirth.

Anterior The front, or ventral, surface.

Anterior cord syndrome Collection of symptoms seen after the compression, death, or transection of the anterior portion of the spinal cord.

Anthrax An acute bacterial infection caused by inhalation, contact, or ingestion of *Bacillus anthracis* organisms. Three forms of anthrax disease may occur depending on the route of exposure. Inhalational anthrax disease occurs after the inhalation of anthrax spores. Cutaneous anthrax disease is the most common form and occurs after the exposure of compromised skin to anthrax spores. Gastrointestinal anthrax disease occurs after the ingestion of live *B. anthracis* in contaminated meat.

Antiarrhythmic Medications used to correct irregular heartbeats and slow hearts that beat too fast.

Antibacterial Medication that kills or limits bacteria.

Antibiotic In common medical terms, a drug that kills bacteria.

Antibody Agents produced by B lymphocytes that bind to antigens, thus killing or controlling them and slowing or stopping an infection; also called *immunoglobulin*.

Antidiuretic hormone (ADH) A hormone released in response to detected loss of body water; prevents further loss of water through the urinary tract by promoting the reabsorption of water into the blood.

Antidote A substance that can reverse the adverse effects of a poison.

Antifungal Agent that kills fungi.

Antigen A marker on a cell that identifies the cell as "self" or "not self"; antigens are used by antibodies to identify cells that should be attacked as not self.

Antihistamine Medication that reduces the effects of histamine.

Antiinflammatory mediators Protein entities, often produced in the liver, that act as modulators of the immune response to the proinflammatory response to injury; also called *cytokines*.

Antipyretic medication A medication that reduces or eliminates a fever.

Antisepsis Prevention of sepsis by preventing or inhibiting the growth of causative microorganisms; in the field, the process used to cleanse local skin areas before needle puncture with products that are alcohol or iodine based.

Antivenin A substance that can reverse the adverse effects of a venom by binding to it and inactivating it.

Antiviral Medication that kills or impedes a virus.

Antonym A root word, prefix, or suffix that has the *opposite* meaning of another word.

Anucleated Cells of the body that do not have a central nucleus, such as those in cardiac muscle.

Anus The end of the anal canal.

Anxiety The sometimes vague feeling of apprehension, uneasiness, dread, or worry that often occurs without a specific source or cause identified. It is also a normal response to a perceived threat.

Aorta Delivers blood from the left ventricle of the heart to the body.

Aortic valve Semilunar valve on the left of the heart; separates the left ventricle from the aorta.

Apex Tip.

Apex of the heart Lower portion of the heart, tip of the ventricles (approximately the level of the fifth left intercostal space); points leftward, downward, and forward.

Apgar score A scoring system applied to an infant after delivery; key components include appearance, pulse, grimace, activity, and respiration.

Aphasia Loss of speech.

Apnea Respiratory arrest.

Apnea monitor A technologic aid used to warn of cessation of breathing in a premature infant; also may warn of bradycardia and tachycardia.

Apocrine glands Sweat glands that open into hair follicles, including in and around the genitalia, axillae, and anus; secrete an organic substance (which is odorless until acted upon by surface bacteria) into the hair follicles.

Appendicitis A tubular process that extends from the colon.

Appendicular region Area that includes the extremities (e.g., arms, pelvis, and legs).

Appendicular skeleton Consists of all the bones not within the axial skeleton: upper and lower extremities, the girdles, and their attachments.

Appendix Accessory structure of the cecum.

Application of principles The step at which the paramedic applies critical thinking in a clinical sense and arrives at a field impression or a working diagnosis.

Aqueous humor Fluid that fills the anterior chamber of the eye; maintains intraocular pressure.

Arachnoid mater Second layer of the meninges.

Arachnoid membrane Weblike middle layer of the meninges.

Areolar connective tissue A loose tissue found in most organs of the body; consists of weblike collagen, reticulum, and elastin fibers.

Arnold-Chiari malformation A complication of spina bifida in which the brainstem and cerebellum extend down through the foramen magnum into the cervical portion of the vertebrae.

Arrector pili Smooth muscle that surrounds each follicle; responsible for "goose bumps," which pull the hair upwards.

Arrhythmia Term often used interchangeably with dysrhythmia; any disturbance or abnormality in a normal rhythmic pattern; any cardiac rhythm other than a sinus rhythm.

Arterial puncture Accidental puncture into an artery instead of a vein.

Arterioles Small arterial vessels; supply oxygenated blood to the capillaries.

Arteriosclerosis A chronic disease of the arterial system characterized by abnormal thickening and hardening of the vessel walls.

Arthritis Inflammation of a joint that results in pain, stiffness, swelling, and redness.

Artifact Distortion of an ECG tracing by electrical activity that is noncardiac in origin (e.g., electrical interference, poor electrical conduction, patient movement).

Artificial anchors The use of specially designed hardware to create anchors where good natural anchors do not exist.

Arytenoid cartilages Six paired cartilages stacked on top of each other in the larynx.

Ascending colon Part of the large intestine.

Ascites Marked abdominal swelling from a buildup of fluid in the peritoneal cavity.

Asepsis Sterile; free from germs, infection, and any form of life.

Asphyxiants Chemicals that impair the body's ability to either get or use oxygen.

Aspiration Inhalation of foreign contents into the lungs.

Aspiration pneumonitis Inflammation of the bronchi and alveoli caused by inhaled foreign objects, usually acids such as stomach acid.

Assault A threat of imminent bodily harm to another person by someone with the obvious ability to carry out the threat.

Assay A test of a substance to determine its components.

Assessment-based management Taking the information you obtain from your assessment and using it to treat the patient.

Asthma Allergic response of the airways causing wheezing and dyspnea.

Asynchronous pacemaker Fixed-rate pacemaker that continuously discharges at a preset rate regardless of the patient's intrinsic activity.

Asystole A total absence of ventricular electrical activity.

Ataxia Inability to control voluntary muscle movements; unsteady movements and staggering gait.

Atelectasis An abnormal condition characterized by the collapse of alveoli, preventing the respiratory exchange of carbon dioxide and oxygen in a part of the lungs.

Atherosclerosis A form of arteriosclerosis in which the thickening and hardening of the vessel walls are caused by a buildup of fatty deposits in the inner lining of large and middle-sized muscular arteries (from *athero*, meaning gruel or paste, and *sclerosis*, meaning hardness).

Atlas First cervical vertebra.

Atopic A genetic disposition to an allergic reaction that is different from developing an allergy after one or more exposures to a drug or substance.

Atresia Absence of a normal opening.

Atria Two receiving chambers of the heart; singular form is *atrium*.

Atrial kick Remaining 20% to 30% of blood forced into the right ventricle during atrial contraction.

Atrioventricular junction The atrioventricular node and the nonbranching portion of the bundle of His.

Atrioventricular node A group of cells that conduct an electrical impulse through the heart; located in the floor of the right atrium immediately behind the tricuspid valve and near the opening of the coronary sinus.

Atrioventricular sequential pacemaker Type of dual-chamber pacemaker that stimulates first the atrium, then the ventricle, mimicking normal cardiac physiology.

Atrioventricular valve Valve located between each atrium and ventricle; the tricuspid separates the right atrium from the right ventricle, and the mitral (bicuspid) separates the left atrium from the left ventricle.

Atrophy Decrease in cell size that negatively affects function.

Attenuated vaccine A vaccine prepared from a live virus or bacteria that has been physically or chemically weakened to produce an immune response without causing the severe effects of the disease.

Attributes Qualities or characteristics of a person.

Auditory ossicles Three small bones (malleus, incus, and stapes) that articulate with each other to transmit sounds waves to the cochlea.

Augmented limb lead Leads aVR, aVL, and aVF; these leads record the difference in electrical potential at one location relative to zero potential rather than relative to the electrical potential of another extremity, as in the bipolar leads.

Aura Sensory disturbances caused by a partial seizure; may precede a generalized seizure.

Auricle Outer ear; also called the *pinna*.

Auscultation The process of listening to body noises with a stethoscope.

Authority having jurisdiction The local agency having legal authority for the type of rescue and the location at which it occurs.

Autoantibodies Antibodies produced by B cells that mistakenly attack and destroy "self" cells belonging to the patient; autoantibodies are the pathophysiologic agent of most autoimmune disorders.

Autografting Transplanting organs or tissues within the same person.

Autoignition point The temperature at which a material ignites and burns without an ignition source.

Autologous skin grafting The transplantation of skin of one patient from its original location to that of a wound on the same patient, such as a burn. Autologous means "derived from the same individual."

Automatic location identification Telephone technology used to identify the location of a caller immediately.

Automatic number identification Telephone technology that provides immediate identification of the caller's 10-digit telephone number.

Automaticity Ability of cardiac pacemaker cells to initiate an electrical impulse spontaneously without being stimulated from another source (such as a nerve).

Autonomic dysreflexia Massive sympathetic stimulation unbalanced by the parasympathetic nervous system because of spinal cord injury, usually at or above T6.

Autonomic dysreflexia syndrome A condition characterized by hypertension superior to an SCI site caused by overstimulation of the sympathetic nervous system.

Autonomic nervous system Provides unconscious control of smooth muscle organ and glands.

AVPU Mnemonic for *a*wake, *v*erbal, *p*ain, *u*nresponsive; used to evaluate a patient's mental status.

Axial compression (loading) The application of a force of energy along the axis of the spine, often resulting in compression fractures of the vertebrae.

Axial loading Application of excessive pressure or weight along the vertical axis of the spine.

Axial region Area that includes the head, neck, thorax, and abdomen.

Axial skeleton Part of the skeleton composed of the skull, hyoid bone, vertebral column, and thoracic cage.

Axis Imaginary line joining the positive and negative electrodes of a lead.

Axon Branching extensions of the neuron where impulses exit the cell.

Azotemia The increase in nitrogen-containing waste products in the blood secondary to renal failure.

B lymphocytes Cells present in the lymphatic system that mediate humoral immunity (also known as *B cells*).

B pillar The structural roof support member on a vehicle located at the rear edge of the front door; also referred to as the *B post*.

Babinski's sign An abnormal finding indicated by the presence of great toe extension with the fanning of all other toes on stimulation of the sole of the foot when it is stroked with a semi-sharp object from the heel to the ball of the foot.

Bacillus anthracis A gram-positive, spore-forming bacterium that causes anthrax disease in human beings and animals.

Bacteremia The presence of bacteria in the blood. This condition could progress to septic shock. Fever, chills, tachycardia, and tachypnea are common manifestations of bacteremia.

Bacteria Prokaryotic microorganisms capable of infecting and injuring patients; however, some bacteria, as part of the normal flora, assist in the processes of the human body.

Bacterial tracheitis A potentially serious bacterial infection of the lower portions of the upper airway: larynx, trachea, and bronchi.

Band A range of radio frequencies.

Bargaining A stage of the grieving process. The individual may attempt to "cut a deal" with a higher power to accomplish a specific goal or task.

Bariatric ambulance Ambulance designed to transport morbidly obese patients.

Barotrauma An injury resulting from rapid or extreme changes in pressure.

Barrier device A thin film of material placed on the patient's face used to prevent direct contact with the patient's mouth during positive-pressure ventilation.

Base of the heart Top of the heart; located at approximately the level of the second intercostal space.

Baseline Straight line recorded on ECG graph paper when no electrical activity is detected.

Bases Materials with a pH value greater than 7.0 (e.g., sodium hydroxide, potassium hydroxide).

Basilar skull fracture Loss of integrity to the bony structures of the base of the skull.

Basophils Type of granulocyte (white blood cell or leukocyte) that releases histamine.

Battery Touching or contact with another person without that person's consent.

Battle's sign Significant bruising around the mastoid process (behind the ears).

Beck's triad Classic signs of cardiac tamponade that include jugular venous distention, hypotension, and muffled heart sounds.

Behavior The conduct and activity of a person that is observable by others.

Behavioral emergency Actions or ideations by the patient that are harmful or potentially harmful to the patient or others.

Belay A safety technique used to safeguard personnel exposed to the risk of falling; the belayer is the person responsible for operation of the belay.

Bell's palsy An inflammation of the facial nerve (cranial nerve VII) that often is preceded by a viral upper respiratory tract infection.

Benchmarking Comparison of operating policies, procedures, protocols, and performance with those of other agencies in an effort to improve results.

Benzodiazepine Any of a group of minor tranquilizers with a common molecular structure and similar pharmacologic activity, including antianxiety, sedative, hypnotic, amnestic, anticonvulsant, and muscle-relaxing effects.

Beriberi Disease caused by a deficiency of thiamine and characterized by neurologic symptoms, cardiovascular abnormalities, and edema.

Beta particle A negatively charged particle emitted by certain radioactive materials.

Bevel The slanted tip at the end of the needle.

Bicuspid valve Left atrioventricular valve in the heart; also called the *mitral valve*.

Bile salts Manufactured in the liver; composed of electrolytes and iron recovered from red blood cells when they die.

Bilevel positive airway pressure (BiPAP) The delivery of two (bi) levels of positive-pressure ventilation; one during inspiration (to keep the airway open as the patient inhales) and the other (lower) pressure during expiration to reduce the work of exhalation.

Bilevel positive airway pressure (BiPAP) device Breathing device that can be set at one pressure for inhaling and a different pressure for exhaling.

Bioassay A test that determines the effects of a substance on an organism and compares the result with some agreed standard.

Bioavailability The speed with which and how much of a drug reaches its intended site of action.

Bioburden Accumulation of bacteria in a wound; does not necessarily imply an infection is present.

Biologic agent A disease-causing pathogen or a toxin that may be used as a weapon to cause disease or injury to people.

Biot respirations Irregular respirations varying in rate and depth and interrupted by periods of apnea; associated with increased intracranial pressure, brain damage at the level of the medulla, and respiratory compromise from drug poisoning.

Biphasic Waveform that is partly positive and partly negative.

Bipolar disorder An illness of extremes of mood, alternating between periods of depression and episodes of mania (type I) or hypomania (type II).

Bipolar limb lead ECG lead consisting of a positive and negative electrode; a pacing lead with two electrical poles that are external from the pulse generator; the negative pole is located at the extreme distal tip of the pacing lead, and the positive pole is located several millimeters proximal to the negative electrode. The stimulating pulse is delivered through the negative electrode.

Birth canal Part of the female reproductive tract through which the fetus is delivered; includes the lower part of the uterus, the cervix, and the vagina.

Blast lung syndrome Injuries to the body from an explosion, characterized by anatomic and physiologic changes from the force generated by the blast wave hitting the body's surface and affecting primarily gas-containing structures (lungs, gastrointestinal tract, and ears).

Bleeding Escape of blood from a blood vessel.

Blister agent A chemical used as a weapon designed specifically to injure the body tissue internally and externally of those exposed to its vapors or liquid; the method of injury is to cause painful skin blisters or tissue destruction of the exposed surface area (e.g., mustard, lewisite).

Blocked premature atrial complex Premature atrial contraction not followed by a QRS complex.

Blocking A position that places the emergency vehicle at an angle to the approaching traffic, across several lanes of traffic if necessary; this position begins to shield the work area and protects the crash scene from some of the approaching traffic.

Blood Liquid connective tissue; allows transport of nutrients, oxygen, and waste products.

Blood agents Chemicals absorbed into the body through the action of breathing, skin absorption, or ingestion (e.g., hydrogen cyanide, cyanogen chloride).

Blood alcohol content Milligrams of ethanol per deciliter of blood divided by 100; a fairly standard measure of how intoxicated a person is.

Blood-brain barrier A layer of tightly adhered cells that protects the brain and spinal cord from exposure to medications, toxins, and infectious particles.

Blood pressure Force exerted by the blood against the walls of the arteries as the ventricles of the heart contract and relax.

Bloody show Passage of the protective blood and mucus plug from the cervix; often is an early sign of labor.

Body mass index A calculation strongly associated with subcutaneous and total body fat and with skinfold thickness measurements.

Body surface area (BSA) Area of the body covered by skin; measured in square meters.

Boiling liquid expanding vapor explosion An explosion that can occur when a vessel containing a pressurized liquid ruptures.

Boiling point The temperature at which the vapor pressure of the material being heated equals atmospheric pressure (760 mm Hg); water boils to steam at 100° C (212° F).

Bone Hard connective tissue; consists of living cells and a matrix made of minerals.

Borborygmi Hyperactivity of bowel sounds.

Borderline personality disorder Cluster B disorder marked by unstable emotions, relationships, and attitudes.

Botulism A severe neurologic illness caused by a potent toxin produced by *Clostridium botulinum* organisms; the three forms are food borne, wound, and infant (also called intestinal) botulism.

Bowel sounds The noises made by the intestinal smooth muscles as they squeeze fluids and food products through the digestive tract.

Bowman's capsule Located in the renal corpuscle.

Boyle's law Gas law that demonstrates that as pressure increases, volume decreases; explains the pain that can occur in flight in the teeth and ears and barotrauma in the gastrointestinal tract.

Bradycardia Heart rate slower than 60 beats/min (from *brady,* meaning "slow").

Bradykinesia Abnormal slowness of muscular movement.

Bradypnea A respiratory rate that is persistently slower than normal for age; in adults, a rate slower than 12 breaths/min.

Brain injury A traumatic insult to the brain capable of producing physical, intellectual, emotional, social, and vocational changes.

Brainstem Part of the brain that connects it to the spinal cord; responsible for many of the autonomic functions the body requires to survive (also called *vegetative functions*).

Brake bar rack A descending device consisting of a U-shaped metal bar to which several metal bars are attached that create friction on the rope. Some racks are limited to use in personal rappelling, whereas others also may be used for lowering rescue loads.

Braxton-Hicks contractions (false labor) Benign and painless contractions that usually occur after the third month of pregnancy.

Breach of duty Violation by the defendant of the standard of care applicable to the circumstances.

Breech presentation Presentation of the buttocks or feet of the fetus as the first part of the infant's body to enter the birth canal.

Bronchioles Smallest of the air passages.

Bronchiolitis An acute, infectious, inflammatory disease of the upper and lower respiratory tracts that results in obstruction of the small airways.

Bronchitis Inflammation of the lower airways, usually with mucus production. Often chronic and related to tobacco abuse.

Bronchopulmonary dysplasia (BPD) Respiratory condition in infants usually arising from preterm birth.

Bronchospasm Wheezing.

Brown-Séquard syndrome Group of symptoms that develop after the herniation or transection of half of the spinal cord manifested with unilateral damage.

Bruit The blowing or swishing sound created by the turbulence within a blood vessel.

Bubonic Relating to an inflamed, enlarged lymph gland.

Buccal An administration route in which medication is placed in the mouth between the gum and the mucous membrane of the cheek and absorbed into the bloodstream.

Buffer systems Compensatory mechanisms that act together to control pH.

Bulbourethral glands Pair of small glands that manufacture a mucous-type secretion that unites with the prostate fluid and spermatozoa to form sperm.

Bulimia nervosa Eating disorder consisting of a pattern of eating large amounts of food in one sitting (binging) and then forcing oneself to regurgitate (purging), with associated guilt and depression.

Bulk containers Large containers and tanks used to transport large quantities of hazardous materials.

Bulla A localized, fluid-filled lesion usually greater than 0.5 cm.

Bundle branch block (BBB) Abnormal conduction of an electrical impulse through either the right or left bundle branches.

Bundle of His Fibers located in the upper portion of the interventricular septum that conduct an electrical impulse through the heart.

Burnout Exhaustion to the point of not being able to perform one's job effectively.

Bursitis Chronic or acute inflammation of the small synovial sacs known as bursa.

Burst Three or more sequential ectopic beats; also referred to as a *salvo* or *run*.

Cadaveric transplantation Transplantation of organs from an already deceased person to a living person.

Calibration Regulation of an ECG machine's stylus sensitivity so that a 1-mV electrical signal will produce a deflection measuring exactly 10 mm.

Call processing time The elapsed time from the moment a call is received by the communications center to the time the responding unit is alerted.

Cancer A group of diseases that allow unrestrained growth of cells in one or more of the body organs or tissues.

Capacitance vessels Venules that have the capability of holding large amounts of volume.

Capillaries Tiny vessels that connect arterioles to venules; deliver blood to each cell in the body.

Capillary leak Loss of intravascular fluid (plasma, water) from a loss of capillary integrity or an opening of gap junctions between the cells of the capillaries.

May be caused by thermal injury to capillaries or the intense inflammatory reaction to burn injury, infection, or physical trauma.

Caplet A tablet with an oblong shape and a film-coated covering.

Capnograph A device that provides a numerical reading of exhaled CO_2 concentrations and a waveform (tracing).

Capnography Continuous analysis and recording of CO_2 concentrations in respiratory gases.

Capnometer A device used to measure the concentration of CO_2 at the end of exhalation.

Capnometry A numeric reading of exhaled CO_2 concentrations without a continuous written record or waveform.

Capsid Layer of protein enveloping the genome of a virion; composed of structural units called the capsomeres.

Capsule A membranous shell surrounding certain microorganisms, such as the pneumococcus bacterium.

Capture Ability of a pacing stimulus to depolarize successfully the cardiac chamber being paced; with one-to-one capture, each pacing stimulus results in depolarization of the appropriate chamber.

Carbamate A pesticide that inhibits acetylcholinesterase.

Carbon dioxide narcosis Condition mostly seen in patients with chronic obstructive pulmonary disease, in whom carbon dioxide is excessively retained, causing mental status changes and decreased respirations.

Carboys Glass or plastic bottles commonly used to transport corrosive products.

Carbuncle A series of abscesses in the subcutaneous tissues that drain through hair follicles.

Cardiac arrest Absence of cardiac mechanical activity confirmed by the absence of a detectable pulse, unresponsiveness, and apnea or agonal, gasping respirations.

Cardiac cycle Period from the beginning of one heartbeat to the beginning of the next; normally consisting of PQRST waves, complexes, and intervals.

Cardiac output Amount of blood pumped into the aorta each minute by the heart.

Cardiac rupture An acute traumatic perforation of the ventricles or atria.

Cardiac sphincter Circular muscle that controls the movement of material into the stomach.

Cardiogenic shock A condition in which heart muscle function is severely impaired, leading to decreased cardiac output and inadequate tissue perfusion.

Cardiomyopathy A disease of the heart muscle.

Cardiovascular disorders A collection of diseases and conditions that involve the heart (cardio) and blood vessels (vascular).

Carina Area in the bronchial tree that separates into the right and left mainstem bronchi.

Carotid bruit The noise made when blood in the carotid arteries passes over plaque buildups.

Carpal tunnel syndrome A medical condition in which the median nerve is compressed at the wrist (within the carpal tunnel), resulting in pain and numbness of the hand.

Carpopedal spasm Spasm of the muscles of the hand when a blood pressure cuff is inflated. Can occur in the feet if the cuff is placed on the leg. A result of hyperventilation.

Cartilage Connective tissue composed of chondrocytes; exact makeup depends on the location and function in the body.

Cartilaginous joint Unites two bones with hyaline cartilage or fibrocartilage.

Case law Interpretations of constitutional, statutory, or administrative law made by the courts; also known as *common law* or *judge-made law.*

Catabolic Refers to the metabolic breakdown of proteins, lipids, and carbohydrates by the body to produce energy.

Catabolism Process of breaking down complex substances into more simple ones.

Catalepsy Abnormal state characterized by a trancelike level of consciousness and postural rigidity; occurs in hypnosis and in certain organic and psychological disorders such as schizophrenia, epilepsy, and hysteria.

Cataract A partial or complete opacity on or in the lens or lens capsule of the eye, especially one impairing vision or causing blindness.

Catatonia A state of psychologically induced immobility with muscular rigidity, at times interrupted by agitation.

Catatonic schizophrenia A form of schizophrenia characterized by alternating periods of extreme withdrawal and extreme excitement. During the withdrawal stage stupor, waxy flexibility, muscular rigidity, mutism, blocking, negativism, and catalepsy may be seen; during the period of excitement, purposeless and impulsive activity may range from mild agitation to violence. See *Catatonia.*

Cathartics Substances that decrease the time a poison spends in the gastrointestinal tract by increasing bowel motility.

Catheter shear/catheter fragment embolism Breaking off the tip of the intravenous catheter inside the vein, which then travels through the venous system; it can lodge in pulmonary circulation as a pulmonary embolism.

Cation A positively charged ion.

Cauda equina Peripheral nerve bundles descending through the spinal column distal to the conus medullaris. Cauda equina are not spinal nerves.

Cauda equina syndrome A group of symptoms associated with the compression of the peripheral nerves still within the spinal canal below the level of the first lumbar vertebra, characterized by lumbar back pain, motor and sensory deficits, and bowel or bladder incontinence.

Caudal A position toward the distal end of the body; usually inferior.

Causation In a negligence case, the negligence of the defendant must have caused or created the harm sustained by the plaintiff; also referred to as *proximate cause.*

Caustic A substance with a pH above 7.0; also known as a *base* or *alkali.*

Cecum First segment of the large intestine; the appendix is its accessory structure.

Cell body Portion of the neuron containing the organelles, where essential cellular functions are performed.

Cell-mediated immunity Form of acquired immunity; results from activation of T lymphocytes that were previously sensitized to a specific antigen.

Cellular swelling Swelling of cellular tissues, usually from injury.

Cellulitis An inflammation of the skin.

Cementum A layer of tough tissue that anchors the root of a tooth to the periodontal membrane/ligament.

Central cord syndrome Collection of symptoms seen after the death of the central portion of the spinal cord.

Central nervous system The brain and spinal cord.

Central neurogenic hyperventilation Similar to Kussmaul respirations; characterized as deep, rapid breathing; associated with increased intracranial pressure.

Central retinal artery occlusion A condition in which the blood supply to the retina is blocked because of a clot or embolus in the central retinal artery or one of its branches.

Central vein A major vein of the chest, neck, or abdomen.

Central venous catheter A catheter through a vein to end in the superior vena cava or right atrium of the heart for medication or fluid administration.

Centrioles Paired, rodlike structures that exist in a specialized area of the cytoplasm known as the centrosome.

Centrosome Specialized area of the cytoplasm; plays an important role in the process of cell division.

Cephalic A position toward the head; usually superior.

Cerebellum Area of the brain involved in fine and gross coordination; responsible for interpretation of actual movement and correction of any movements that interfere with coordination and the body's position.

Cerebral contusion A brain injury in which brain tissue is bruised in a local area but does not puncture the pia mater.

Cerebral palsy Neuromuscular condition in which the patient has difficulty controlling the voluntary muscles because of damage to a portion of the brain.

Cerebral perfusion pressure Pressure inside the cerebral arteries and an indicator of brain perfusion; calculated by subtracting intracranial pressure from mean arterial pressure (CPP = MAP − ICP).

Cerebrospinal fluid (CSF) Fluid that bathes, protects, and nourishes the central nervous system.

Cerebrovascular accident (CVA) Blockage or hemorrhage of the blood vessels in the brain, usually causing focal neurologic deficits; also known as a *stroke.*

Cerebrum Largest part of the brain, divided into right and left hemispheres.

Certification An external verification of the competencies that an individual has achieved and typically involves an examination process; in healthcare these processes are typically designed to verify that an individual has achieved minimal competency to ensure safe and effective patient care.

Certified Flight Paramedic (FP-C) A certification obtained by paramedics on successful completion of the Flight Paramedic Examination.

Certified Flight Registered Nurse (CFRN) A nurse who has completed education, training, and certification beyond a registered nurse with a focus on air medical transport of potentially critically ill or injured patients.

Cerumen Earwax.

Ceruminous glands Glands lining the external auditory canal; produce cerumen or earwax.

Cervical spondylosis Degeneration of two or more cervical vertebrae, usually resulting in a narrowing of the space between the vertebrae.

Cervical vertebrae First seven vertebrae in descending order from the base of the skull.

Cervix Inferior portion of the uterus.

Chalazion A small bump on the eyelid caused by a blocked oil gland.

Charles' law Law stating that oxygen cylinders can have variations in pressure readings in different ambient temperatures.

Chelating agent A substance that can bind metals; used as an antidote to many heavy metal poisonings.

Chemical Abstracts Services (CAS) number Unique identification number of chemicals, much like a person's Social Security number.

Chemical asphyxiants Chemicals that prevent the transportation of oxygen to the cells or the use of oxygen at the cellular level.

Chemical name A precise description of a drug's chemical composition and molecular structure.

Chemical restraints Agents such as sedatives that can suppress a patient's neurologic and/or motor capabilities and reduce the threat to the paramedic; also known as *pharmacologic restraints*.

Cheyne-Stokes respirations A pattern of gradually increasing rate and depth of breathing that tapers to slower and shallower breathing with a period of apnea before the cycle repeats itself; often described as a crescendo-decrescendo pattern or periodic breathing.

Chief complaint The reason the patient has sought medical attention.

Child maltreatment An all-encompassing term for all types of child abuse and neglect, including physical abuse, emotional abuse, sexual abuse, and neglect.

Chloracetophenone Tear gas; commercially known as *Mace*.

Choanal atresia Narrowing or blockage of one or both nares by membranous or bony tissue.

Choking agent An industrial chemical used as a weapon to kill those who inhale the vapors or gases; the method of injury is asphyxiation resulting from lung damage from hydrochloric acid burns (e.g., chlorine, phosgene); also known as a pulmonary agent.

Cholangitis Inflammation of the bile duct.

Cholecystitis Inflammation of the gallbladder.

Choledocholithiasis The presence of gallstones in the common bile duct.

Cholelithiasis The presence of stones in the gallbladder.

Cholinergic Having the characteristics of the parasympathetic division of the autonomic nervous system.

Cholinesterase inhibitor A chemical that blocks the action of acetylcholinesterase; thus the neurotransmitter acetylcholine is allowed to send its signals continuously to innervate nerve endings.

Chordae tendineae Fibrous bands of tissue in the valves that attach to each part or cusp of the valve.

Chorioamnionitis Infection of the amniotic sac and its contents.

Choroid Vascular layer of the eyeball.

Choroid plexus Group of specialized cells in the ventricles of the brain; filters blood through cerebral capillaries to create the cerebrospinal fluid.

Chromatin Material within a cell nucleus from which the chromosomes are formed.

Chromosomes Any of the threadlike structures in the nucleus of a cell that function in the transmission of genetic information; each consists of a double strand of DNA attached to proteins called histones.

Chronic Long, drawn out; applied to a disease that is not acute.

Chronic exposure An exposure to low concentrations over a long period.

Chronic obstructive pulmonary disease (COPD) A progressive and irreversible condition characterized by diminished inspiratory and expiratory capacity of the lungs.

Chronic renal failure The gradual, long-term deterioration of kidney function.

Chronology The arrangement of events in time.

Chronotropism A change in heart rate.

Chute time The time required to get a unit en route to a call from dispatch.

Chyme Semifluid mass of partly digested food expelled by the stomach into the duodenum.

Ciliary body Consists of muscles that change the shape of the lens in the eye; includes a network of capillaries that produce aqueous humor.

Circadian A daily rhythmic activity cycle based on 24-hour intervals or events that occur at approximately 24-hour intervals, such as certain physiologic occurrences.

Circadian rhythm The 24-hour cycle that relates to work and rest time.

Circumflex artery Division of the left coronary artery.

Circumoral paresthesia A feeling of tingling around the lips and mouth caused by hyperventilation.

Circumstantial thinking Adding detours and extra details to conversations but eventually returning to the main topic.

Cirrhosis A chronic degenerative disease of the liver.

Civil law A branch of law that deals with torts (civil wrongs) committed by one individual, organization, or group against another.

Clarification Asking to speaker to help you understand.

Classic heat stroke Heat stroke caused by environmental exposure that results in core hyperthermia greater than 40°C. (104°F).

Clean To wash with soap and water.

Cleft lip Incomplete closure of the upper lip.

Cleft palate Incomplete closure of the hard and/or soft palate of the mouth.

Clinical performance indicator A definable, measurable, skilled task completed by the dispatcher that has a significant impact on the delivery of patient care.

Clitoris Small, erectile structure at the entrance to the vagina.

Closed-ended questions A form of interview question that limits a patient's response to simple, brief words or phrases (e.g., "yes or no," "sharp or dull").

Closed fracture Fracture of the bone tissue that has not broken the skin tissue.

Clostridium botulinum A bacterium that produces a powerful toxin that causes botulism disease in human beings, waterfowl, and cattle.

Cluster A personality disorders Odd and eccentric type of personality disorders, including paranoid, schizoid, and schizotypal; characterized by social isolation and odd thought processes.

Cluster B personality disorders Emotional and dramatic type of personality disorders, including histrionic, borderline, antisocial, and narcissistic; characterized by impulsive, unpredictable behavior, and manipulation of others.

Cluster C personality disorders Anxious and fearful type of personality disorders, including avoidant, dependent, and compulsive; marked by anxiety, shyness, and avoidance of conflict.

Cluster headache A migraine-like condition characterized by attacks of intense unilateral pain. The pain occurs most often over the eye and forehead and is accompanied by flushing and watering of the eyes and nose. The attacks occur in groups, with a duration of several hours.

CNS-PAD An acronym for *c*entral *n*ervous *s*ystem padding: *p*ia matter, *a*rachnid matter, *d*ura matter.

Coagulation Formation of blood clots with the associated increase in blood viscosity.

Coagulation cascade A set of interactions of the circulating clotting factors.

Coagulation necrosis Dead or dying tissue that forms a scar or eschar.

Cocaine hydrochloride Fine, white powdered form of cocaine, a powerful central nervous system stimulant; typically snorted intranasally.

Coccyx (coccygeal vertebrae) Terminal end of the spinal column; a tail-like bone composed of three to five vertebra. No nerve roots travel through the coccyx.

Cochlea Bony structure in the inner ear resembling a tiny snail shell.

Code of ethics A guide for interactions between members of a specific profession (such as physicians) and the public.

Codependence A psychological concept defined as exhibiting too much and often inappropriate caring behavior.

Cognition Operation of the mind by which one becomes aware of objects of thought or perception; includes all aspects of perceiving, thinking, and remembering.

cognitive disability An impairment that affects an individual's awareness and memory as well as his or her ability to learn, process information, communicate, and make decisions.

Cognitive phase In the phases of immune response, the stage at which a foreign antigen is recognized to be present.

Cold diuresis The occurrence of increased urine production on exposure to cold.

Cold protective response The mechanism associated with cold water in which individuals can survive extended periods of submersion.

Cold zone A safe area isolated from the area of contamination; also called the *support zone*. This zone has safe and easy access. It contains the command post and staging areas for personnel, vehicles, and equipment. EMS personnel are stationed in the cold zone.

Collagen A fibrous protein that provides elasticity and strength to skin and the body's connective tissue.

Collapsed lung See *Pneumothorax*.

Colostomy Incision in the colon for the purpose of making a temporary or permanent opening between the bowel and the abdominal wall.

Combination deployment Using a mix of geographic coverage and demand posts to best serve the community given the number of ambulances available at any one time.

Combining form A word root followed by a vowel.

Combining vowel A vowel that is added to a word root before a suffix.

Comfort care Medical care intended to provide relief from pain and discomfort, such as the control of pain with medications.

Command post The location from which incident operations are directed.

Comminuted skull fracture Breakage of a bone or bones of the skull into multiple fragments.

Communicable period The period after infection during which the diease may be transmitted to another host.

Communication The exchange of thoughts, messages, and information.

Compartment syndrome (CS) A condition in which compartment pressures increase in an injured extremity to the point that capillary circulation is stopped; often only correctable through surgical opening of the compartment.

Compensatory pause Pause for which the normal beat after a premature complex occurs when expected; also called a *complete pause*.

Complete abortion Passage of all fetal tissue before 20 weeks of gestation.

Complex Several waveforms.

Complex partial seizure A seizure affecting only one part of the brain that does alter consciousness.

Compliance The resistance of the patient's lung tissue to ventilation.

Compound presentation Presentation of an extremity beside the major presenting fetal part.

Compound skull fracture Open skull fracture.

Compound word Word that contains more than one root.

Computer-aided dispatch (CAD) A computer-aided system that automates dispatching by enhanced data collection, rapid recall of information, dispatch mapping, as well as unit tracking and the ability to track and dispatch resources.

Concealment To hide or put out of site; provides no ballistic protection.

Concept formation The initial formation of an overall concept of care for a particular patient begins when the paramedic arrives on location of the incident.

Conception The act or process of fertilization; beginning of pregnancy.

Concurrent medical direction Consultation with a physician or other advanced health care professional by telephone, radio, or other electronic means, permitting the physician and paramedic to decide together on the best course of action in the delivery of patient care.

Concussion A brain injury with a transient impairment of consciousness followed by a rapid recovery to baseline neurologic activity.

Conducting arteries Large arteries of the body (e.g., aorta and the pulmonary trunk); have more elastic tissue and less smooth muscle; stretch under great pressures and then quickly return back to their original shapes.

Conduction system A system of pathways in the heart composed of specialized electrical (pacemaker) cells.

Conductive hearing loss Type of deafness that occurs where there is a problem with the transfer of sound from the outer to the inner ear.

Conductivity Ability of a cardiac cell to receive an electrical stimulus and conduct that impulse to an adjacent cardiac cell.

Confidentiality Protection of patient information in any form and the disclosure of that information only as needed for patient care or as otherwise permitted by law.

Confined space By Occupational Safety and Health Administration (OSHA) definition, a space large enough and configured so that an employee can enter and perform assigned work but has limited or restricted means for entry or exit (e.g., tanks, vessels, silos, storage bins, hoppers, vaults, and pits are spaces that may have limited means of entry); not designed for continuous employee occupancy.

Confrontation Focusing on a particular point made during the interview.

Congenital Present at or before birth.

Conjunctiva Thin, transparent mucous membrane that covers the inner surface of the eyelids and the outer surface of the sclera.

Conjunctivitis Inflammation of the conjunctiva.

Connective tissue Most abundant type of tissue in the body; composed of cells that are separated by a matrix.

Conscious sedation A medication or combination of medications that allows a patient to undergo what could be an unpleasant experience by producing an altered level of consciousness but not complete anesthesia. The goal is for the patient to breathe spontaneously and maintain his or her own airway.

Consensus formula Formula used to calculate the volume of fluid needed to properly resuscitate a burn patient. The formula is 2 to 4 mL/kg/% total body surface area burned. This is the formula currently regarded by the American Burn Association as the standard of care in adult burn patients. Several other, similar formulas exist that also may be used.

Consent Permission.

Constricted affect Emotion shown in degrees less than expected.

Contamination The deposition or absorption of chemical, biologic, or radiologic materials onto personnel or other materials.

Contamination reduction zone See *Warm zone.*

Continuing education (CE) Lifelong learning.

Continuous positive airway pressure (CPAP) The delivery of slight positive pressure throughout the respiratory cycle to prevent airway collapse, reduce the work of breathing, and improve alveolar ventilation.

Continuous positive airway pressure (CPAP) device Breathing device that allows delivery of slight positive pressure to prevent airway collapse and improve oxygenation and ventilation in spontaneously breathing patients.

Continuous quality improvement (CQI) Programs designed to improve the level of care; commonly driven by quality assurance.

Contractility Ability to shorten in length actively.

Contraction Rhythmic tightening of the muscular uterine wall that occurs during normal labor and leads to expulsion of the fetus and placenta from the uterus.

Contraction interval The time from the beginning of one contraction to the beginning of the next contraction.

Contraction time The time from the beginning to the end of a single uterine contraction.

Contraindication Use of a drug for a condition when it is not advisable.

Contrecoup injury An injury at another site, usually opposite the point of impact.

Contributory negligence An injured plaintiff's failure to exercise due care that, along with the defendant's negligence, contributed to the injury.

Conus medullaris Terminal end of the spinal cord.

Conus medullaris syndrome Complications resulting from injury to the conus medullaris.

Conventional silo A vertical structure used to store ensiled plant material in a aerobic environment.

Cor pulmonale Right-sided heart failure caused by pulmonary disease.

Core body temperature The measured body temperature within the core of the body; generally measured with an esophageal probe; normal is 98.6° F.

Cornea Avascular, transparent structure that permits light through to the interior of the eye.

Coronary artery disease Disease of the arteries that supply the heart muscle with blood.

Coronary heart disease Disease of the coronary arteries and their resulting complications, such as angina pectoris or acute myocardial infarction.

Coronary sinus Venous drain for the coronary circulation into the right atrium.

Corrosive A substance able to corrode tissue or metal (e.g., acids and bases).

Corticosteroids See *Adrenocortical steroids.*

Cosmesis Of or referring to the improvement of physical appearance.

Costal angle The angle formed by the margins of the ribs at the sternum.

Costochondritis Inflammation of the cartilage in the anterior chest that causes chest pain.

Coughing A protective mechanism usually induced by mucosal irritation; the forceful, spastic expiration experienced during coughing aids in the clearance of the bronchi and bronchioles.

Coup contrecoup An injury most often associated with a blow to the skull in which the force of the impact is transmitted through the skull bones to the opposite side of the head, where the bruise, fracture, or other sign of injury appears.

Coup injury An injury directly below the point of impact.

Couplet Two consecutive premature complexes.

Cover A type of concealment that hides the body and offers ballistic protection.

Crack cocaine Solid, brownish-white crystal form of cocaine, a powerful central nervous system stimulant; typically smoked.

Crackles (rales) As the name implies, when fluid accumulates in the smaller airway passages, air passing through the fluid creates a moist crackling or popping sound heard on inspiration.

Cranial nerve Twelve pairs of nerves that exit the brain and innervate the head and face; some also are part of the visceral portion of the peripheral nervous system.

Cranium The vaultlike portion of the skull, behind and above the face.

Creatinine End product of creatine metabolism; released during anaerobic metabolism. Elevated levels of creatinine are common in advanced stages of renal failure.

Creatine kinase An enzyme in skeletal and cardiac muscles that is released into circulation as a result of tissue damage. Can be used as a laboratory indicator of muscle damage.

Credentialing A local process by which an individual is permitted by a specific entity (e.g., medical director) to practice in a specific setting (e.g., EMS agency).

Crepitation A crackling sound indicative of bone ends grinding together.

Crepitus The grating, crackling, or popping sounds and sensations experienced under skin and joints.

Cricoid cartilage Most inferior cartilage of the larynx; only complete ring in the larynx.

Cricothyroid membrane A fibrous membrane located between the cricoid and thyroid cartilages.

Cricothyrotomy An emergency procedure performed to allow rapid entrance to the airway (by the cricothyroid membrane) for temporary oxygenation and ventilation.

Crime scene A location where any part of a criminal act has occurred or where evidence relating to a crime may be found.

Criminal law A branch of law in which the federal, state, or local government prosecutes individuals on behalf of society for violating laws designed to safeguard society.

Cross tolerance Decreasing responsiveness to the effects of a drug in a drug classification (such as narcotics) and the likelihood of development of decreased responsiveness to another drug in that classification.

Crossmatch The process by which blood compatibility is determined by mixing blood samples from the donor and recipient.

Croup A viral infection of the upper airway that is notorious for causing a "seal bark" cough.

Crown The visible part of a tooth.

Crowning The appearance of the first part of the infant at the vaginal opening during delivery.

Crush points Formed when two objects are moving toward each other or when one object is moving toward a stationary object and the gap between the two is decreasing.

Crush syndrome Renal failure and shock after crush injuries.

Crust A collection of cellular debris or dried blood; often called a *scab.*

Cryogenic Pertaining to extremely low temperatures.

CSM A mnemonic for *c*irculation, *s*ensation, and *m*ovement.

Cullen's sign Yellow-blue ecchymosis surrounding the umbilicus.

Cultural beliefs Values and perspectives common to a racial, religious, or social group of people.

Cultural imposition The tendency to impose your beliefs, values, and patterns of behavior on an individual from another culture.

Cumulative action Increased intensity of drug action evident after administration of several doses.

Current Flow of electrical charge from one point to another.

Current health status Focus on the environmental and personal habits of the patient that may influence the patient's general state of health.

Cushing syndrome Disorder caused by the overproduction of corticosteroids; characterized by a "moon face," obesity, fat accumulation on the upper back, increased facial hair, acne, diabetes, and hypertension.

Cushing's triad Characteristic pattern of vital signs during rising intracranial pressure, presenting as rising hypertension, bradycardia, and abnormal respirations.

Customs A practice or set of practices followed by a group of people.

Cyanogen chloride A highly toxic blood agent.

Cyanosis A bluish coloration of the skin as a result of hypoxemia, or deoxygenation of hemoglobin.

Cyclohexyl methyl phosphonofluoridate G nerve agent. The G agents tend to be nonpersistent, volatile agents.

Cyclothymia A less-severe form of bipolar disorder marked by more frequently alternating periods of a dysphoric mood that does not meet the criteria for depression and hypomania.

Cylinders Nonbulk containers that normally contain liquefied gases, nonliquified gases, or mixtures under pressure; cylinders also may contain liquids or solids.

Cyst A walled cavity that contains fluid or purulent material.

Cystic fibrosis (CF) Genetic disease marked by hypersecretion of glands, including mucus glands in the lungs.

Cystic medial degeneration A connective tissue disease in which the elastic tissue and smooth muscle fibers of the middle arterial layer degenerate.

Cystitis Infection isolated in the bladder.

Cytokines Protein molecules produced by white blood cells that act as chemical messengers between cells.

Cytoplasm Fluid-like material in which the organelles are suspended; lies between the plasma membrane and the nucleus.

Cytoplasmic membrane Encloses the cytoplasm and its organelles; forms the outer border of the cell.

Cytosol Liquid medium of the cytoplasm.

Dalton's law (law of partial pressure) Law relating to the partial pressure of oxygen during transport; defines that it is more difficult for oxygen to transfer from air to blood at lower pressures.

Damages Compensable harm or other losses incurred by an injured party (plaintiff) because of the negligence of the defendant.

Data interpretation The step that uses all the data gathered in the concept formation stage with the paramedic's knowledge of anatomy, physiology, and pathophysiology to continue the decision-making process.

Daughter cells Two cells that result from mitosis.

Dead air space Not all the air inspired during a breath participates in gas exchange and can be further classified as anatomic or physiologic dead space. In the average adult male this equates to approximately 150 mL. Anatomic dead space includes airway passages such as the trachea and bronchi, which are incapable of participating in gas exchange. Alveoli that have the potential to participate in gas exchange but do not because of disease or obstruction, as in chronic obstructive pulmonary disease (COPD) or atelectasis, are referred to as physiologic dead space.

Deafness A complete or partial inability to hear.

Debridement Removal of foreign material or dead tissue from a wound (pronounced *da brēd'*).

Decannulation Removal of a tracheostomy tube.

Decompensated shock A clinical state of tissue perfusion that is inadequate to meet the body's metabolic demands; accompanied by hypotension; also called *progressive* or *late shock.*

Decompression sickness An illness occurring during or after a diving ascent that results when nitrogen in compressed air converts back from solution to gas, forming bubbles in tissues and blood.

Decontamination The process of removing dangerous substances from the patient; may involve removing substances from the skin (external decontamination) and/or removing substances from the gastrointestinal tract (internal decontamination).

Deep fascia Fibrous, nonelastic connective tissue that forms the boundaries of muscle compartments.

Deep partial-thickness burn A burn in which the mid- or deeper dermis is injured. Results in injury to the deeper hair follicle, glandular, nerve, and blood vessel structures.

Deep venous thrombosis (DVT) A blood clot that forms in the deep venous system of the pelvis or legs; may progress to a pulmonary embolism.

Defamation The publication of false information about a person that tends to blacken the person's character or injure his or her reputation.

Defendant The person or institution being sued; also called the *respondent.*

Defibrillation Therapeutic use of electric current to terminate lethal cardiac dysrhythmias.

Degenerative joint disease See *Osteoarthritis.*

Dehydration A state in which the body has an excessive water loss from the tissues.

Delayed reaction A delay between exposure and onset of action.

Delirium Short-term and temporary mental confusion and fluctuating level of consciousness, often caused by intoxication from various substances, hypoglycemia, or acute psychiatric episodes.

Delirium tremens (DT) The most severe form of ethanol withdrawal, including hallucinations, delusions, confusion, and seizures.

Delta wave Slurring of the beginning portion of the QRS complex caused by preexcitation.

Delusion False perception and interpretation of situations and events that a person believes to be true no matter how convincing evidence is to the contrary.

Delusions of reference A belief that ordinary events have a special, often dangerous, meaning to the self.

Demand pacemaker Synchronous pacemaker that discharges only when the patient's heart rate drops below the preset rate for the pacemaker.

Dementia Long-term decline in mental faculties such as memory, concentration, and judgment; often seen with degenerative neurologic disorders such as Alzheimer's disease.

Dendrite Branchlike projections from a neuron that receive impulses or sensory information.

Denial A common defense mechanism that presents with feelings of disbelief, such as "no, that can't be right" when a life-threatening or terminal diagnosis is received; one of the stages of the grief response.

Denominator The number or mathematic expression below the line in a fraction; the denominator is the sum of the parts.

Dentin A hard but porous tissue found under the enamel and cementum of a tooth.

Deoxyribonucleic acid (DNA) Specialized structure within the cell that carries genetic material for reproduction.

Depersonalization A sudden sense of the loss of one's identity.

Deployment Matching production capacity of an ambulance system to the changing patterns of call demand.

Depolarization Movement of ions across a cell membrane, causing the inside of the cell to become more positive; an electrical event expected to result in contraction.

Depressed skull fracture A fracture of the skull with inward displacement of bone fragments.

Depression Sorrow and lack of interest in the things that previously produced pleasure.

Derealization A sudden feeling that one's surroundings are not real, as if one is watching a movie or television, not reality.

Dermatomes Areas of the body innervated by specific sensory spinal nerves; also a device used to remove healthy skin from somewhere on the body of the burn patient for the purpose of transplanting (grafting) at another site, such as an excised burn wound or other open wound.

Dermis Located below the epidermis and consists mainly of connective tissue containing both collagen and elastin fibers; contains specialized nervous tissue that provides sensory information, pain, pressure, touch, and temperature, to the central nervous system; also contains hair follicles, sweat and sebaceous glands, and a large network of blood vessels.

Descending colon Part of the large intestine.

Desired action The intended beneficial effect of a drug.

Developmental disabilities Disabilities that involve some degree of impaired adaptation in learning, social adjustment, or maturation.

Diabetes insipidus (DI) Disorder caused by insufficient production of ADH in the posterior pituitary gland, causing a larger than normal increase in the secretion of free water in the urine and poor absorption of water into the bloodstream.

Diabetic ketoacidosis (DKA) Condition found in diabetic patients caused by the lack or absence of insulin, leading to an increase of ketone bodies and acidosis in the blood.

Dialysis The process of diffusing blood across a semipermeable membrane to remove substances that the kidney would normally eliminate.

Dialysis shunt Shunt composed of two plastic tubes (one inserted into an artery, the other into a vein) that stick out of the skin to allow easy access and attachment to a dialysis machine for filtering waste products from the blood.

Diapedesis Migration of phagocytes through the endothelial wall of the vasculature into surrounding tissues.

Diaphragm Muscle that separates the thoracic cavity from the abdominal cavity.

Diaphragmatic hernia Protrusion of the abdominal contents into the chest cavity through a opening in the diaphragm.

Diaphysis Shaft of the bone where marrow is found that forms red and white blood cells.

Diastole Phase of the cardiac cycle in which the atria and ventricles relax between contractions and blood enters these chambers; when the term is used without reference to a specific chamber of the heart, the term implies ventricular diastole.

Diastolic blood pressure The pressure exerted against the walls of the large arteries during ventricular relaxation.

Diencephalon Portion of the brain between the brainstem and cerebrum; contains the thalamus and hypothalamus and the temperature regulatory centers for the body.

Differential diagnosis The list of problems that could produce the patient's chief complaint.

Differentiation Process of cell maturation; the cell becomes specialized for a specific purpose, such as a cardiac cell versus a bone cell.

Diffuse axonal injury (DAI) A type of brain injury caused by shearing forces that occur between different parts of the brain as a result of rotational acceleration.

Diffusion Spreading out of molecules from an area of higher concentration to an area of lower concentration.

Digestion Chemical breakdown of food material into smaller fragments that can be absorbed into the circulatory system.

Digestive tract Series of muscular tubes designed to move food and liquid.

Digoxin A medication derived from digitalis that acts by increasing the force of myocardial contraction and the refractory period and decreasing the conduction rate of the atrioventricular node; used to treat heart failure, most supraventricular tachycardias, and cardiogenic shock.

Dilation Spontaneous opening of the cervix that occurs as part of labor.

Diplomacy Tact and skill in dealing with people.

Direct (closed-ended) questions Questions that can be answered with short responses such as "yes" or "no."

Direct communication Method of intercellular communication in which one cell communicates with the cell adjacent to it by using minerals and ions.

Dirty bomb A conventional explosive device used as a radiologic agent dispersal device.

Disaster An incident involving 100 or more persons.

Disaster Medical Assistance Team (DMAT) Field-deployable hospital teams that include physicians, nurses, emergency medical technicians, and other medical and nonmedical support personnel.

Disaster Mortuary Operations Teams Teams composed of forensic and mortuary professionals trained to deal with human remains after disaster situations.

Discrimination Treatment or consideration based on class or category rather than individual merit.

Disease period The interval between the first appearance of symptoms and resolution.

Disinfect To clean with an agent that should kill many of, or most, surface organisms.

Disinfection Process of cleaning the ambulance, the cot, and equipment; disinfectant substances are toxic to body tissues.

Disorganized schizophrenia A subtype of schizophrenia characterized by an earlier age of onset, usually at puberty, and a more severe disintegration of personality than occurs in other forms of the disease; symptoms include incoherence, loose associations, gross disorganization or behavior, and flat or inappropriate affect.

Dispatch A central location that receives information and collects, disseminates, and transmits the information to the proper resources.

Dispatch factors Training and education of communications personnel, rapid call taking, call prioritization (selecting the most appropriate resources to respond), managing out-of-chute times (getting crews on the road quickly), and providing crews with route selection assistance.

Dispatch life support The provision of clinically approved, scripted instructions by telephone by a trained and certified emergency medical dispatcher.

Disseminated intravascular coagulation (DIC) A complex, systemic, thrombohemorrhagic disorder involving the generation of intravascular fibrin and the consumption of procoagulants and platelets.

Dissociatives Substances that cause feelings of detachment (dissociation) from one's surroundings and self; includes PCP, ketamine, and dextromethorphan.

Distal A position farthest away from a limb to the trunk.

Distracting injury An injury that occupies the patient's attention and focus. The injury causes significant enough pain that the patient may not feel pain from other injuries, particular spine injuries.

Distraction A self-defense measure that creates diversion in a person's attention.

Distress Stress that is perceived as negative; it may be seen as physical or mental pain or suffering.

Distributing arteries Blood vessels that have well-defined adventitia layers and larger amounts of smooth muscle; capable of altering blood flow.

Distribution The movement of drugs from the bloodstream to target organs.

Distributive shock Inadequate tissue perfusion as a result of fluid shifts between body compartments. Burn shock is a distributive shock in which plasma and water are lost from the vascular tree into the surrounding tissues. This shock also is seen in the setting of sepsis, in which a similar fluid redistribution occurs.

Diuretic An agent that promotes the excretion of urine.

Diversity Differences of any kind such as race, class, religion, gender, sexual preference, personal habitat, and physical ability.

Diverticulitis Inflammation of a diverticulum, especially of the small pockets in the wall of the colon that fill with stagnant fecal material and become inflamed.

Diverticulosis A condition of the colon in which outpouches develop.

Documentation Written information to support actions that lead to conclusive information; written evidence.

Donor skin site A site on the body from which healthy skin is removed for the purpose of grafting a burn or other open wound.

Do not resuscitate (DNR) orders Orders limiting cardiopulmonary resuscitation or advanced life support treatment in the case of a cardiac arrest. These orders may be individualized in that they may allow for differing levels of interventions. When individualized, they usually grant or deny permission for chest compressions, intubation or ventilation, and life-saving medications.

Dorsal Referring to the back of the body; posterior.

Dosage The amount of medication that can be safely given for the average person for a specified condition. Also the administration of a therapeutic agent in prescribed amounts.

Dose The exact amount of medication to be given or taken at one time.

Down syndrome A genetic syndrome characterized by varying degrees of mental retardation and multiple physical defects.

Downregulation The process by which a cell decreases the number of receptors exposed to a given substance to reduce its sensitivity to that substance.

Dromotropism The speed of conduction through the atrioventricular junction.

Drop (or drip) factor The number of drops per milliliter that an intravenous administration set delivers.

Drowning A process resulting in primary respiratory impairment from submersion or immersion in a liquid medium.

Drug Any substance (other than a food or device) intended for use in the diagnosis, cure, relief, treatment, or prevention of disease or intended to affect the structure or function of the body of human beings or animals.

Drug allergy The reaction to a medication with an adverse outcome.

Drug antagonism The interaction between two drugs in which one partially or completely inhibits the effects of the other.

284

Drug dependence A physical need or adaptation to the drug without the psychological need to take the drug.

Drug interaction The manner in which one drug and a second drug (or food) act on each other.

Drug overdose Internalization of more than the safe amount of a medication or drug; often associated with illegal drugs when a user administers too great an amount of substance; may be used to commit suicide.

Drug-food interaction Changes in a drug's effects caused by food or beverages ingested during the same period.

Dual-chamber pacemaker Pacemaker that stimulates the atrium and ventricle.

Dual-stage airbags An airbag with two inflation charges inside; only one of the two charges may deploy during the initial crash, causing the bag to inflate; the second charge of the dual-stage airbag may remain.

Ductus arteriosus Blood vessel that connects the pulmonary trunk to the aorta in a fetus.

Ductus deferens Also known as *vas deferens;* tubes that extend from the end of the epididymis and through the seminal vesicles.

Ductus venosus Fetal blood vessel that conects the umbilical vein and the inferior vena cava.

Due process The constitutional guarantee that laws and legal proceedings must be fair regarding an individual's legal rights.

Due regard Principle used when driving an emergency vehicle of ensuring that all other vehicles and citizens in the area see and grant the emergency vehicle the right of way.

Duodenum First part of the small intestine; has important accessory structures that help digest various types of nutrients.

Duplex A radio system that allows transmitting and receiving at the same time through two different frequencies.

Dura mater Toughest layer of the meninges; top layer.

Durable power of attorney for health care A type of advanced directive that allows an individual to appoint someone to make health care decisions for him or her if the person's ability to make these decisions or communicate wishes is lost.

Duty to act A legal obligation (created by statute, contract, or voluntarily) to provide services.

Dysarthria An articulation disorder in which the patient is not able to produce speech sounds.

Dyspareunia Pain during sexual intercourse.

Dyspepsia Epigastric discomfort often occurring after meals.

Dysphagia Difficulty swallowing.

Dysphoric mood (dysphoria) An unpleasant emotional state characterized by sadness, irritability, or depression.

Dysplasia Abnormal cell growth; cells take on an abnormal size, shape, and organization as a result of ongoing irritation or inflammation.

Dyspnea An uncomfortable awareness of one's breathing that may be associated with a change in the breathing rate, effort, or pattern.

Dysrhythmia An abnormal heart rhythm.

Dysthymia A constant, chronic, low-grade form of depression.

Dystonia Impairment of muscle tone, particularly involuntary muscle contractions of the face, neck, and tongue; often caused by a reaction to certain antipsychotic medications.

Ebola A viral hemorrhagic fever illness caused by the Ebola virus (Filovirus family); seen mostly in Africa; transmitted by person-to-person contact with body fluids of infected individuals; no specific treatment is available, and it often is fatal within several days.

Ecchymosis Collection of blood within the skin that appears blue-black, eventually fading to a greenish-brown and yellow. Commonly called a *bruise.*

Eclampsia A life-threatening condition of pregnancy and the postpartum period characterized by hypertension, edema, and seizures.

Economic abuse Preventing others from having or keeping a job; forcing control of another's paycheck; restricting access or forcing conditions on others to receive an allowance; stealing money; not allowing others to know about or have access to economic assets.

Ecstasy (MDMA) A synthetic, hallucinogenic stimulant drug similar to both methamphetamine and mescaline.

Ectopic Impulse(s) originating from a source other than the sinoatrial node.

Ectopic pregnancy A pregnancy that implants outside the uterus, usually in the fallopian tube.

Eczema A disorder of the skin characterized by inflammation, itching, blisters, and scales.

Edema A collection of water in the interstitial space.

Effector The muscle, gland, or organ on which the autonomic nervous system exerts an effect; target organ.

Effector phase In phases of immunity, the stage at which the infection is eradicated.

Efferent division Nerve fibers that send impulses from the central nervous system to the periphery.

Efficacy The ability of a drug to produce a physiologic response after attaching to a receptor.

Efflux Flowing out of.

Ejection fraction Fraction (expressed as a percentage) of blood ejected from the ventricle of the heart with each contraction. Generally at least 60% of the blood entering the ventricle should be forced to the lungs or systemic circulation.

Elasticity Ability of muscle to rebound toward its original length after contraction.

Electrical alternans A beat-to-beat change in waveform amplitude on the ECG.

Electrodes Adhesive pads that contain a conductive gel and are applied at specific locations on the patient's chest wall and extremities and connected by cables to an ECG machine.

Electrolytes Elements or compounds that break into charged particles (ions) when melted or dissolved in water or another solvent.

Elevated mood (euphoria) Exaggerated sense of happiness and joy; a feeling of being on top of the world.

Elimination The process of removing a drug from the body.

Elixir A clear, oral solution that contains the drug, water, and some alcohol.

Emancipated minor A self-supporting minor. This status often depends on the minor receiving an actual court order of emancipation.

Embryo The developing egg from approximately 2 weeks after fertilization until approximately 8 weeks of pregnancy.

Emergency decontamination The process of decontaminating people exposed to and potentially contaminated with hazardous materials by rapidly removing most of the contamination to reduce exposure and save lives, with secondary regard for completeness of decontamination.

Emergency medical dispatching (EMD) The science and skills associated with the tasks of an emergency medical dispatcher.

Emergency medical responder (EMR) An EMS professional who provides initial basic life-support care to patients who access the EMS system; formerly called *first responder.*

Emergency Medical Treatment and Active Labor Act (EMTALA) A federal law that requires a hospital to provide a medical screening examination to anyone who comes to that hospital and to provide stabilizing treatment to anyone with an emergency medical condition without considering the patient's ability to pay.

Emergency operations center A gathering point for strategic policymakers during an emergency incident.

Emergency service function (ESF) A grouping of government and certain private sector capabilities into an organizational structure to provide the support, resources, program implementation, and services most likely to be needed to save lives, protect property and the environment, restore essential services and critical infrastructure, and help victims and communities return to normal, when feasible, after domestic incidents.

Emesis Vomiting.

Emotional/mental impairment Impaired intellectual functioning (such as mental retardation), which results in an inability to cope with normal responsibilities of life.

Empathy Identification with and understanding of another's situation, feelings, and motives.

Emphysema Lung disease in which destruction of the alveoli creates dyspnea; often associated with tobacco abuse.

Empyema A collection of pus in the pleural cavity.

EMS Emergency medical services.

EMS system A network of resources that provides emergency care and transportation to victims of sudden illness or injury.

Emulsification The breakdown of fats on the skin surface by alkaloids, creating a soapy substance; penetrates deeply.

Emulsion A water and oil mixture containing medication.

Enabling behavior Behavior that allows another individual to continue to stay ill.

Enamel Hard, white outer surface of a tooth.

Encephalitis Inflammation and usually infection of brain tissue.

Encephalopathy A condition of disturbances of consciousness and possible progression to coma.

Endocardium Innermost layer of the heart that lines the inside of the myocardium and covers the heart valves.

Endocrine communication Method of intercellular communication in which one cell communicates with target cells throughout the body by using hormones.

Endocrine gland Where hormones are manufactured.

Endogenous Produced within the organism.

Endolymph Fluid that fills the labyrinth.

Endometriosis Growth of endometrial tissue outside the uterus, often causing pain.

Endometritis Infection of the endometrium.

Endometrium Innermost tissue lining of the uterus that is shed during menstruation.

Endoplasmic reticulum (ER) Chain of canals or sacs that wind through the cytoplasm.

Endorphins Neurotransmitters that function in the transmission of signals within the nervous system.

Endothelial cells A thin layer of flat epithelial cells that lines serous cavities, lymph vessels, and blood vessels.

Endotoxin A substance contained in the cell wall of gram-negative bacteria, generally released during the destruction of the bacteria by either the host organism's defense mechanisms or by treatment with medications.

Endotracheal (ET) Within or through the trachea.

Endotracheal intubation An advanced airway procedure in which a tube is placed directly into the trachea.

End-stage renal disease (ESRD) When the kidneys function at 10% to 15% of normal and dialysis or transplantation is the only option for the patient's survival.

Enlargement Implies the presence of dilation or hypertrophy or both.

Enteral A drug given for its systemic effects that passes through the digestive tract.

Enteric-coated tablets Tablets that have a special coating so they break down in the intestines instead of the stomach.

Enteral drug One that is given and passed through any portion of the digestive tract.

Entrapment A state of being pinned or entrapped.

Envenomation The process of injecting venom into a wound; venomous animals include snakes, insects, and marine creatures.

Environmental emergency A medical condition caused or exacerbated by weather, terrain, atmospheric pressure, or other local environmental factors.

Environmental hazards Hazards related to the weather and time of day, including extremes of heat, cold, wetness, dryness, and darkness, that increase risks to crews and patients.

Enzyme A large molecule (protein) that performs a biochemical reaction in the cell.

Eosinophils Type of granulocyte (white blood cell, or leukocyte) involved in immune response to parasites as well as in allergic responses.

Epicardium Also known as the *visceral pericardium;* the external layer of the heart wall that covers the heart muscle.

Epidemiologist Medical professional who studies the causes, distribution, and control of disease in populations.

Epidemiology The study of the causes, patterns, prevalence, and control of disease in groups of people.

Epidermis The outermost layer of the skin; made of tightly packed epithelial cells.

Epididymis Convoluted series of tubes located in the posterior portion of the scrotum; final maturation of sperm occurs here.

Epidural hematoma A collection of blood between the skull and dura mater.

Epidural space Potential area above the dura mater; contains arterial vessels.

Epiglottitis An inflammation of the epiglottis.

Epilepsy Group of neurologic disorders characterized by recurrent seizures, often of unknown cause.

Epiphyseal plate Found in children who are still generating bone growth; also known as the *growth plate.*

Epiphysis Either end of the bone where bone growth occurs during the developmental years.

Epistaxis Bloody nose.

Epithelial tissue Covers most of the internal and external surfaces of the body.

Epithelialization Migration of basal cells across a wound and the growth of skin over a wound.

Eponym A word that derives its name from the specific person (or place or thing) for whom (or which) it is named.

Erosion A partial focal loss of epidermis. This lesion is depressed, moist, and does not bleed; usually heals without scarring.

Erythema multiforme An internal (immunologic) reaction in the skin characterized by a variety of lesions.

Erythrocytes Red blood cells.

Erythropoiesis The development and differentiation of red blood cells; typically occurs in the bone marrow.

Erythropoietin A hormone that stimulates peripheral stem cells in the bone marrow to produce red blood cells.

Escape Term used when the sinus node slows or fails to initiate depolarization and a lower pacemaker site spontaneously produces electrical impulses, assuming responsibility for pacing the heart.

Eschar A thick wound covering that consists of necrotic or otherwise devitalized tissue or cellular components. In a burn wound, this is the burned tissue or skin of the wound.

Esophageal atresia (EA) A condition in which the section of the esophagus from the mouth and the section of the esophagus from the stomach end as a blind pouch without connecting to each other.

Esophagitis Inflammation of the esophagus.

Esophagoduodenoscopy Medical procedure in which an endoscope is used to look at the esophagus, stomach, and duodenum.

Esophagus Tube surrounded by smooth muscle that propels material into the stomach.

Essential hypertension High blood pressure for which no cause is identifiable; also called *primary hypertension.*

Estimated date of confinement The due date of the fetus.

Estrogen A female hormone produced mainly by the ovaries from puberty to menopause that is responsible for the development of secondary sexual characteristics and cyclic changes in the thickness of the uterine lining during the first half of the menstrual cycle.

Ethanol (ETOH) Colorless, odorless alcohol found in alcoholic beverages such as beer, wine, and liquor.

Ethics Expectations established by the community at large reflecting their views of the conduct of a profession.

Ethnocentrism Viewing your life as the most desirable, acceptable, or best and to act in a superior manner to another culture's way of life.

Eukaryotes One of the two major classes of cells found in higher life forms (more complex in structure).

Eustachian tube A small tube connecting the middle ear to the posterior nasopharynx; allows the ear to adjust to atmospheric pressure.

Eustress Stress that occurs from events, people, or influences that are perceived as good or positive. Eustress can increase productivity and performance.

Euthymic mood A normal, baseline emotional state.

Evaluation of treatment A reassessment of the patient overall and specifically the body system(s) affected by that treatment to answer two critical questions: Did the treatment work as intended? What is the clinical condition of the patient after the treatment?

Evasive tactic A self-defense measure in which the moves and actions of an aggressor are anticipated and unconventional pathways are used during retreat for personal safety.

Excision In reference to burn surgery, this is the sharp, surgical removal of burned tissue that will never regain function. Excision is carried out before skin grafting.

Excitability Ability to respond to a stimulus.

Excited delirium Acute and sudden agitation, paranoia, aggression, hyperthermia, dramatically increased strength, and decreased sensitivity to pain related to long-term use of stimulant drugs; often ends in sudden death.

Excoriation A linear erosion created by scratching. It is a hollowed out area that is sometimes crusted.

Excretion Removal of waste products from the body.

Exertional heat stroke A condition primarily affecting younger, active persons characterized by rapid onset (developing in hours) and frequently associated with high core temperatures.

Exhaled CO_2 detector A capnometer that provides a noninvasive estimate of alveolar ventilation, the concentration of exhaled CO_2 from the lungs, and arterial carbon dioxide content; also called an *end-tidal CO₂ detector.*

Exhaustion The last stage of the stress response and the body's inability to respond appropriately to subsequent stressors.

Exhaustion stage Occurs when the body's resistance to a stressor (decreased reaction to the stress, tolerance) and the ability to adapt fail; the ability to respond appropriately to other stressors may then fail; the immune system can be affected, and the individual may be at risk physically or emotionally.

Exogenous Produced outside the organism.

Exotoxin Proteins released during the growth phase of the bacteria that may cause systemic effects.

Expiratory reserve volume Amount of gas that can be forcefully expired at the end of a normal expiration.

Explanation Sharing objective information related to a message.

Explosive Any chemical compound, mixture, or device, the primary or common purpose of which is to function by detonation or rapid combustion (i.e., with substantial instantaneous release of gas and heat); found in liquid or solid forms (e.g., dynamite, TNT, black powder, fireworks, ammunition).

Exposure When blood or body fluids come in contact with eyes, mucous membranes, nonintact skin, or through a needlestick; it also can occur through inhalation and ingestion.

Expressed consent Permission given by a patient or his or her responsible decision maker either verbally or through some physical expression of consent.

Exsanguinate Near complete loss of blood; not conducive with life.

Exsanguination Bleeding to death.

Extensibility Ability to continue to contract over a range of lengths.

Extension posturing (decerebrate) Occurs as a result of an injury to the brainstem; presents as the patient's arms at the side with wrists turned outward.

External anal sphincter Muscle under voluntary control that allows a controlled bowel movement.

External auditory canal Tube from the external ear to the middle ear; lined with hair and ceruminous glands.

External bleeding Observable blood loss.

External ear Includes the auricle and external auditory canal.

External respiration The exchange of gases between the alveoli of the lungs and the blood cells traveling through the pulmonary capillaries.

External urinary sphincter Ring of smooth muscle in the urethra under voluntary control.

Extracellular Outside the cell or cytoplasmic membrane.

Extracellular fluid (ECF) The fluid found outside of the cells.

Extubation Removal of an endotracheal tube from the trachea.

Exudate Drainage from a vesicle or pustule.

Eyebrows Protect the eyes by providing shade and preventing foreign material (sweat, dust, etc.) from entering the eyes from above.

Eyelids Protect the eyes from foreign objects.

Facilitated diffusion Movement of substances across a membrane by binding to a helper protein integrated into the cell wall and highly selective about the chemicals allowed to cross the membrane.

Facilitated transport The transport of substances through a protein channel carrier with no energy input.

Facilitation Encouraging the patient to provide more information.

Factitious disorder Condition in which patients intentionally produce signs and symptoms of illness to assume the sick role.

Fainting (syncope) A brief loss of consciousness caused by a temporary decrease in blood flow to the brain.

Fallopian tube Paired structures extending from each side of the uterus to each ovary; they provide a way for the egg to reach the uterus.

False imprisonment Confinement or restraint of a person against his or her will or without appropriate legal justification.

False motion Abnormal movement of a bone or joint typically associated with a fracture or dislocation.

Fascia Anatomically, the tough connective tissue covering of the muscles of the body. Fascia contains the muscles within a compartment.

Fascicle Small bundle of nerve fibers.

Fasciotomy A surgical incision into the muscle fascia to relieve intracompartmental pressures; the emergency treatment for compartment syndrome.

Fear Physical and emotional reaction to a real or perceived threat.

Febrile seizure Seizure caused by too rapid of a rise in body temperature; rarely seen after age 2 years.

Fecalith A hard impacted mass of feces in the colon.

Feces Undigested food material that has been processed in the colon.

Federal Communication Commission (FCC) An independent U.S. government agency, directly responsible to Congress, established by the Communications Act of 1934; it regulates interstate and international communications by radio, television, wire, satellite, and cable. The FCC's jurisdiction covers the 50 states, the District of Columbia, and U.S. possessions.

Fetus The term used for an infant from approximately 8 weeks of pregnancy until birth.

Fibrin A threadlike protein formed during the clotting process that crisscrosses the wound opening and forms a matrix that traps blood cells and platelets, thereby creating a clot. Fibrin is formed by the action of thrombin and fibrinogen.

Fibrinolysis The breakdown of fibrin, the main component of blood clots.

Fibrinolytic agent Clot-busting drug; used in very early treatment of acute myocardial infarction, stroke, deep vein thrombosis, pulmonary embolism, and peripheral arterial occlusion.

Fibroblasts A cell that gives rise to connective tissue.

Fibrous connective tissue Composed of bundles of strong, white collagenous fibers (protein) in parallel rows; tendons and ligaments are composed of this type of tissue; relatively strong and inelastic.

Fibrous joints Two bones united by fibrous tissue that have little or no movement.

Fibrous tunic Layer of the eye that contains the sclera and the cornea.

Fick principle Describes the components needed for the oxygenation of the body's cells.

Finance officer The person responsible for providing a cost analysis of an incident.

Fine ventricular fibrillation Ventricular fibrillation with fibrillatory waves less than 3 mm in height.

FiO$_2$ Fraction of inspired oxygen.

"First on the Scene" program An educational program that teaches people what to do and what not to do when they come upon an injury emergency.

First-degree burn Superficial burn involving only the epidermis, such as a minor sunburn.

First-pass effect The breakdown of a drug in the liver and walls of the intestines before it reaches the systemic circulation.

First responder unit The closest trained persons and vehicle assigned to respond to a call; often the closest available fire department vehicle.

Fissure A vertical loss of epidermis and dermis with sharply defined walls (sometimes called a *crack*).

Fistula An abnormal tunnel that has formed from within the body to the skin.

Fixed positioning Establishing a single location in a central point to station an emergency vehicle, such as a fire station.

Fixed-rate pacemaker Asynchronous pacemaker that continuously discharges at a preset rate regardless of the patient's heart rate.

Fixed-station deployment Deployment method of using only geographically based stations.

Fixed-wing aircraft Airplanes used for longer distance medical flights; they can travel higher and faster than rotor-wing aircraft.

Flail segment A free-floating section of the chest wall that results when two or more adjacent ribs are fractured in two or more places or when the sternum is detached.

Flammable The capacity of a substance to ignite.

Flammable gases Any compressed gas that meets requirements for lower flammability limit, flammability limit range, flame projection, or flame propagation as specified in CFR Title 49, Sec. 173.300(b) (e.g., acetylene, butane, hydrogen, propane).

Flammable range The concentration of fuel and air between the lower flammable limit or lower explosive limit and the upper flammable limit or upper explosive limit; the mixture of fuel and air in the flammable range supports combustion.

Flammable solid A solid material other than an explosive that is liable to cause fires through friction or retained heat from manufacturing or processing or that can be ignited readily; when ignited, it burns so vigorously and persistently that it creates a serious transportation hazard (e.g., phosphorus, lithium, magnesium, titanium, calcium resinate).

Flash electrical burn A burn resulting from indirect contact with an electrical explosion.

Flashpoint The minimal temperature at which a substance evaporates fast enough to form an ignitable mixture with air near the surface of the substance.

Flat affect A complete or near-complete lack of emotion.

Flat bones Specialized bones that protect vital anatomic structures (e.g., ribs and bones of the skull).

Flexible deployment See *System status management.*

Flexion posturing (decorticate) Occurs from an injury to the cerebrum; presents as a bending of the arms at the elbow, the patient's arms pulled upwards to the chest, and the hands turned downward at the wrists.

Flight of ideas Moving quickly from topic to topic during conversation but without any connection or transition.

Flow rate The number of drops per minute an intravenous administration set will deliver.

Fluctuance A wavelike motion felt between two fingertips when palpating a fluid-filled structure such as a subcutaneous abscess.

Fluctuant nodule A movable and compressible mass; typically a pocket of pus or fluid within the dermis.

Focal atrial tachycardia Atrial tachycardia that begins in a small area (focus) within the heart.

Focal deficit Alteration or lack of strength or sensation in the body caused by a neurologic problem.

Focal injury An injury limited to a particular area of the brain.

Follicle Small, tubelike structure in which hair grows; contains a small cluster of cells known as the hair papilla.

Follicles Vesicles within the cortex of the ovary.

Folliculitis Inflammation of the follicle; localized to hair follicles and is more common in immunocompromised patients; usually are multiple and measure 5 mm or less in diameter; erythematous, pruritic, and frequently have a central pustule on top of a raised lesion, often with a central hair.

Fontanelles Membranous spaces at the juncture of an infant's cranial bones that later ossify.

Foramen Open passage.

Foramen magnum Opening in the floor of the cranium where the spinal cord exits the skull.

Foramen ovale The opening in the interatrial septum in a fetal heart.

Foreign body Any object or substance found in a organ or tissue where it does not belong under normal circumstances.

Form of thought Ability to compose thoughts in a logical manner.

Formed elements Located in the bloodstream; erythrocytes, leukocytes, and thrombocytes, or platelets.

Formulary A book that contains a list of medicinal substances with their formulas, uses, and methods of preparation.

Fractile response time Method used to determine the time at which 90% all requests for service receive a response; considered a more definitive measure of performance than averages.

Francisella tularensis A hardy, slow-growing, highly infectious, aerobic organism; human infection may result in tularemia, also known as *rabbit fever* or *deer fly fever.*

Free nerve endings Most common type of dermal nerve ending; responsible for sensing pain, temperature, and pressure.

Free radical A molecule containing an extra electron, which allows it to form potentially harmful bonds with other molecules.

Frontal lobe Section of cerebrum important in voluntary motor function and the emotions of aggression, motivation, and mood.

Frontal plane Imaginary straight line that divides the body into anterior (ventral) and posterior (dorsal) sections.

Frostbite A condition in which the skin and underlying tissue freeze.

Frostnip Reversible freezing of superficial skin layer marked by numbness and whiteness of the skin.

Fully deployed Assigning ambulances to a street corner post.

Fulminant Sudden, intense occurrence.

Functional reserve capacity At the end of a normal expiration, the volume of air remaining in the lungs.

Fundus Superior aspect of the uterus.

Fungi Plantlike organisms that do not contain chlorophyll; the two classes of fungi are yeasts and molds.

Furuncles Inflammatory nodules that involve the hair follicle (e. g., boils).

Gag reflex A normal neural reflex elicited by touching the soft palate or posterior pharynx; the responses are symmetric elevation of the palate, retraction of the tongue, and contraction of the pharyngeal muscles.

Gagging A reflex caused by irritation of the posterior pharynx that can result in vomiting.

Gamma A type of electromagnetic radiation.

Gamma-hydroxybutyrate (GHB) A drug structurally related to the neurotransmitter gamma-aminobutyric acid, usually dissolved in liquid, that causes profound central nervous system depression.

Gamma rays A type of electromagnetic radiation that can travel great distances; can be stopped by heavy shielding, such as lead.

Gamow bag Portable hyperbaric chamber that can help with altitude sickness emergencies.

Ganglion The junction between the preganglionic and postganglionic nerves.

Gangrenous necrosis Tissue death over a large area.

Gases Substances inhaled and absorbed through the respiratory tract.

Gasoline and electric hybrid vehicle Vehicle designed to produce low emissions by combining a smaller than normal internal combustion gasoline engine with a special electric motor to power the vehicle.

Gasping Inhaling and exhaling with quick, difficult breaths.

Gastric The route used when a tube is placed into the digestive tract, such as a nasogastric, orogastric, or gastrostomy tube.

Gastric distention Swelling of the abdomen caused by an influx of air or fluid.

Gastric lavage A procedure commonly known as "stomach pumping" in which the stomach is flushed with water; typically used to treat overdose or poisoning.

Gastritis Inflammation of the stomach.

Gastroenteritis Inflammation of the stomach and the intestines.

Gastrostomy tube A tube placed in a person's stomach that allows continuous feeding for an extended time.

Gay-Lussac's law A gas law sometimes combined with Charles' law that deals with the relation between pressure and temperature; in an oxygen cylinder, as the ambient temperature decreases, so does the pressure reading.

Gel cap Soft gelatin shell filled with liquid medication.

Gene The biologic unit of inheritance, consisting of a particular nucleotide sequence within a DNA molecule that occupies a precise locus on a chromosome and codes for a specific polypeptide chain.

Generalized anxiety disorder Condition characterized by excessive worries about everyday life.

Generalized seizure Excessive electrical activity in both hemispheres of the brain at the same time.

Generic name The name proposed by the first manufacturer when a drug is submitted to the FDA for approval; often an abbreviated form of the drug's chemical name, structure, or formula.

Geospatial demand analysis Understanding the different locations of demand within a community.

Germ theory Controversial theory developed in the 1600s in which microorganisms were first identified as the possible cause of some disease processes.

Germinativum Basal layer of the epidermis where the epidermal cells are formed.

Gestation or gestational age The number of completed weeks of pregnancy from the last menstrual period.

Glasgow Coma Scale (GCS) Neurologic assessment of a patient's best verbal response, eye opening, and motor function.

Glaucoma Increased intraocular pressure caused by a disruption in the normal production and drainage of aqueous humor; causes often are unknown.

Global positioning system (GPS) A satellite-based geographic locating system often placed on an ambulance to track its exact location.

Glomerulus Network of capillaries in the renal corpuscle.

Glottis The true vocal cords and the space between them.

Gluconeogenesis Creation of new glucose in the body by using noncarbohydrate sources such as fats and proteins.

Glycogenolysis Breakdown of glycogen to glucose in the liver.

Glycolysis Process by which glucose and other sugars are broken down to yield lactic acid (anaerobic glycolysis) or pyruvic acid (aerobic glycolysis). The breakdown releases energy in the form of adenosine triphosphate.

Glycoside A compound that yields a sugar and one or more other products when its parts are separated.

Golgi apparatus Substance that concentrates and packages material for secretion out of the cell.

Gomphoses Joint in which a peg fits into a socket.

Gout A metabolic disease in which uric acid crystals are deposited onto the cartilaginous surfaces of a joint, resulting in pain, swelling, and inflammation.

Graft Connection by a surgeon of a piece of the patient's saphenous vein to an artery and vein; in lieu of using the patient's own blood vessel, a cow's artery or a synthetic graft may be used.

Graham's law Law stating that gases move from a higher pressure or concentration to an area of lower pressure or concentration; takes into consideration the effect of simple diffusion at a cellular level.

Gram-negative bacteria Bacteria that do not retain the crystal violet stain used in Gram's stain and that take the color of the red counterstain.

Gram-positive bacteria Bacteria that retain the crystal violet stain used in Gram's stain.

Grandiose delusions Dramatically inflated perceptions of one's own worth, power, or knowledge.

Granulocyte A form of leukocyte that attacks foreign material in the wound.

Gravida Number of pregnancies.

Gravidity The number of times a patient has been pregnant.

Great vessels Large vessels that carry blood to and from the heart; superior and inferior venae cavae, pulmonary veins, aorta, and pulmonary trunk.

greenstick fracture The incomplete fracturing of an immature bone.

Grey-Turner's sign Bruising along the flanks that may indicate pancreatitis or intraabdominal hemorrhage.

Ground effect The cushion of air created by downdraft when a helicopter is in a low hover. Ground effect benefits the helicopter flight because it increases lift capacity, meaning less power is required for the helicopter to hover. When the helicopter has ground effect, it is said to be in ground effect. If a helicopter does not have ground effect, it is said to be operating out of ground effect.

Ground electrode Third ECG electrode (the first and second are the positive and negative electrodes), which minimizes electrical activity from other sources.

Grunting A short, low-pitched sound heard at the end of exhalation that represents an attempt to generate positive end-expiratory pressure by exhaling against a closed glottis, prolonging the period of oxygen and carbon dioxide exchange across the alveolar-capillary membrane; a compensatory mechanism to help maintain patency of small airways and prevent atelectasis.

Guarding The contraction of abdominal muscles in the anticipation of a painful stimulus.

Guidelines For emergency medical dispatchers, an unstructured, subjective, unscripted method of telephone assessment and treatment; a less-effective process than protocols.

Guillain-Barré syndrome Autoimmune neurologic disorder marked by weakness and paresthesia that usually travel up the legs.

Gum Plant residue used for medicinal or recreational purposes.

Gurgling Abnormal respiratory sound associated with collection of liquid or semisolid material in the patient's upper airway.

Gurney Stretcher or cot used to transport patients.

Gustation Sense of taste.

Hair papilla Small cluster of cells within a follicle; growth of hair starts in this cluster of cells, which is hidden in the follicle.

Half duplex A radio system that use two frequencies: one to transmit and one to receive; however, like a simplex system, only one person can transmit at a time.

Half-life The time required to eliminate half of a substance from the body.

Hallucination A false sensory perception originating inside the brain, such as hearing the voices of people who are not present.

Hallucinogen Substance that cause hallucinations and intense distortions and perceptions of reality; includes LSD, psilocybin mushrooms, peyote, and mescaline.

Hamman's sign A crunching sound occasionally heard on auscultation of the heart when air is in the mediastinum.

Hangman's fracture A fracture of the axis, the second cervical vertebra. This may occur with or without axis dislocation.

Hazard Communication Standard (HAZCOM) Occupational Safety and Health Administration standard regarding worker protection when handling chemicals.

Hazardous materials A substance (solid, liquid, or gas) capable of posing an unreasonable risk to health, safety, environment, or property.

Hazardous Waste Operations and Emergency Response (HAZWOPER) Occupational Safety and Health Administration and Environmental Protection Agency regulations regarding worker safety when responding to hazardous materials emergencies.

Head bobbing Indicator of increased work of breathing in infants; the head falls forward with exhalation and comes up with expansion of the chest on inhalation.

Head injury A traumatic insult to the head that may result in injury to the soft tissue or bony structures of the head and/or brain injury.

Headache A pain in the head from any cause.

Health A state of complete physical, mental, and social well-being, not merely the absence of disease or infirmity.

Health Insurance Portability and Accountability Act (HIPAA) Rules governing the protection of a patient's identifiable information.

Healthcare professional An individual who has special skills and knowledge in medicine and adheres to the standards of conduct and performance of that medical profession.

Healthcare A business associated with the provision of medical care to individuals.

Heart disease A broad term referring to conditions affecting the heart.

Heart failure A condition in which the heart is unable to pump enough blood to meet the metabolic needs of the body.

Heartbeat Organized mechanical action of the heart.

Heat emergencies Conditions in which the body's thermoregulation mechanisms begin to fail in response to ambient heat, causing illness.

Hematemesis Vomiting of bright red blood.

Hematochezia Bright red blood in the stool.

Hematocrit A measure of the relative percentage of blood cells (mainly erythrocytes) in a given volume of whole blood; also called *volume of packed red cells* or *packed cell volume.*

Hematoma Collection of blood beneath the skin or within a body compartment.

Hematuria Blood found in the urine.

Hemiparesis Muscle weakness of one half of the body.

Hemiplegia Paralysis of one side of the body.

Hemoglobin A protein found on red blood cells that is rich in iron.

Hemolytic anemia Anemia that results from the destruction of red blood cells.

Hemopoietic tissue Connective tissue found in the marrow cavities of bones (mainly long bones).

Hemoptysis The coughing up of blood.

Hemorrhage Heavy bleeding.

Hemorrhagic anemia Anemia caused by hemorrhage.

Hemorrhagic stroke Rupture of a blood vessel in the brain causing decreased perfusion and potentially leading to rising intracranial pressure.

Hemorrhoids Swollen, distended veins in the anorectal area.

Hemostasis Stopping a hemorrhage.

Hemothorax Blood within the thoracic cavity, a potentially life-threatening injury.

Henry's law Law associated with decompression sickness that deals with the solubility of gases in liquids at equilibrium.

Hepatic artery The artery that supplies the liver with blood and nutrients from the circulatory system.

Hepatic duct Connects the gallbladder to the liver; secretes bile into the gallbladder.

Hepatitis Inflammation of the liver.

Hering-Breuer reflex A reflex that limits inspiration to prevent overinflation of the lungs in a conscious, spontaneously breathing person; also called the *inhibito-inspiratory reflex.*

Hernia Protrusion of any organ through an abdominal opening in the muscle wall of the cavity that surrounds it.

Herniated disc A condition in which an intervertebral disc weakens and protrudes out of position, often affecting adjacent nerve roots.

Herniation Protrusion of the brain through an abnormal opening, often the foramen magnum.

Heroin (diacetylmorphine) The most popular, powerful, and addictive member of the opioids.

Herpes simplex A skin eruption caused by the herpes simplex virus, divided into two types; HSV-1 causes oral infection and HSV-2 causes genital infections.

Herpes zoster A skin eruption that follows a particular nerve distribution (dermatome); caused by the varicella zoster virus in persons who have had varicella sometime in their lives (also called *shingles*).

Hiatus A gap or a cleft.

Hiccup (hiccoughing) Intermittent spasm of the diaphragm resulting in sudden inspiration with spastic closure of the glottis; usually annoying and serves no known physiologic purpose.

High angle An environment in which the load is predominately supported by the rope rescue system.

High voltage Greater than 1000 V.

High-altitude cerebral edema The most severe high-altitude illness, characterized by increased intracranial pressure.

High-altitude pulmonary edema A high-altitude illness characterized by increased pulmonary artery pressure and edema, leading to cough and fluid in the lungs (pulmonary edema).

High-angle terrain (vertical terrain) A steep environment such as a cliff or building side where hands must be used for balance when ascending.

Hilum Point of entry for bronchial vessels, bronchi, and nerves in each lung.

Hilus Indentation through which the renal artery, vein, lymphatic vessels, and nerves enter and leave the kidney.

Hippocampi Structures within the limbic system that filter incoming information, determine what stimuli is important, and commit the experiences to memory.

His-Purkinje system Portion of the conduction system consisting of the bundle of His, bundle branches, and Purkinje fibers.

Histamine A substance released by mast cells that promotes inflammation.

History of present illness A narrative detail of the symptoms the patient is experiencing.

Hollow organ An organ (a part of the body or group of tissues that performs a specific function) that contains a channel or cavity within it, such as the large and small intestines.

Homan's sign Pain and tenderness in the calf muscle on dorsiflexion of the foot.

Home care The provision of health services by formal and informal caregivers in the home to promote, restore, and maintain a person's maximal level of comfort, function, and health, including care toward a dignified death.

Homeostasis A state of equilibrium in the body with respect to functions and composition of fluids and tissues.

Homeotherm Organism with a stable independent body temperature; an organism whose stable body temperature generally is independent of the surrounding environment.

Homonyms Terms that sound alike but are spelled differently and have different meanings.

Honeymoon phase A period of remorse by the abuser characterized by the abuser's denial and apologies.

Hordeolum A common acute infection of the glands of the eyelids.

Hormones Chemicals within the body that reach every cell through the circulatory system.

Hospice A care program that provides for the dying and their special needs.

Hospital Incident Command System An emergency management system that uses a logical management structure, defined responsibilities, clear reporting channels, and a common nomenclature to help unify hospitals with other emergency responders.

Hospital off-load time The time necessary for a crew to become available once they arrive at a hospital.

Hot load Loading a patient into a helicopter while the rotors are spinning.

Hot zone The primary danger zone around a crash scene that typically extends approximately 50 feet in all directions from the wreckage.

Hover The condition in which a helicopter remains fairly stationary over a given point, moving neither vertically nor horizontally.

Hub The plastic piece that houses a needle and fits onto a syringe.

Human immunodeficiency virus (HIV) The virus that can cause AIDS.

Human leukocyte antigen Leukocyte antigen that transplant surgeons attempt to match to prevent incompatibility.

Humoral immunity Immunity from antibodies in the blood.

Humoral Pertaining to elements in the blood or other body fluids.

Huntington's disease Programmed cell death of certain neurons in the brain, leading to behavioral abnormalities, movement disorders, and a decline in cognitive function.

Hydration Process of taking in fluids with the normal daily output.

Hydraulic A water hazard caused when water moves over a uniform obstruction to flow.

Hydraulic injection injuries High-pressure fluid that leaks from hydraulic hoses and is injected into the body.

Hydrocarbon A member of a large class of chemicals belonging to the petroleum derivative family; they have a variety of uses, such as solvents, oils, reagents, and fuels.

Hydrocele Collection of fluid in the scrotum or along the spermatic cord.

Hydrocephalus An excessive amount of cerebrospinal fluid.

Hydrogen cyanide A highly toxic blood agent.

Hydrogen ion concentration Concentration of hydrogen ions in a given solution, such as water or blood; used to calculate the pH of a substance.

Hydrogen sulfide A hazardous gas produced by the decomposition of organic material prevalent when manure is stored in a liquid form for an extended period.

Hydrophilic Attracts water molecules.

Hydrophobic Repels water molecules.

Hydrostatic pressure Pressure exerted by a fluid from its weight.

Hydroxylysine An amino acid found in collagen.

Hymen Thin of layer of tissue that covers the vaginal orifice in virgins.

Hypercalcemia A state in which the body has an abnormally high level of calcium.

Hypercapnia An increased amount of carbon dioxide in the blood; may be a result of hypoventilation.

Hypercarbia An excess of CO_2 in the blood.

Hyperdynamic Excessively forceful or energetic. Term is used to describe shock states in which the heart is pumping aggressively to make up for fluid losses, such as in burn or septic shock.

Hyperextension Extension beyond a joint's normal range of motion.

Hyperflexion Flexion beyond a joint's normal range of motion.

Hyperkalemia A state in which the body has an abnormally elevated potassium level.

Hypermagnesemia A state in which the body has an abnormally elevated concentration of magnesium in the blood.

Hypermetabolic A state or condition of the body characterized by excessive production and utilization of energy molecules such as protein.

Hyperopia Farsightedness; difficulty seeing objects close to the person.

Hyperosmolar hyperglycemic nonketotic coma (HHNC) Condition caused by a relative insulin insufficiency that leads to extremely high blood sugar levels while still allowing for normal glucose metabolism and an absence of ketone bodies.

Hyperplasia Abnormal cell division that increases the number or a specific type of cell.

Hyperpnea Increased respiratory rate or deeper than normal breathing.

Hyperresonant A high-pitched sound.

Hypersensitivity disorder A disorder in which the immune system responds inappropriately and excessively to an antigen (in this response, known as allergens).

Hypersensitivity pneumonitis Inflammation in and around the tiny air sacs (alveoli) and smallest airways (bronchioles) of the lung caused by an allergic reaction to inhaled organic dusts or, less commonly, chemicals; also called *extrinsic allergic alveolitis, allergic interstitial pneumonitis,* or *organic dust pneumoconiosis.*

Hypersensitivity reaction An immune response that is excessive beyond the bounds of normalcy to a point that it leads to damage (as with endotoxins) or is potentially damaging to the individual.

Hypersensitivity An altered reactivity to a medication that occurs after prior sensitization; response is independent of the dose.

Hypertension Elevated blood pressure.

Hypertensive emergencies Situations that require rapid (within 1 hour) lowering of blood pressure to prevent or limit organ damage.

Hypertensive urgencies Significant elevations in blood pressure with nonspecific symptoms that should be corrected within 24 hours.

Hyperthermia A core body temperature greater than 98.6° F.

Hypertonic In a membrane, the side with the higher concentration in an imbalance in the ionic concentration from one side to the other.

Hypertrophic scar Scar that forms with excessive amounts of scar tissue. The scar remains contained by the wound boundaries but may be slightly raised and can impair function.

Hypertrophy Enlargement or increase in the size of a cell(s) or tissue.

Hyperventilation Blowing off too much carbon dioxide.

Hyphema Blood in the anterior chamber of the eye.

Hypocalcemia A state in which the body has an abnormally low calcium level.

Hypocarbia An inadequate amount of carbon dioxide in the blood.

Hypokalemia A state in which the level of potassium in the serum falls below 3.5 mEq/L.

Hypomagnesemia A state in which the body has an abnormally low serum concentration of magnesium.

Hypomania An episode of a lesser form of mania that may transition into mania or alternate with depression.

Hypoperfusion The inadequate circulation of blood through an organ or a part of the body; shock.

Hypotension Low blood pressure significant enough to cause inadequate perfusion.

Hypothalamus Interface between the brain and the endocrine system; provides control for many autonomic functions.

Hypothermia A core body temperature below 95° F (35° C).

Hypotonic In a membrane, the side with the lower concentration when an imbalance exists in the ionic concentration from one side to the other.

Hypoventilation Occurs when the volume of air that enters the alveoli and takes part in gas exchange is not adequate for the body's metabolic needs.

Hypovolemic shock Inadequate tissue perfusion caused by inadequate vascular volume.

Hypoxemia An abnormal deficiency in the concentration of oxygen in arterial blood.

Hypoxia Inadequate oxygenation of the cells.

Iatrogenic drug response An unintentional disease or drug effect produced by a physician's prescribed therapy; *iatros* means "physician," and *-genic* is a word root meaning "produce."

Icterus Jaundice.

Idiosyncrasy The unexpected and usually individual (genetic) adverse response to a drug.

Ileostomy Surgical creation of a passage through the abdominal wall into the ileum.

Ileum Last segment of the small intestine; area of decreased absorption where is prepared for entry into the large intestine.

Ileus Decreased peristaltic movement of the colon.

Immediately dangerous to life or health concentrations (IDHLs) Maximal environmental air concentration of a substance from which a person could escape within 30 minutes without symptoms of impairment or irreversible health effects.

Immersion To be covered in water or other fluid.

Immunity Protection from legal liability in accordance with applicable laws.

Immunodeficiency Deficit in the immune system and its response to infection or injury.

Immunoglobulin See *Antibody.*

Impetigo A highly contagious infection caused by staphylococcal or streptococcal bacteria. A superficial vesicopustular skin infection that primarily occurs on exposed areas of the face and extremities from scratching infected lesions; usually begins at a traumatized region of the skin, where a combination of vesicles and pustules develops; the pustules rupture and crust, leaving a characteristic thick, golden or honeylike appearance.

Implied consent The presumption that a patient who is ill or injured and unable to give consent for any reason would agree to the delivery of emergency health care necessitated by his or her condition.

Incarcerated hernia Hernia of intestine that cannot be returned or reduced by manipulation; it may or may not become strangulated.

Incendiary device A device designed to ignite a fire.

Incidence The rate at which a certain event occurs, such as the number of new cases of a specific disease occurring during a certain period in a population at risk.

Incidence rate The rate of contraction of a disease versus how many are currently sick with the disease.

Incident commander The person responsible for the overall management of an emergency scene.

Incident scene hazards Hazards directly related to the specific incident scene, including control of crowds, traffic, the danger of downed electrical wires, the presence of hazardous materials, and the location of an emergency.

Incomplete abortion An abortion in which the uterus retains part of the products of the pregnancy.

Incomplete cord transaction A partial cutting (severing) of the spinal cord in which some cord function remains distal to the injury site.

Incontinence Inability to control excretory functions; usually refers to the involuntary passage of urinary or fecal matter.

Incubation period The time between exposure to a disease pathogen and the appearance of the first signs or symptoms.

Incus The anvil-shaped bone located between the malleus and stapes in the middle ear.

Index of suspicion The expectation that certain injuries or patterns of injuries have resulted to a body part, organ, or system based on the mechanism of injury and the force of impact to the patient.

Indication The appropriate use of a drug when treating a disease or condition.

Indicative change ECG changes seen in leads looking directly at the wall of the heart in an infarction.

Induration Hardened mass within the tissue typically associated with inflammation.

Infarction Death of tissue because of an inadequate blood supply.

Inferior Toward the feet; below a point of reference in the anatomic position.

Inferior vena cava Vessels that return venous blood from the lower part of the body to the right atrium.

Infiltration Complication of intravenous therapy when the catheter tip is outside the vein and the intravenous solution is dispersed into the surrounding tissues.

Inflammation A tissue reaction in an injury, infection, or insult.

Influx Flowing into.

Ingestion Process of bringing food into the digestive tract.

Inhalants Substances such as aerosols, fuels, paints, and other chemicals that produce fumes at room temperature; they are breathed in, producing a high.

Inhalation A route in which the medication is aerosolized and delivered directly to the lung tissue.

Injury Intentional or unintentional damage to a person resulting from acute exposure to thermal, mechanical, electrical, or chemical energy or from the absence of such essentials as heat or oxygen.

Injury risk A real or potential hazardous situation that puts individuals at risk for sustaining an injury.

Injury surveillance An ongoing systematic collection, analysis, and interpretation of injury data essential to the planning, implementation, and evaluation of public health practice, closely integrated with the timely dissemination of the data to those who need to know.

Inner ear Location of the sensory organs for hearing and balance.

Inotropic Relating to the force of cardiac contraction.

Inotropism A change in myocardial contractility.

Inspiratory reserve volume Amount of gas that can be forcefully inspired in addition to a normal breath's tidal volume.

Integrity Doing the right thing even when no one is looking.

Integumentary system The largest organ system in the body, consisting of the skin and accessory structures (e.g., hair, nails, glands).

Intense affect Heated and passionate emotional responses.

Intentional injury Injuries and deaths self-inflicted or perpetrated by another person, usually involving some type of violence.

Intentional tort A wrong in which the defendant meant to cause the harmful action.

Interatrial septum Septum dividing the atria in the heart.

Intercalated discs The cell-to-cell connection with gap junctions between cardiac muscle cells.

Interference The ability of one drug to limit the physiologic function of another drug.

Intermittent claudication Pain, cramping, muscle tightness, fatigue, or weakness of the legs when walking or during exercise.

Internal anal sphincter Muscle under autonomic control; has stretch receptors that provide the sensation of the need to defecate.

Internal bleeding Escape of blood from blood vessels into tissues and spaces within the body.

Internal respiration The exchange of gases between blood cells and tissues.

Internal urinary sphincter Ring of smooth muscle in the urethra that is under autonomic control.

International medical surgical response teams Specialty surgical teams that can respond both in the United States and internationally.

Interoperability Describes a radio system that can use the components of several different systems; it can use specialized equipment to connect several different radio systems and components together and have them communicate with each other.

Interpretation Stating the conclusions you have drawn from the information.

Interstitial compartment Area consisting of fluid outside cells and outside the circulatory system.

Interstitium Extravascular and extracellular milieu; also known as the *third space.*

Interval Waveform and a segment; in pacing, the period, measured in milliseconds, between any two designated cardiac events.

Interventricular septum Septum dividing the ventricles in the heart.

Intimal In reference to blood vessels, the innermost lining of an artery; composed of a single layer of cells.

Intimate partner violence and abuse Formerly called *domestic violence,* this is a learned pattern of assaultive and controlling behavior, including physical, sexual, and psychological attacks as well as economic control, which adults or adolescents use against their intimate partners to gain power and control.

Intimate space The area within 1.5 feet of a person.

Intoxication Being under the effect of a toxin or drug; common terminology (nonmedical) refers to intoxication as being under the effect of alcohol or illegal drugs.

Intracardiac The injection of a drug directly into a ventricle of the heart during cardiac arrest.

Intracellular Inside of the cell or cytoplasmic membrane.

Intracellular fluid (ICF) Fluid found within cells.

Intracerebral hematoma Bleeding within the brain tissue itself.

Intracerebral hemorrhage Bleeding within the brain tissue, often from smaller blood vessels.

Intracranial pressure (ICP) Pressure inside the brain cavity; should be very low, usually less than 15 mm Hg.

Intradermal Route of the injection of medication between the dermal layers of skin.

Intralingual Direct injection into the underside of the tongue with a small volume of medication.

Intramuscular (IM) An injection of medication directly into the muscle.

Intranasal The route that offers direct delivery of medications into the nasal passages and sinuses.

Intraosseous An administration route used in emergency situations when peripheral venous access is not established; a needle is passed through the cortex of the bone and the medication is infused into the capillary network within the bone matrix.

Intraosseous infusion The process of infusing medications, fluids, and blood products into the bone marrow cavity for subsequent delivery to the venous circulation.

Intraperitoneal Abdominopelvic organs surrounded by the peritoneum.

Intrathecal The direct deposition of medication into the spinal canal.

Intravascular compartment Area consisting of fluid outside cells but inside the circulatory system; the majority of intravascular fluid is plasma, which is the fluid component of blood.

Intravenous (IV) Administration route offering instantaneous and nearly complete absorption through peripheral or central venous access.

Intravenous (IV) bolus The delivery of a drug directly into an infusion port on the administration set using a syringe.

Intravenous cannulation Placement of a catheter into a vein to gain access to the body's venous circulation.

Intravenous therapy Administration of a fluid into a vein.

Intrinsic rate Rate at which a pacemaker of the heart normally generates impulses.

Intussusception Invagination of a part of the colon into another part of the colon; also referred to as *telescoping*.

Invasion of privacy Disclosure or publication of personal or private facts about a person to a person or persons not authorized to receive such information.

Invasive wound infection An infection involving the deeper tissues of a wound that may be destructive to blood vessels and other structures of the skin and soft tissues.

Investigational drug A drug not yet approved by the Food and Drug Administration.

Involuntary consent The rendering of care to a person under specific legal authority, even if the patient does not consent to the care.

Ion Electrically charged particle.

Ionizing radiation Particles or pure energy that produces changes in matter by creating ion pairs.

Iris Colored part of the eye; ring of smooth muscle that surrounds the pupil; controls the size (diameter) of the pupil.

Irregular bones Unique bones with specialized functions not easily classified into the other types of bone (e.g., vertebrae).

Ischemia Decreased supply of oxygenated blood to a body part or organ.

Ischemic phase Vascular response to shock when precapillary and postcapillary sphincters constrict, halting blood to distal tissues.

Ischemic stroke Lack of perfusion to an area of brain tissue; caused by a thrombus or embolus.

Islets of Langerhans Groups of cells located in the pancreas that produce insulin, glucagon, somatostatin, and pancreatic polypeptide.

Isoelectric line Absence of electrical activity; observed on the ECG as a straight line.

Isografting Transplanting tissue from a genetically identical person (i.e., identical twin).

Isolation The seclusion of individuals with an illness to prevent transmission to others.

Isotonic A balance in the ionic concentration from one side of the membrane to the other.

Jacking the dash Making cuts into the front pillar and A pillar and lifting the dash, instrument panel, steering wheel, column, and even the pedals off a trapped driver or front seat passenger.

Jejunum Second part of the small intestine; major site of nutrient absorption.

Joint dislocation Disruption of articulating bones from their normal location.

Joints Point where two or more bones make contact to allow movement and provide mechanical support.

J-point Point where the QRS complex and ST segment meet.

Jugular venous distension (JVD) The presence of visually enlarged external jugular neck veins.

Jump kit A hard- or soft-sided bag used by paramedics to carry supplies and medications to the patient's side.

Junctional bradycardia A rhythm that begins in the atrioventricular junction with a rate of less than 40 beats/min.

Jurisprudence The theory and philosophy of law.

Kehr's sign Acute left shoulder pain caused by the presence of blood or other irritants in the peritoneal cavity.

Keloid An excessive accumulation of scar tissue that extends beyond the original wound margins.

Keratinized Accumulation of the protein keratin within the cytoplasm of skin cells. These cells comprise the epidermis of the skin. These dead cells function as the first defense against invaders and minor trauma.

Keratinocytes Epidermal cells.

Keratitis Inflammation and swelling of the cornea.

Kernicterus Excessive fetal bilirubin; associated with hemolytic disease.

Ketonemia The presence of ketones in the blood.

Kinetic energy M [mass] × $^1/_2$ V [velocity]^2; also called the *energy of motion.*

Knee bags Airbags mounted low on the instrument panel designed to deploy against the driver's and front seat passenger's knees in a frontal collision.

Korotkoff sounds The noise made by blood under pressure tumbling through the arteries.

Kussmaul respirations An abnormal respiratory pattern characterized by deep, gasping respirations that may be slow or rapid.

Kwashiorkor A form of malnutrition caused by inadequate protein intake compared with the total needed or required calorie intake.

Kyphosis Abnormally increased convexity in the curvature of the thoracic spine as viewed from the side; also called *hunchback.*

Labeling The application of a derogatory term to a patient on the basis of an event, habit, or personality trait that may not be accurate about the underlying condition.

Labia majora Rounded folds of external adipose tissue of the external female genitalia.

Labia minora Thinner, pinkish folds of skin that extend anteriorly to form the prepuce of the external female genitalia.

Labile Affect that changes frequently and rapidly.

Labor The process by which the fetus and placenta are expelled from the uterus. Usually divided into three stages, starting with the first contraction and ending with delivery of the placenta.

Labyrinth Series of bony tunnels inside the inner ear.

Labyrinthitis An inflammation of the structures in the inner ear.

Lacrimal ducts Small openings at the medial edge of the eye; drain holes for water from the surface of the eye.

Lacrimal fluid Watery, slightly alkaline secretion that consists of tears and saline that moisten the conjunctiva.

Lacrimal gland One of a pair of glands situated superior and lateral to the eye bulb; secretes lacrimal fluid.

Lacrimation Tearing of the eyes.

Lactic acid Byproduct of anaerobic metabolism.

Landing zone An area used to land a helicopter that is 100 feet × 100 feet and free of overhead wires.

Large intestine Organ where a large amount of water and electrolytes is absorbed and where undigested food is concentrated into feces.

Laryngoscope An instrument used to examine the interior of the larynx; during endotracheal intubation the device is used to visualize the glottic opening.

Laryngotracheobronchitis Croup.

Larynx Lies between the pharynx and the lungs; outer case of nine cartilages that protect and support the vocal cords.

Lassa fever A viral hemorrhagic fever illness caused by the Lassa virus (Arenavirus family).

Latent period Period during and after infection in which the disease is no longer transmissable.

Lateral A position away from the midline of the body.

Lateral recumbent Lying on either the right or left side.

Lead Electrical connection attached to the body to record electrical activity.

Left A position toward the left side of the body.

Left coronary artery Vessel that supplies oxygenated blood to the left side of the heart muscle.

Legally blind Less than 20/200 vision in at least one eye or a extremely limited field of vision (such as 20 degrees at its widest point).

Lens Transparent, biconvex elastic disc suspended by ligaments.

Leptomeningitis Inflammation of the inner brain coverings.

Lesions A wound, injury, or pathologic change in body tissue; any visible, local abnormality of the tissues of the skin, such as a wound, sore, rash, or boil.

Lethal concentration 50% (LC50) The air concentration of a substance that kills 50% of the exposed animal population; also commonly noted as LCt50; this denotes the concentration and the length of exposure time that results in 50% fatality in the exposed animal population.

Lethal dose 50% (LD50) The oral or dermal exposure dose that kills 50% of the exposed animal population in 2 weeks.

Leukocytes White blood cells.

Leukocytosis An increase in the number of white blood cells in the blood; typically results from infection, hemorrhage, fever, inflammation, or other factors.

Leukopenia A decrease in the total number of white blood cells in the blood.

Liability The legal responsibility of a party for the consequences of his or her acts or omissions.

Libel False statements about a person made in writing that blacken the person's character or injure his or her reputation.

Lice Wingless insects that live in human hair.

Licensure Permission granted to an individual by a governmental authority, such as a state, to perform certain restricted activities.

Life-threatening conditions A problem to the circulatory, respiratory, or nervous system that will kill a patient within minutes if not properly managed.

Ligaments Fibrous connective tissue that connects bones to bones, forming joint capsules.

Limbic system The part of the brain involved in mood, emotions, and the sensation of pain and pleasure.

Linear laceration Laceration that generally has smooth margins, although not as precise as those of an incision.

Linear skull fracture A line crack in the skull.

Lipid accumulation Accumulation of lipids in cells, usually as a result of the failure or inadequate performance of the enzyme that metabolizes fats.

Lipid peroxidation Process of cellular membrane destruction from exposure of the membrane to oxygen free radicals.

Lipophilic Substances that tend to seek out and bind to fatty substances.

Liquefaction necrosis Dead or dying tissue in which the necrotic material becomes softened and liquefied.

Liver Largest internal organ in the body; serves as a major detoxifier in the body.

Living will A type of advanced directive with written and signed specific instructions to health care providers about the individual's wishes regarding what types of health care measures or treatments should be undertaken to prolong life.

Loaded airbag An airbag that has not deployed during the initial crash.

Local damage Damage present at the point of chemical contact.

Local effect The effects of a drug at the site where the drug is applied or in the surrounding tissues.

Lock out, tag out An industrial workplace safety term describing actions taken to shut off power to a device, appliance, machine, or vehicle and to ensure that power remains off until work is completed.

Logistics officer The person responsible for assembling supplies used during an incident.

Long bones Bones that are longer than they are wide, have attachments for muscles to allow movement, and are found in limbs (e.g., the femur).

Looseness of associations (LOA) Going off track during conversation to varying degrees.

Low-angle terrain An environment in flat or mildly sloping areas in which rescuers primarily support themselves with their feet on the terrain surface.

Low vision Level of visual impairment in which an individual is unable to read a newspaper at the usual viewing distance even if wearing glasses or contact lenses. It is not limited to distance vision and can be a severe visual impairment.

Low voltage Less than 1000 V.

Lower airway Portion of the respiratory tract below the glottis.

Lower airway inhalation injury Injury to the anatomic portion of the respiratory tree below the level of the glottis. Generally caused by the inhalation of the toxic by products of combustion.

Lower flammable limit The minimal concentration of fuel in the air that will ignite; below this point too much oxygen and not enough fuel are present to burn (too lean); also called the *lower explosive limit*.

Ludwig's angina A bacterial infection of the floor of the mouth resulting from an infection in the root of the teeth, an abscessed tooth, or an injury to the mouth.

Lumbar vertebrae Vertebrae of the lower back that do not attach to any ribs and are superior to the pelvis.

Lumen An opening in the bevel of a needle.

Lungs Organs that allow the mechanical movement of air to and from the respiratory membrane.

Lymph Fluid within the lymphatic system.

Lymph nodes Filter out foreign materials and collect infection-fighting cells that kill pathogens.

Lymphadenopathy Swelling of lymph nodes.

Lymphatic system The network of vessels, ducts, nodes, valves, and organs involved in protecting and maintaining the internal fluid environment of the body; part of the circulatory system.

Lymphatic vessels Unidirectional tubes that carry fluid or lymph within the lymphatic system.

Lymphedema Edema that follows when lymphatic pathways are blocked and fluid accumulates in the interstitial space.

Lymphocyte A form of leukocyte.

Lyse To destroy a cell.

Lysergic acid diethylamide (LSD) A powerful synthetic hallucinogen, often called *acid* and found on small squares of blotter paper.

Lysosomes Membrane-walled structures that contain enzymes.

Macrophages A monocyte that has matured and localized in one particular type of tissue; active in the immune system by activating agents that kill pathogens, absorbing foreign materials, and slowing infections and infectious agents.

Macule A flat, circumscribed, discolored lesion (e.g., freckle) measuring less than 1 cm.

Mainstem bronchi Each of two main breathing tubes that lead from the trachea into the lungs. There is one right mainstem bronchus and one left mainstem bronchus.

Malaise General feeling of illness without any specific symptoms.

Malfeasance Performing a wrongful act.

Malignant Highly dangerous or virulent; often used to describe a deadly form of cancer or a spreading of cancer.

Malignant hypertension Severe hypertension with signs of acute and progressive damage to end organs such as the heart, brain, and kidneys.

Malingering Faking illness for a tangible gain (missing work, avoiding incarceration, etc.).

Malleus Hammer-shaped bone located at the front of the middle ear; receives vibrations from the tympanic membrane.

Malocclusion The condition in which the teeth of the upper and lower jaws do not line up.

Mammary glands Female organs of milk production; located within the breast tissue.

Mania An excessively intense enthusiasm, interest, or desire; a craze.

Manure gas A name used for several different gases formed by decomposition of manure (methane, carbon dioxide, ammonia, hydrogen sulfide, and hydrogen disulfide); in certain concentrations all are toxic to animals and human beings.

Marasmus A form of nutritional deficiency from an overall lack of calories that results in wasting.

Marburg A viral hemorrhagic fever illness caused by the Marburg virus (Filovirus family).

Margination Process of phagocytes adhering to capillary and venule walls in the early phases of inflammation.

Marijuana Dried mixture of shredded leaves, stems, and seeds of the hemp plant that usually are smoked and contain many psychoactive compounds, most notably tetrahydrocannabinol (THC).

Mark 1 antidote kit Self-injected nerve agent antidote kit consisting of atropine and 2-pralidoxime (2-PAM).

Mast cells Connective tissue cell that contains histamine; important in initiating the inflammatory response.

Material safety data sheet (MSDS) A document that contains information about the specific identity of a hazardous chemical; information includes exact name and synonyms, health effects, first aid, chemical and physical properties, and emergency telephone numbers.

Matrix Nonliving material that separates cells in the connective tissue.

Mechanical processing Physical manipulation and breakdown of food.

Mechanism of action The manner in which a drug works to produce its intended effect.

Mechanism of injury The way an injury occurs on the body.

Meconium A dark green substance that represents the infant's first bowel movement.

Medial A position toward the midline of the body.

Median lethal dose The dose that kills 50% of the drug-tested population.

Mediastinitis Infection of the mediastinum; a serious medical condition.

Mediastinoscopy Surgical procedure of looking into the mediastinum with an endoscope.

Mediastinum Area that includes the trachea, esophagus, thymus gland, heart, and great vessels.

Medical asepsis Medically clean, not sterile; the goal in prehospital care because complete asepsis is not always possible.

Medical direction Physician oversight of paramedic practice; also called *medical control.*

Medical director A physician responsible for the oversight of the EMS system and the actions of the paramedics; also known as a *physician advisor.*

Medical ethics A field of study that evaluates the decisions, conduct, policies, and social concerns of medical activities.

Medical practice act Legislation that governs the practice of medicine; may prescribe how and to what extent a physician may delegate authority to a paramedic to perform medical acts; varies from state to state.

Medical terminology Greek- and Latin-based words (typically) that function as a common language for the medical community.

Medically clean Disinfected.

Medulla Most inferior part of the brainstem; responsible for some vegetative functions.

Medulla oblongata Lowest portion of brain tissue and the interface between the brain and the spinal cord; responsible for maintenance of basic life functions such as heart rate and respirations.

Meissner corpuscle Encapsulated nerve endings in the superficial dermis responsible for sensing vibrations and light touch.

Melancholy An episode of dysphoric mood with disruptions of homeostasis, including alterations in appetite, activities, and sleep patterns; also called *major* or *severe depression.*

Melena Foul-smelling, dark, and tarry stools stained with blood pigments or with digested blood, often indicating gastrointestinal bleeding.

Melting point The temperature at which a solid changes to a liquid (e.g., ice melting to water at $0°C$ ($32°F$).

Membrane potential Difference in electrical charge across the cell membrane.

Menarche A girl's first menstruation.

Meninges Covering of the brain and spinal cord; layers include the dura mater, arachnoid, and pia mater.

Meningitis Irritation of the connective tissue covering the central nervous system, often from infection or hemorrhage.

Meningocele A type of spina bifida in which the spinal cord develops normally but a saclike cyst that contains the meninges and cerebrospinal fluid protrudes from an opening in the spine, usually in the lumbosacral area.

Meningomyelocele The severest form of spina bifida in which the meninges, cerebrospinal fluid, and a portion of the spinal cord protrude from an opening in the spine and are encased in a sac covered by a thin membrane; also called *myelomeningocele.*

Menopause Cessation of menstruation in the human female.

Menstruation Shedding of endometrial lining.

Mental illness Any form of psychiatric disorder.

Mental retardation Developmental disability characterized by a lower than normal IQ.

Merocrine glands Sweat glands that open directly to the surface of the body; produce a fluid (mainly water) when the temperature rises that allows the body to dispel large amounts of heat through the evaporation process.

Mesentery Layers of connective tissue found in the peritoneal cavity.

Metabolism Sum of all physical and chemical changes that occur within an organism.

Metabolites The smaller molecules from the breakdown that occurs during metabolism.

Metaplasia The transformation of one type of mature differentiated cell into another type of mature differentiated cell.

Metastatic Spread of cancerous cells to a distant site.

Metered-dose inhaler (MDI) A handheld device that disperses a measured dose of medication in the form of a fine spray directly into the airway.

Methamphetamine A powerful, highly addictive central nervous system stimulant found in either a white powder form or a clear crystal form ("crystal meth").

Methemoglobinemia The oxidation of hemoglobin from the ferrous iron to the ferric iron state.

Methicillin-resistant Staphylococcus aureus Any of several bacterial strains of *S. aureus* resistant to methicillin (a penicillin) and related drugs; typically acquired in the hospital.

Micturition Urination.

Midbrain Lies below the diencephalon and above the pons; works with the pons to route information from higher within the brain to the spinal cord and vice versa.

Middle ear Air-filled chamber within the temporal bone; contains the auditory ossicles.

Migraine headache A recurring vascular headache characterized by unilateral onset, severe pain, sensitivity to light, and autonomic disturbances during the acute phase, which may last for hours or days.

Milliampere (mA) Unit of measure of electrical current needed to elicit depolarization of the myocardium.

Millivolt (mV) Difference in electrical charge between two points in a circuit.

Minor In most states, a person younger than 18 years.

Minute volume Amount of gas moved in and out of the respiratory tract per minute. Tidal volume multiplied by ventilatory rate equals minute volume. The minute volume is the true measurement of a patient's ventilatory status and is vital in assessing pulmonary function. It ascertains the ventilatory rate and the depth of each inhalation.

Miosis Pinpoint pupils.

Miscarriage (spontaneous abortion) Loss of the products of conception before the fetus can survive on its own.

Misfeasance Performing a legal act in a harmful manner.

Mitochondria Power plant of the cell and body; site of aerobic oxidation.

Mitosis Process of division and multiplication in which one cell divides into two cells.

Mitral valve Left atrioventricular valve in the heart; also called the *bicuspid valve.*

Mittelschmerz Pain occurring at time of ovulation.

Mixed episode A period of manic-like energy and agitation coupled with the pessimism and dysphoria of severe depression.

Mobile data computer A device used in an ambulance or first responder vehicle to retrieve and send call information; has its own memory storage and processing capability.

Mobile data terminal A device used like a mobile data computer but without its own memory storage and processing capability.

Mobile radio A radio installed in an emergency vehicle; usually transmits by higher wattage than a portable radio.

Modern deployment Deployment that considers workload and how available resources can achieve a balance among coverage, response times, and crew satisfaction.

Mold A multicellular type of fungus that grows hyphae.

Monoblasts Immature monocytes.

Monocytes Type of white blood cell (leukocyte) designed to consume foreign material and fight pathogens; generally become macrophages within a few days after release into the bloodstream.

Monomorphic Having the same shape.

Mons pubis A hair-covered fat pad overlying the symphysis pubis.

Mood The dominant and sustained emotional state of a patient; the emotional lens through which a patient views the world.

Morals Social standards that help a person define right (what a person ought to do) versus wrong (what a person ought not to do).

Morbid obesity Having a body mass index of 40 or more; equates to approximately 100 lb more than ideal weight.

Morbidity A disease state.

Mortality Death.

Mortality rate The number of patients who have died from a disease in a given period.

Motor cortex Area of brain tissue on the frontal lobe that controls voluntary movements.

Mucosa Layer of cells lining body cavities or organs (e.g., the lining of the mouth and digestive tract); generally implies a moist surface.

Multiformed atrial rhythm Cardiac dysrhythmia that occurs because of impulses originating from various sites, including the sinoatrial node, the atria, and/or the atrioventricular junction; requires at least three different P waves seen in the same lead for proper diagnosis.

Multipara A woman who has given birth multiple times.

Multiple-casualty incident An incident involving 26 to 99 persons.

Multiple organ dysfunction syndrome Altered organ function in an acutely ill person in whom homeostasis cannot be maintained without intervention.

Multiple-patient incident An incident involving two to 25 persons.

Multiple sclerosis (MS) Autoimmune disorder in which the immune system attacks the myelin sheath surrounding neurons, causing widespread motor problems and pain.

Multiplex This system allows the crew to transmit voice and data at the same time, enabling the crew to call in a patient report while transmitting an ECG strip to the hospital.

Murphy's sign An inspiratory pause when the right upper quadrant is palpated.

Muscle tissue Contractile tissue that is the basis of movement.

Muscular dystrophy (MD) Hereditary condition causing malformation of muscle tissue and leading to malformation of the musculoskeletal system and physical disability.

Mutate To change in an unusual way.

Mutism A condition in which a person will not speak.

Myasthenia gravis Autoimmune disorder affecting acetylcholine receptors throughout the body, causing widespread muscle weakness.

Mycoses Diseases caused by fungi.

Mydriasis Dilation of the pupils.

Myelomeningocele Developmental anomaly of the central nervous system in which a hernial sac containing a portion of the spinal cord, the meninges, and cerebrospinal fluid protrudes through a congenital cleft in the vertebral column; occurs in approximately two of every 1000 live births, is readily apparent, and is easily diagnosed at birth.

Myocardial cells Working cells of the myocardium that contain contractile filaments and form the muscular layer of the atrial walls and the thicker muscular layer of the ventricular walls.

Myocardial depressant factor An inflammatory mediator (cytokine) produced as a result of significant burn injury; known to affect the contractile function of the cardiac ventricles.

Myocardial infarction (MI) Necrosis of some mass of the heart muscle caused by an inadequate blood supply.

Myocarditis Inflammation of the middle and thickest layer of the heart, the myocardium.

Myocardium Middle and thickest layer of the heart; contains the cardiac muscle fibers that cause contraction of the heart as well as the conduction system and blood supply.

Myoglobin A pigment in muscle tissue that serves as an oxygen carrier (also known as *myohemoglobin*).

Myoglobinuria Presence of myoglobin in the urine; almost always a result of a pathologic (disease) state such as widespread muscle injury.

Myometrium Muscular region of the uterus.

Myopia Nearsightedness; difficulty seeing objects at a distance.

Myositis A rare muscle disease in which the body's immune system is activated, resulting in inflammation and pain of muscle tissue.

Myotomes Areas of the body controlled by specific motor spinal nerves.

Myxedema Severe form of hypothyroidism characterized by hypothermia and unresponsiveness.

N-95 particulate mask (medical) A facial mask worn over the nose and mouth that removes particulates from the inspired and expired air.

Nasal flaring Widening of the nostrils on inhalation; an attempt to increase the size of the airway and increase the amount of available oxygen.

Nasal polyps Small, saclike growths consisting of inflamed nasal mucosa.

Nasogastric The administration route used when a nasogastric tube is in place; bypasses the voluntary swallowing reflex.

Nasogastric tube A tube placed by way of the nose into the stomach.

Nasolacrimal duct Opening at the medial corner of the eye that drains excess fluid into the nasal cavity.

Natal Connected with birth.

National Disaster Medical System An organized response to an event that includes field units, coordination of patient transportation, and provision of hospital beds. The field component is composed of many volunteer teams of medical professionals.

National Fire Protection Association (NFPA) International voluntary membership organization that promotes improved fire protection and prevention and establishes safeguards against loss of life and property by fire; writes and publishes national voluntary consensus standards.

National Flight Paramedics Association (NFPA) Association established in 1984 to differentiate the critical care paramedic from the flight paramedic; has developed a position statement recommending the training considered necessary to perform the duties of a flight paramedic.

National Highway Traffic Safety Administration (NHTSA) An agency within the U.S. Department of Transportation that was first given the authority to develop EMS systems, including the development of curriculum.

National Medical Response Team Quick response specialty teams trained and equipped to provide mass casualty decontamination and patient care after the release of a chemical, biologic, or radiologic agent.

National Registry of EMTs (NREMT) A national organization developed to ensure that graduates of EMS training programs have met minimal standards by measuring competency through a uniform testing process.

National Standard Curriculum (NSC) Document providing information or course planning and structure, objectives, and detailed lesson plans. It also suggests hours of instruction for the EMT-A.

Natural immunity Nonspecific immunity that mounts a generalized response to any foreign material or pathogen (e.g., inflammation).

Natural killer cells Specialized lymphocytes capable of killing infected or malignant cells.

Nebulizer A machine that turns liquid medication into fine droplets in aerosol or mist form.

Necrosis Death of an area of tissue.

Necrotizing Causing the death (necrosis) of tissue.

Negative battery cable An electrical power cable that allows the vehicle's electrical system to be grounded or neutral as an electrical circuit.

Negative pressure Pressure that acts as a vacuum, pulling more fluid from the vascular space at a faster rate than before, further depleting the intravascular volume; also known as *inhibition pressure*.

Neglect Failure to provide for a child's basic needs; can be physical, educational, or emotional.

Negligence The failure to act as a reasonably prudent and careful person would under similar circumstances.

Negligence per se Conduct that may be declared and treated as negligent without having to prove what would be reasonable and prudent under similar circumstances, usually because the conduct violates a law or regulation.

Nematocyst The stinging cells many marine creatures use to envenomate and immobilize prey.

Neonatal abstinence syndrome Withdrawal symptoms that occur in newborns born to opioid-addicted mothers.

Neonate An infant from birth to 1 month of age.

Neoplasm Cancerous growth; a tumor that may be malignant or benign.

Neovascularization New blood vessel growth to support healing tissue.

Nephron Functional unit of the kidney.

Nephrotoxic Chemicals, medications, or other substances that can be toxic to the kidneys.

Nerve Neurons and blood vessels wrapped together with connective tissue; the body's information highways.

Nervous tissue Tissue that can conduct electrical impulses.

Neural tube defects Congenital anomalies that involve incomplete development of the brain, spinal cord, and/or their protective coverings.

Neuralgia Pain caused by chronic nerve damage.

Neuroeffector junction Interface between a neuron and its target tissue.

Neurogenic shock Shock with hypotension caused by a sudden loss of control over the sympathetic nervous system. Loss can be caused by a variety of mechanisms from traumatic injury to disease and infection.

Neuroglia Supporting cells of nervous tissue; functions include nourishment, protection, and insulation.

Neurons Conducting cells of nervous tissue; composed of a cell body, dendrites, and axon.

Neuropeptide A protein that may interact with a receptor after circulation through the blood.

Neuroses Mental diseases related to upbringing and personality in which the person remains "out of touch" with reality.

Neurotransmitters A chemical released from one nerve that crosses the synaptic cleft to reach a receptor.

Neutralizing agent A substance that counteracts the effects of acids or bases; brings the pH of a solution back to 7.0.

Neutron radiation Penetrating radiation that can result in whole-body irradiation.

Neutrophils A form of granulocyte that is short lived but often first to arrive at the site of injury; capable of phagocytosis.

Newborn asphyxia The inability of a newborn to begin and continue breathing at birth.

Newly born An infant in the first minutes to hours after birth; also called *newborn*.

Nodule An elevated, solid lesion in the deep skin or subcutaneous tissues.

Noncardiogenic pulmonary edema Fluid collection in the alveoli of the lung that does not result from heart failure.

Nonfeasance Failure to perform a required act or duty.

Nonproprietary name Generic name.

Nonsteroidal antiinflammatory drug (NSAID) Medications used primarily to treat inflammation, mild to moderate pain, and fever.

Nonverbal cues Expressions, motions, gestures, and body language that may be used to communicate other than with words.

Normal flora Nonthreatening bacteria found naturally in the human body that, in some cases, are necessary for normal function.

Nuclear envelope The outer boundary between the nucleus and the rest of the cell to the endoplasmic reticulum for protein synthesis.

Nuclear membrane Membrane in the cell that surrounds the nucleus.

Nucleoplasm Protoplasm of the nucleus as contrasted with that of the cell.

Nucleus Area within a cell where the genetic material is stored.

Nullipara A woman who has not borne a child.

Numerator The number or mathematic expression written above the line in a fraction; the numerator is a portion of the denominator.

Nystagmus Involuntary rapid movement of the eyes in the horizontal, vertical, or rotary planes of the eyeball.

Obesity An excessively high amount of body fat or adipose tissue in relation to lean body mass.

Objective information Verifiable findings, such as information seen, felt, or heard by the paramedic.

Obsessive-compulsive disorder (OCD) An anxiety disorder marked by frequent, intrusive, unwanted, and bothersome thoughts (obsessions) and repetitive rituals (compulsions).

Obstructed lane +1 Blocking with an emergency vehicle to stop the flow of traffic in the lane in which the damaged vehicle is positioned plus one additional lane or the shoulder of the roadway.

Occipital lobe Most rearward portion of the cerebrum; mainly responsible for processing the sense of sight.

Occupational Safety and Health Administration (OSHA) A unit of the U.S. Department of Labor that establishes protective standards, enforces those standards, and reaches out to employers and employees through technical assistance and consultation programs.

Official name A drug's name as listed in the *United States Pharmacopoeia*.

Offline medical direction Prospective and retrospective medical direction.

Oils In medicine, substances extracted from flowers, leaves, stems, roots, seeds, or bark for use therapeutic treatments.

Olfactory Sense of smell.

Olfactory fatigue Desensitization of the sense of smell.

Olfactory tissue Located within the nasopharynx; contains receptors that enable the ability of smell (olfaction).

Omphalocele Protrusion of abdominal organs into the umbilical cord.

Oncotic pressure The net effect of opposing osmotic pressures in the capillary beds.

Online medical direction Direct voice communication by a medical director (or designee) to a prehospital professional while he or she is attending to the patient; also called *direct medical direction*.

Oocyte The female gamete; product of the female reproductive system.

Oogenesis Egg production.

Open-ended questions A form of interview question that allows patients to respond in narrative form so that they may feel free to answer in their own way and provide details and information that they believe to be important.

Open fracture Fracture of the bone tissue that breaks the skin and may or may not still be exposed.

Open pneumothorax Injury to the thoracic cavity in which the cavity is breached, allowing air into the space between the lung and the chest wall.

Operations Carries out the tactical objectives of the incident commander.

Ophthalmic Route of administration in which medications are applied to the eye, such as antibiotic eye drops.

Ophthalmoscope An instrument used to examine the inner parts of the eye; consists of an adjustable light and multiple magnification lenses.

Opioids Powerful pain-relieving drugs derived from the seed pods of the poppy plant or drugs that are similar in molecular structure.

Oral A route of administration in which the medication is placed in the mouth and swallowed; the drug is absorbed through the gastrointestinal tract.

Oral cavity First part of the gastrointestinal tract; includes salivary glands, teeth, and tongue.

Organ A structure composed of two or more kinds of tissues organized to perform a more complex function than any one tissue alone can.

Organ of Corti Organ of hearing located in the cochlea.

Organ systems The coordination of several organs working together.

Organelles Numerous structures within the cell.

Organic An etiology of an illness that stems from a biologic cause, such as a stroke or electrolyte imbalance.

Organism An entity composed of cells and capable of carrying on life functions.

Organophosphate A pesticide that inhibits acetylcholinesterase.

Orogastric (OG) tube A tube placed by way of the mouth into the stomach.

Oropharynx Starts at the uvula; back of the oral cavity that extends down to the epiglottis.

Orphan drugs Products developed for the diagnosis and/or treatment of rare diseases or conditions, such as sickle cell anemia and cystic fibrosis.

Orthopnea Dyspnea relieved by a change in position (either sitting upright or standing).

Orthostatic vital signs Serial measurements of the patient's pulse and blood pressure taken with the patient recumbent, sitting, and standing. Results are used to assess possible volume depletion; also called the *tilt test* or *postural vital signs.*

Osmolarity The number, or concentration, of solute per liter of water.

Osmosis The passive movement of water from a higher to a lower concentration.

Osmotic gradient The difference in the concentration from one side of a membrane to the other in the presence of an imbalance in the ionic concentration.

Osmotic pressure The pressure exerted by the concentration of the solutes in a given space.

Osteoarthritis A disorder in which the cartilaginous covering of the joint surface starts to wear away, resulting in pain and inflammation of a joint; also known as *degenerative joint disease.*

Osteomyelitis An infection of bone.

Osteoporosis Reduction in the amount of bone mass, which leads to fractures after minimal trauma.

Ostomy Hole; usually refers to a surgically made hole in some part of the body (e.g., tracheostomy, gastrostomy, colostomy).

Otic Route of administration in which medications are applied to the ear, such as antibiotic drops.

Otitis externa A condition manifested by redness and irritation of the external auditory canal; also called *swimmer's ear.*

Otosclerosis Abnormal growth of bone that prevents structures in the ear from working properly; thought to be a hereditary disease.

Otoscope An instrument used to examine the inner ear; consists of a light source and magnifying lens; the tip is covered with a disposable cone.

Oval window A membranous structure that separates the middle ear from the inner ear.

Ovarian follicle The ovum and its surrounding cells.

Ovarian medulla Inner portion of the ovary.

Ovarian torsion Twisting of an ovary on its axis such that the venous flow to the ovary is interrupted.

Ovaries Site of egg production in females.

Overdose The accidental or intentional ingestion of an excess of a substance with the potential for toxicity.

Over-the-counter (OTC) Drugs that can be purchased without a prescription.

Overweight State of increased body weight in relation to height.

Ovulation Mid-cycle release of an ovum during the menstrual cycle.

Ovum (oocyte) Human egg that, when fertilized, implants in the lining of the uterus and results in pregnancy.

Oxidation A normal chemical process in the body caused by the release of oxygen atoms created during normal cell metabolism.

Oxidation ability The ability of a substance to readily release oxygen to stimulate combustion.

Oxygen-limiting silo A vertical structure used to store ensiled plant material in an anaerobic environment.

Oxyhemoglobin Hemoglobin that has oxygen molecules bound to it.

P wave First wave in the cardiac cycle; represents atrial depolarization and the spread of the electrical impulse throughout the right and left atria.

Pacemaker Artificial pulse generator that delivers an electrical current to the heart to stimulate depolarization.

Pacemaker cells Specialized cells of the heart's electrical conduction system capable of spontaneously generating and conducting electrical impulses.

Packaging Placing the injured or ill patient in a litter and securing him or her for evacuation.

Painful stimulus Any stimulus that causes discomfort to the patient, triggering some sort of response.

Palliative care Provision of comfort measures (physical, social, psychological, and spiritual) to terminally ill patients.

Pallor Pale, washed-out coloration of skin. Often a result of extreme anemia or chronic illness. A patient with pallor can be referred to as pallid.

Palpation The process of applying pressure against the body with the intent of gathering information.

Palpitations An unpleasant awareness of one's heartbeat.

Pancreatitis Inflammation of the pancreas.

Pandemic A disease that affects the majority of the population of a single region or that is epidemic at the same time in many different regions.

Panic attack A sudden, paralyzing anxiety reaction characterized by an overwhelming sense of fear, anxiety, and impending doom, often with physical symptoms such as chest pain and difficulty breathing.

Papillary dermis Section of the dermis composed of loose connective tissue that contains vasculature that feeds the epidermis.

Papillary muscles Muscles attached to the chordae tendineae of the heart valves and the ventricular muscle of the heart.

Papule An elevated, solid lesion usually less than 0.5 centimeters in diameter; may arise from the epidermis, dermis, or both.

Para The number of pregnancies carried to term.

Paracrine communication Method of intercellular communication in which cells communicate with cells in close proximity through the release of paracrine factors, or cytokines.

Paradoxic motion (of a segment of the chest wall) Part of the chest moves in an opposite direction from the rest during respiration.

Paranoid delusions False perceptions of persecution and the feeling that one is being hunted or conspired against; this is the most common type of delusion.

Paranoid schizophrenia A form of schizophrenia characterized by persistent preoccupation with illogical, absurd, and changeable delusions, usually of a persecutory, grandiose, or jealous nature, accompanied by related hallucinations.

Paraphimosis Tight, constricting band caused by the foreskin when it is retracted behind the glans penis.

Paraplegia Paralysis of the lower limbs and trunk.

Parasites An organism that lives within or on another organism (the host) but does not contribute to the host's survival.

Parasympathetic division A division of the autonomic nervous system; responsible for the relaxed state of the body known as "feed and breed."

Parasympathetic nervous system The subdivision of the autonomic nervous system usually involved in activating vegetative functions, such as digestion, defecation, and urination.

Parasympatholytics Drugs that block or inhibit the function of the parasympathetic receptors.

Parasympathomimetics Drugs that mimic the parasympathetic division of the autonomic nervous system.

Parenteral Administration route used for systemic effects and given by a route other than the digestive tract.

Paresthesia Abnormal sensation described as numbness, tingling, or pins and needles.

Parietal lobe Section of the cerebrum responsible for the integration of most sensory information from the body.

Parietal pleura Lining of the pleural cavity attached tightly to the interior of the chest cage.

Parity The number of pregnancies that have resulted in a viable infant.

Parkinson's disease Progressive movement disorder caused by dysfunction in the cerebellum; rigidity, tremor, bradykinesia, and postural instability are characteristic.

Parkmedic A National Park Service ranger who has undergone additional wilderness medical training and who operates in certain parks under the medical direction of emergency physicians from University of Southern California–Fresno; scope of practice lies between a traditional EMT-Intermediate and EMT-Paramedic, with additional wilderness medical training.

Paroxysmal atrial tachycardia Atrial tachycardia that starts or ends suddenly.

Paroxysmal nocturnal dyspnea (PND) A sudden onset of difficulty breathing that awakens the patient from sleep.

Paroxysmal supraventricular tachycardia (PSVT) A regular, narrow QRS tachycardia that starts or ends suddenly.

Partial agonist A drug that when bound to a receptor may elicit a physiologic response, but it is less than that of an agonist; may also may block the response of a competing agonist.

Partial pressure The pressure exerted by an individual gas in a mixture.

Partial seizure A seizure confined to one area of the brain.

Partial-thickness burn Burns that involve any layer of the dermis. The depth of these burns varies and depends on location, so they are further subcategorized as superficial partial-thickness or deep partial-thickness burns. Also called *second-degree burns.*

Partially sighted Level of vision in persons who have some type of visual problem and may need assistance.

Passive immunity Induced immunity that only lasts as long as the injected immune agents are alive and active (e.g., immunoglobulin injection).

Passive range of motion Degree of movement at a joint determined when the examiner causes the movement with the patient at rest.

Passive transport The ability of a substance to traverse a barrier without any energy input; generally occurs from a higher to a lower concentration.

Past medical history A summary of all past health-related events.

Patch A flat, circumscribed, discolored lesion.

Pathologic fracture Fractures that occur as a result of an underlying disease process that weakens the mechanical properties of the bone.

Pathophysiology Functional changes that accompany a particular syndrome or disease.

Patients with terminal illness Patients with advanced stage of illness or disease with an unfavorable prognosis and no known cure.

Pattern recognition Gathering patient information, relating it to the health care professional's knowledge of pathophysiology and the signs and symptoms of illnesses and injuries, and determining whether the patient's presentation fits a particular pattern.

Pattern response Anticipating the equipment and emergency care interventions needed on the basis of the patient's history and physical examination findings.

Patterned injuries Those that leave a distinctive mark, indicating that an object was used in the assault (e.g., cigarette burns, electrical cord whipping, human bites, glove injuries, attempted strangulation, and slaps).

Peak expiratory flow The greatest rate of airflow that can be achieved during forced expiration beginning with the lungs fully inflated.

Peak flow meter A device used to assess the severity of respiratory distress.

Pediculosis Human infestation with lice.

Pelvic inflammatory disease (PID) An infection of a woman's reproductive organs, usually from a bacterial infection, that spreads from the vagina to the upper parts of the reproductive tract.

Penetrating trauma Any mechanism of injury that causes a cut or piercing of skin.

Penis Male sex organ with three columns of erectile tissue; transfers sperm during copulation.

Percussion A diagnostic technique that uses tapping on the body to differentiate air, solids, and fluids.

Performance-based response system A contractual agreement between the EMS provider and the government authority to provide ambulance response to a particular municipality or region with time requirements for each response and total responses on a monthly basis.

Perfusion Circulation of blood through an organ or a part of the body.

Pericardial cavity The potential space between the two layers of the pericardium.

Pericardial effusion An increase in the volume and/or character of pericardial fluid that surrounds the heart.

Pericardial tamponade Life-threatening injury in which blood collects within the pericardium until the increasing pressure prevents the heart from filling with blood, causing death.

Pericardiocentesis A procedure in which a needle is inserted into the pericardial space and the excess fluid is drawn out (aspirated) through the needle.

Pericarditis Inflammation of the double-walled sac (pericardium) that encloses the heart.

Pericardium Two-layer serous membrane lining the pericardial cavity.

Perinatal From the twenty-eighth week of gestation through the first 7 days after delivery.

Perineal body See *Perineum.*

Perineum The tissue between the mother's vaginal and rectal openings; may be torn during delivery.

Periodontal membrane/ligament Ligamentous attachment between the root of a tooth and the socket of the bone within which it sits.

Periosteum Fibrous connective tissue rich in nerve endings that envelops bone.

Peripheral nervous system All the nerves outside the central nervous system.

Peripheral vein A vein outside the chest or abdomen, such as the veins of the upper and lower extremities.

Peripherally inserted central catheter (PICC) line A thin tube inserted into a peripheral vein (usually the arm) and threaded into the superior vena cava to allow fluid or medication administration.

Peristalsis The wavelike contraction of the smooth muscle of the gastrointestinal tract.

Peritoneal cavity The space between the parietal and visceral peritoneum; also called the *peritoneal space.*

Peritoneum Double-layered serous membrane that lines the abdominal cavity and covers the organs located in it.

Peritonitis Inflammation of the peritoneum, typically caused by infection or in response to contact with blood or digestive fluids.

Peritonsillar abscess (PTA) An infection of tissue between the tonsil and pharynx, usually the result of a significant infection in the tonsils.

Permeability Ability of a membrane channel to allow passage of electrolytes once it is open.

Permissible exposure limit Allowable air concentration of a substance in the workplace as established by the Occupational Safety and Health Administration; these values are legally enforceable.

Permit-required confined space A confined space with one or more of the following characteristics: (1) contains or has a potential to contain a hazardous atmosphere; (2) contains a material with the potential for engulfing an entrant; (3) has an internal configuration such that an entrant could be trapped or asphyxiated by inwardly converging walls or by a floor that slopes downward and tapers to a smaller cross-section; or (4) contains any other recognized serious safety or health hazard.

Personal protective equipment (PPE) Equipment used to protect personnel; includes items such as gloves, eyewear, masks, respirators, and gowns.

Personal space The area around an individual that the person perceives as an extension of himself or herself. In the United States, personal distance is 1.5 to 4 feet.

Personality disorders Patterns of interacting with others and the world that are rigid and harmful, causing social and occupational problems.

Pertinent negative In a patient assessment, the signs and symptoms found not to be present that support a working diagnosis.

Pertinent positive In a patient assessment, the signs and symptoms found to be present that support a working diagnosis.

Pesticide A chemical material used to control a pest (insect, weed, etc.).

Petechiae A tiny pinpoint rash on the upper area of the neck and the face; may indicate near strangulation or suffocation; caused by an occlusion of venous return from the head while arterial pressure remains normal; may be present in mothers after childbirth; reddish-purple nonblanchable discolorations in the skin less than 0.5 cm in diameter.

pH A numeric assignment used to define the hydrogen ion concentration of a given chemical. The lower the pH, the higher the hydrogen ion concentration and the more acidic the solution.

Phagocyte Cells that are part of the body's immune system that play a predominant role in the destruction of invading microorganisms.

Phagocytosis Ingestion and digestion of foreign materials by phagocytes (cells, such as macrophages, designed to perform this function).

Pharmaceutics The science of preparing and dispensing drugs.

Pharmacogenetics The study of inherited differences (variation) in drug metabolism and response.

Pharmacokinetics The process by which a drug is absorbed, distributed, metabolized, and eliminated by the body.

Pharmacologic restraints Agents such as sedatives that can suppress a patient's neurologic and/or motor capabilities so that the threat to the paramedic is reduced; also known as *chemical restraints*.

Pharmacology The study of drugs, including their actions and effects on the host.

Pharmacopeia A book describing drugs, chemicals, and medicinal preparations in a country or specific geographic area, including a description of the drug, its formula, and dosage.

Phases of rescue The training and organizational concept that groups all the activities that take place at a typical vehicle crash with entrapment into four categories, with each known as a phase of rescue.

Phlebitis Inflammation of a vein.

Phobia An intense fear of a particular object or situation.

Phosphate A salt of phosphoric acid that is important in the maintenance of the acid-base balance of the blood.

Phospholipid bilayer A double layer composed of three types of lipid molecules that comprise the plasma membrane.

Photoreceptor cells Rods and cones contained in the sensory part of the retina; they relay impulses to the optic nerve.

Photosensitivity A condition in which the patient's eyes are sensitive or feel pain when exposed to bright light.

Physical abuse Inflicting a nonaccidental physical injury on another person such as punching, kicking, hitting, or biting.

Physical disabilities Disabilities that involve limitation of mobility.

Physical restraints Straps, splints, and other devices that prevent movement of all or part of the patient's body.

Physician advisor A physician responsible for the oversight of the EMS system and the actions of the paramedics; also known as a *medical director.*

Physiology Study of how the body functions.

Pia mater Last meningeal layer; adheres to the central nervous system.

Pierre Robin sequence A congenital anomaly characterized by a very small lower jaw (micrognathia), a tongue that tends to fall back and downward (glossoptosis), and cleft palate.

Pill Dried powder forms of medication in the form of a small pellet; the term "pill" has been replaced with tablet and capsule.

Pinch points A machinery entanglement hazard formed when two machine parts move together and at least one of the parts moves in a circle.

Pinocytosis Absorption or ingestion of nutrients, debris, and fluids by a cell.

Placards Diamond-shaped signs placed on the sides and ends of bulk transport containers (e.g., truck, tank car, freight container) that carry hazardous materials.

Placenta (afterbirth) The organ inside the uterus that exchanges nutrition and waste between mother and fetus.

Placenta previa Placement of the placenta such that it partially or completely covers the cervix.

Placental abruption (abruptio placenta) Separation of part of the placenta away from the wall of the uterus.

Placental barrier Many layers of cells that form between maternal and fetal circulation that protect the fetus from toxins.

Plague An acute infectious disease caused by the anaerobic, gram-negative bacterium *Yersinia pestis;* transmitted naturally from rodents to human beings through flea bites; three common syndromes are bubonic (most likely form of the disease to be seen from naturally occurring infections), pneumonic (most likely form of the disease to result from an act of terrorism), and septicemic plague.

Plaintiff The person who initiates a lawsuit by filing a complaint; also known as a *claimant, petitioner,* or *applicant.*

Planning Supplies past, present, and future information about the incident.

Plaque An elevated, solid lesion usually greater than 0.5 cm in diameter that lacks any deep component.

Plasma Pale, yellow material in the blood; made of approximately 92% water and 8% dissolved molecules.

Plasma level profile The measurement of blood level of a medication versus the dosage administered.

Plasma membrane The outer covering of a cell that contains the cellular cytoplasm; also known as the *cell membrane.*

Platelets One of three formed elements in the blood; also called *thrombocytes.*

Pleura Serous membrane that lines the pleural cavity.

Pleural cavities Areas that contain the lungs.

Pleural effusion Collection of fluid in the pleural space, usually fluid that has seeped through the lung or chest wall tissue.

Pleural friction rub Noise made when the visceral and parietal pleura rub together.

Pleurisy Painful rubbing of the pleural lining.

Plural Amount that refers to more than one person, place, or thing.

Pluripotent Cell line that has the ability to differentiate into multiple different cell lines based on the right physiologic stimulus.

Pneumomediastinum Air entrapped within the mediastinum; a serious medical condition.

Pneumonia An inflammation and infection of the lower airway and lungs caused by a viral, bacterial, parasitic, or fungal organism.

Pneumonia Infection of the lungs.

Pneumothorax A collection of air in the pleural space, usually from either a hole in the lung or a hole in the chest wall.

Pocket mask A clear, semirigid mask designed for mouth-to-mask ventilation of a nonbreathing adult, child, or infant.

Poikilothermic An organism whose temperature matches the ambient temperature.

Point of maximum impulse (PMI) The apical impulse; the site where the heartbeat is most strongly felt.

Poison Any substance that can harm the human body; also known as a *toxin.*

Poisoning Exposure to a substance that is harmful in any dosage.

Poisonous Describes gases, liquids, or other substances of such nature that exposure to a very small amount is dangerous to life or is a hazard to health; also known as *toxic* (e.g., cyanide, arsenic, phosgene, aniline, methyl bromide, insecticides, pesticides).

Polarized state Period after repolarization of a myocardial cell (also called the *resting state*) when the outside of the cell is positive and the interior of the cell is negative.

Poliomyelitis Viral infection that tends to attack the motor roots of the spinal nerves, often leading to physical disability and even paralysis of the diaphragm.

Polydipsia Excessive thirst.

Polymorphic Varying in shape.

Polyphagia Excessive eating.

Polypharmacy The concurrent use of several medications.

Polyuria Excessive urination.

Pons Area of the brainstem that contains the sleep and respiratory centers for the body, which along with the medulla control breathing.

Portable radio Also referred to as a *walkie-talkie.* These radios are carried by emergency personnel and have a lower wattage output than the mobile or base unit. To use these portable radios with a higher watt output, the units can be connected through a repeater system to increase their output, which increases range.

Portal hypertension Increased venous pressure in the portal circulation.

Portal vein A vein composed of a group of vessels that originate from the digestive system.

Positive battery cable Also known as the *hot cable,* this electrical power cable allows a vehicle's electrical system to carry the current or electrical energy from the battery to the electrically powered appliances throughout the vehicle.

Positive end-expiratory pressure (PEEP) The amount of pressure above atmospheric pressure present in the airway at the end of the expiratory cycle. When forcing air into the lungs (positive-pressure ventilation), airway pressure is maintained above atmospheric pressure at the end of exhalation by means of a mechanical device, such as a PEEP valve.

Positive-pressure ventilation Forcing air into the lungs.

Postconcussion syndrome Symptoms of a concussion that persist for weeks to 1 year after an initial injury to the head.

Posterior The back, or dorsal, surface.

Postganglionic neuron The nerve that travels from the ganglia to the desired organ or tissue.

Postictal State that begins at the termination of seizure activity in the brain and ends with the patient returning to a level of normal behavior.

Postnatal The period immediately following the birth of a child and lasting for approximately 6 weeks.

Postpartum Pertaining to the mother after delivery.

Posttraumatic stress disorder (PTSD) An anxiety disorder that occurs after a traumatic, often life-threatening event.

Posture A patient's overall attitude and frame of mind.

Potassium The main intracellular ion (electrolyte), with the chemical designation K+.

Potential difference Difference in electrical charge between two points in a circuit; expressed in volts or millivolts.

Potentiating To augment or increase the action of.

Potentiation A prolongation or increase in the effect of a drug by another drug.

Pounds per square inch (psi) The amount of pressure on an area that is 1 inch square.

Poverty of speech A disorder of thought form characterized by very little spontaneous, voluntary speech and short answers to questions.

Powder Medication ground into a fine substance.

power take-off Element that connects a tractor to an implement; also called a *driveshaft.*

Prearrival instructions Clinically approved instructions provided by telephone by a trained and certified emergency medical dispatcher.

Precapillary sphincters Smooth muscle located at the entrances to the capillaries; responsive to local tissue needs.

Preeclampsia A complication of pregnancy that includes hypertension, swelling of the extremities and, in its most severe form, seizures (see *Eclampsia*).

Preexcitation Term used to describe rhythms that originate from above the ventricles but in which the impulse travels by a pathway other than the atrioventricular node and bundle of His; thus the supraventricular impulse excites the ventricles earlier than normal.

Prefix A sequence of letters that comes before the word root and often describes a variation of the norm.

Preganglionic neuron The nerve that extends from the spinal cord (central nervous system) to the ganglion.

Prehospital care report (PCR) The report written by the paramedic after the call has been completed. The report becomes part of the patient's permanent medical record.

Preload Force exerted by the blood on the walls of the ventricles at the end of diastole.

Premature birth Delivery between the twentieth and thirty-seventh weeks of pregnancy.

Premature complex Early beat occurring before the next expected beat; can be atrial or ventricular.

Premature or preterm infant Infant born before 37 weeks of gestation.

Prenatal Preceding birth.

Preoccupation A topic or theme that consistently recurs in a person's thought process and conversations.

Prepuce A fold formed by the union of the labia minora over the clitoris.

Presbycusis Age-related hearing loss.

Presbyopia Loss of function of the lens to adjust to close reading; usual onset in middle age.

Presenting part The first part of the infant to appear at the vaginal opening, usually the head.

Pressured speech Rapid, loud, and intense speech that often results from racing thoughts and frequently is seen during manic episodes.

Preterm birth Birth before 37 weeks of gestation.

Preterm delivery Delivery between the twentieth and thirty-seventh weeks of pregnancy.

Prevalence rate The fraction of the population that currently has a certain disease.

Priapism A prolonged and painful erection.

Primary apnea The newly born's initial response to hypoxemia consisting of initial tachypnea, then apnea, bradycardia, and a slight increase in blood pressure; if stimulated, responds with resumption of breathing.

Primary blast injury Injuries caused by an explosive's pressure wave.

Primary cord injury A spinal cord injury caused by a direct traumatic blow.

Primary hypertension High blood pressure for which no cause is identifiable; also called *essential hypertension.*

Primary injury prevention Keeping an injury from occurring.

Primary skin lesion A lesion that has not been altered by scratching, rubbing, scrubbing, or other types of trauma.

Primary triage The initial sorting of patients to determine which are most injured and in need of immediate care.

Primary tumor A collection of cells that grow out of control, far in excess of normal rates. A primary tumor is a tumor that develops in one tissue only (e.g., a liver primary tumor originates in the liver).

Primigravida A woman who is pregnant for the first time.

Primipara A woman who has given birth to her first child.

Primum non nocere Latin for "first, do no harm."

Prions Infectious agents composed of only proteins.

Prodromal An early symptom of a disease.

Prodrome A symptom indication the onset of a disease.

Prodrug A substance that is inactive when it is given and is converted to an active form within the body.

Profession A group of similar jobs or fields of interest that involve a responsibility to serve the public and require mastery of specific knowledge and specialized skills.

Professional A person who has special knowledge and skills and conforms to high standards of conduct and performance.

Professional malpractice A type of tort case addressing whether a professional person failed to act as a reasonably prudent and careful person with similar training would act under similar circumstances.

Professionalism Following the standards of conduct and performance for a profession.

Progesterone A female hormone secreted after ovulation has occurred that causes changes in the lining of the uterus necessary for successful implantation of a fertilized egg.

Prokaryotes One of the kingdoms of cells; simpler in structure and found in lower life forms such as bacteria.

Proliferative phase Portion of the menstrual cycle in which the endometrial lining grows under the influence of estrogen.

Prone Position in which the patient is lying on his or her stomach (face down).

Proprioception Ability to sense the orientation, location, and movement of the body's parts relative to other body parts.

Prospective medical direction Physician participation in the development of EMS protocols, procedures, and participation in the education and testing of EMS professionals; a type of offline medical direction.

Prostaglandins A class of fatty acids that has many of the properties of hormones.

Prostate Glandular tissue that produces prostatic fluid and muscular portion that contracts during ejaculation to prevent urine flow; dorsal to the symphysis pubis and the base of the urinary bladder.

Protein Any one of a number of large molecules composed of amino acids that form the structural components of cells or carry out biochemical functions.

Protocols A set of treatment guidelines written for the paramedic to follow.

Protoxin A substance converted to a toxin through a biochemical process in the body; would be harmless if they were not converted (e.g., methanol and ethylene glycol).

Proximal A position nearer to the attachment of a limb to the trunk.

Pruritus Itching of the skin.

Psoriasis A common chronic skin disorder characterized by erythematous papules and plaques with a silver scale.

Psychological abuse The verbal or psychological misuse of another person, including threatening, name calling, ignoring, shaming unfairly, shouting, and cursing; mind games are another form of psychological abuse.

Psychomotor Pertaining to motor effects of cerebral or psychic activity.

Psychomotor agitation Excessive motor activity that is usually nonproductive and tedious, resulting from inner tensions (pacing, fidgeting, hand wringing, etc.)

Psychoses A group of mental disorders in which the individual loses contact with reality; psychosis is thought to be related to complex biochemical disease that disorders brain function. Examples include schizophrenia, bipolar disease (also known as *manic-depressive illness*), and organic brain disease.

Psychosis An abnormal state of widespread brain dysfunction characterized by bizarre thought content, typically delusions and hallucinations.

Psychosocial development The social and psychological changes human beings undergo as they grow and age.

Psychosocial factors Life events that affect a person's emotional state, such as marriage, divorce, or death of a loved one.

Public health The discipline that studies the overall health of populations and intervenes on behalf of those populations rather than on behalf of individuals.

Public Safety Answering Point (PSAP) A dispatch center set up to receive and dispatch 9-1-1 calls.

Pull-in point Machinery entanglement hazard created when an operator attempts to remove material being pulled into a machine.

Pulmonary abscess A collection of pus within the lung itself.

Pulmonary arteries Left and right pulmonary arteries supplying the lungs.

Pulmonary bleb Cavity in the lung much like a balloon; may rupture to create a pneumothorax.

Pulmonary circulation Blood from the right ventricle is pumped directly to the lungs for oxygenation through the pulmonary trunk; blood becomes oxygenated and is then delivered through the pulmonary arteries for the left atrium.

Pulmonary edema A buildup of fluid in the lungs, usually a complication of left ventricular fibrillation.

Pulmonary embolism Movement of a clot into the pulmonary circulation.

Pulmonary embolus A blood clot that has lodged in the pulmonary artery, causing shortness of breath and hypoxia.

Pulmonary trunk Vessels that deliver blood from the right ventricle of the heart to the lungs for oxygenation.

Pulmonary veins Vessels that return blood to the left atrium of the heart.

Pulmonic valve Right semilunar valve; separates the right ventricle and the pulmonary trunk.

Pulp Center of a tooth that contains nerves, blood vessels, and connective tissue.

Pulse deficit A difference between the apical pulse and the peripheral pulse rates.

Pulse generator Power source that houses the battery and controls for regulating a pacemaker.

Pulse oximetry A noninvasive method of measuring the percentage of oxygen-bound hemoglobin.

Pulse pressure The difference between the systolic and diastolic blood pressures.

Pulseless electrical activity (PEA) Organized electrical activity observed on a cardiac monitor (other than ventricular tachycardia) without the patient having a palpable pulse.

Pulsus alternans A beat-to-beat difference in the strength of a pulse (also called *mechanical alternans*).

Pulsus paradoxus A fall in systolic blood pressure of more than 10 mm Hg during inspiration (also called *paradoxic pulse*).

Pupil Central opening in the iris.

Purkinje fibers Fibers found in both ventricles that conduct an electrical impulse through the heart.

Purpura Reddish-purple nonblanchable discolorations greater than 0.5 cm in diameter; large purpura are called ecchymoses.

Pustule A lesion that contains purulent material.

Pyelonephritis Infection of the kidney.

Pyrogenic Substances, such as endotoxins from certain bacteria, that stimulate the body to produce a fever.

Pyrophorics Substances that form self-ignitable flammable vapors when in contact with air.

QRS complex Several waveforms (Q wave, R wave, and S wave) that represent the spread of an electrical impulse through the ventricles (ventricular depolarization).

Quadriplegia Paralysis affecting all four extremities.

Quality assurance Programs designed to achieve a desired level of care.

Quality improvement Programs designed to improve the level of care; commonly driven by quality assurance.

Quality improvement unit (QIU) Trained and certified quality specialists who have the knowledge and skills to measure dispatcher performance against established standards accurately and consistently.

Quarantine The seclusion of groups of exposed but asymptomatic individuals for monitoring.

Quick response unit A type of responder with paramedic-level skills but no transport capability.

R wave On an EGG, the first positive deflection in the QRS complex, representing ventricular depolarization.

Raccoon eyes Bruising around the orbits of the eyes.

Racing thoughts The subjective feeling that one's thoughts are moving so fast that one cannot keep up; often seen during manic episodes.

Radio frequency Channel that allows communication from one specific user to another. For simple communication, both users must be on the same frequency or channel.

Radioactive The ability to emit ionizing radioactive energy.

Radioactive substances Any material or combination of materials that spontaneously emit ionizing radiation and have a specific activity greater than 0.002 mcCi/g (e.g., plutonium, cobalt, uranium 235, radioactive waste).

Radioactivity The spontaneous disintegration of unstable nuclei accompanied by the emission of nuclear radiation.

Range of motion The full and natural range of a joint's movement.

Rapid medical assessment A quick head-to-toe assessment of a medical patient who is unresponsive or has an altered mental status.

Rapid sequence intubation (RSI) The use of medications to sedate and paralyze a patient to achieve endotracheal intubation rapidly.

Rapid trauma assessment A quick head-to-toe assessment of a trauma patient with a significant mechanism of injury.

Rattles (rhonchi) Attributable to inflammation and mucus or fluid in the larger airway passages; descriptive of airway congestion heard on inspiration. Rhonchi are commonly associated with bronchitis or pneumonia.

Red blood cell count The number of red blood cells per liter of blood.

Rebound tenderness Discomfort experienced by the patient that occurs when the pressure from palpation is released.

Receptor A molecule, such as a protein, found inside or on the surface of a cell that binds to a specific substance (such as hormones, antigens, drugs, or neurotransmitters) and causes a specific physiologic effect in the cell.

Reciprocal change Mirror image ECG changes seen in the wall of the heart opposite the location of an infarction.

Reciprocity The ability for an EMS professional to use his or her certification or license to be able to practice in a different state.

Recompression A method used to treat divers with certain diving disorders, such as decompression sickness.

Rectal The drug administration route for suppositories; the drug is placed into the rectum (colon) and is absorbed into the venous circulation.

Rectum End of the sigmoid colon; feces are further compacted into waste here.

Reentry Spread of an impulse through tissue already stimulated by that same impulse.

Referred pain Pain felt at a site distant to the organ of origin.

Reflection Echoing the patient's message using your own words.

Reflection on actions A final step that may involve a personal reflection or a run critique; in certain instances this may be done formally, but in most instances it is accomplished informally.

Refractoriness Period of recovery that cells need after being discharged before they are able to respond to a stimulus.

Refresher education The process of refreshing information and skills previously learned.

Registration The process of entering an individual's name and essential information into a record as a means of verifying initial certification and monitoring recertification.

Regurgitation Backward flow of blood through a valve during ventricular contraction of the heart.

Rejection In terms of organ transplantation, the process by which the body uses its immune system to identify a transplanted organ and kill it; the medical management of posttransplant patients is largely directed at preventing rejection.

Relative refractory period Corresponds with the downslope of the T wave; cardiac cells can be stimulated to depolarize if the stimulus is strong enough.

Relief medic Emergency medical technician who has obtained additional training and certification in disaster and relief medical operations.

Rem Roentgen equivalent man.

Renal calculi Kidney stones formed by substances such as calcium, uric acid, or cystine.

Renal corpuscle Large terminal end of the nephron.

Renal insufficiency A decrease in renal function to approximately 25% of normal.

Renal pyramids Number of divisions in the kidney.

Repeater A system that receives transmissions from a low-wattage radio and rebroadcasts the signal at a higher wattage to the dispatch center.

Reperfusion phenomenon Series of events that result from the reperfusion of tissue damaged in a crush injury or tissue that is profoundly hypoxic; can lead to crush syndrome (rhabdomyolysis).

Repolarization Movement of ions across a cell membrane in which the inside of the cell is restored to its negative charge.

Res ipsa loquitur Latin phrase meaning "the thing speaks for itself." In negligence cases, this doctrine can be imposed when the plaintiff cannot prove all four components of negligence, but the injury itself would not have occurred without negligence (e.g., a sponge left in a patient after surgery).

Rescue The act of delivery from danger or entrapment.

Residual volume After a maximal forced exhalation, the amount of air remaining in the lungs and airway passages not able to be expelled.

Resistance The amount of weight moved or lifted during isotonic exercise. Also the ability of the body to defend itself against disease-causing microorganisms.

Resistance stage The stage of the stress response in which the specific stimulus no longer elicits an alarm reaction.

Respiration The exchange of gases between a living organism and its environment.

respiratory arrest Absence of breathing.

respiratory distress Increased work of breathing (respiratory effort).

Respiratory failure Failure of the ventilation system of the body to provide sufficient oxygen to the body; does not require apnea.

Respiratory membrane Where gas exchange takes place; oxygen is picked up in the bloodstream and carbon dioxide is eliminated through the lungs.

Respiratory syncytial virus A virus linked to bronchiolitis in infants and children.

Respiratory tract Passages to move air to and from the exchange surfaces.

Respondeat superior Latin phrase meaning "let the master answer." Under this legal doctrine, an employer is liable for the acts of employees within their scope of employment.

Response area The geographic area assigned to an emergency vehicle for responding to the sick and injured.

Response assignment plan An approved, consistent plan for responding to each call type.

Response mode A type of response, either with or without lights and sirens use.

Response time The time from when the call is received until the paramedics arrive at the scene.

Restraint Any mechanism that physically restricts an individual's freedom of movement, physical activity, or normal access to his or her body.

Restraint asphyxia Suffocation of a patient stemming from an inability to expand the chest cavity during inspiration because of restraint and immobilization.

Reticular activating system Group of specialized neurons in the brainstem; involved in sleep and wake cycles; maintains consciousness.

Reticular cells The cells forming the reticular fibers of connective tissue; those forming the framework of lymph nodes, bone marrow, and spleen are part of the reticuloendothelial system and under appropriate stimulation may differentiate into macrophages.

Reticular dermis Section of the dermis composed of larger and denser collagen fibers; provides most of the skin's elasticity and strength. This layer contains most of the skin structures located within the dermis.

Reticular formation A cloud of neurons in the brainstem and midbrain responsible for maintaining consciousness.

Retina Outer pigmented area and inner sensory layer that responds to light.

Retinal detachment A condition in which the retina is lifted or pulled from its normal position, resulting in a loss of vision.

Retractions Sinking in of the soft tissues above the sternum or clavicle or between or below the ribs during inhalation.

Retreat Leaving the scene when danger is observed or when violence or indicators of violence are displayed; requires immediate and decisive action.

Retrograde Moving backward or moving in the opposite direction to that which is considered normal.

Retrograde amnesia The inability to remember events or recall memories from before an event in which the head was struck.

Retroperitoneal Abdominopelvic organs found behind the peritoneum.

Retrospective medical direction Physician review of prehospital care reports and participation in the quality improvement process; a type of offline medical direction.

Reuptake Absorption of neurotransmitters from the synapse into the presynaptic neuron to be reused or destroyed.

Review of systems A review of symptoms for each organ system.

Rhabdomyolysis Complex series of events that occur in patients with severe muscle injury (e.g., crush injuries); destruction of the muscle tissues results in a release of cellular material and acidosis that can lead to acute renal failure.

Rheumatoid arthritis A painful, disabling disease in which the body's immune system attacks the joints.

Rhinitis Runny nose; inflammation of the mucous membranes of the nose, usually accompanied by swelling of the mucosa and a nasal discharge.

Rhinorrhea Persistent discharge of fluid (such as blood or cerebrospinal fluid) from the nose.

Rhonchi Rattling or rumbling in the lungs.

Ribonucleic acid (RNA) Specialized structures within the cell that carry genetic material for reproduction.

Ribosome Substance in organelle where new protein is synthesized; forms the framework for the genetic blueprint.

Right A position toward the right side of the body.

Right block or left block Terms describing a responding vehicle arriving on scene and turning at a right or left angle. In this block position, the emergency vehicle acts as a physical barrier between the crash scene work area and approaching traffic.

Right coronary artery Blood vessel that provides oxygenated blood to the right side of the heart muscle.

Risk factors Traits and lifestyle habits that may increase a person's chance of developing a disease.

Risus sardonicus Distorted grinning expression caused by involuntary contraction of the facial muscles.

Roentgens Denote ionizing radiation passing through air.

Rolling the dash Rescue tasks involving strategic cuts to the firewall structure followed by pushing, spreading, or even pulling equipment to move the dash, firewall, steering wheel, column, and pedals away from front seat occupants.

Rollover protective structure A structure mounted on a tractor designed to support the weight of the tractor if an overturn occurs; if a tractor has this structure and the operator wears a seat belt, the operator will stay in the safety zone if the tractor overturns.

Root word In medical terminology, the part of the word that gives the primary meaning.

Rotor-wing aircraft Helicopter that can be used for hospital-to-hospital and scene-to-hospital transports;

usually travels a shorter distance and is used in the prehospital setting for certain types of transport.

Routes of administration Various methods of giving drugs, including oral, enteral, parenteral, and inhalational.

Rovsing's sign Palpation of the abdomen in the left lower quadrant elicits pain in the right lower quadrant.

S1 The sound of the bicuspid and mitral valves closing.

S2 The sound of the closing of the pulmonary and aortic valves.

Sacrum (sacral vertebrae) A heavy, large bone at the base of the spinal cord between the lumbar vertebrae and the coccyx. Roughly triangular in shape, it comprises the back of the pelvis and is made of the five sacral vertebrae fused together.

Safety officer The person responsible for ensuring that no unsafe acts occur during the emergency incident.

Sagittal plane Imaginary straight line that runs vertically through the middle of the body, creating right and left halves.

Saliva Mucus that lubricates material like food that is placed in it; enzymes begin the digestive process of starchy material.

Salivary glands Located in the oral cavity; produce saliva.

Saponification A form of necrosis in which fatty acids combine with certain electrolytes to form soaps.

Sarin A nerve agent.

Saturation of peripheral oxygen The percentage of hemoglobin saturated with oxygen (SpO_2).

Scabies A contagious skin disease of the epidermis marked by itching and small raised red spots caused by the itch mite *(Sarcoptes scabiei)*.

Scale Thick stratum corneum that results from hyperproliferation or increased cohesion of keratinocytes (can include eczema or psoriasis).

Scar A collection of new connective tissue; may be hypertrophic or atrophic and implies dermoepidermal damage.

Schizophrenia A group of disorders characterized by psychotic symptoms, thought disorder, and negative symptoms (social isolation and withdrawal); types include paranoid, disorganized, and catatonic.

Sciatica Pain in the lumbar back and leg caused by irritation and impingement of the sciatic nerve, usually from a herniated disc.

Sclera Firm, opaque, white outer layer of the eye; helps maintain the shape of the eye.

Scope of practice A predefined set of skills, interventions, or other activities that the paramedic is legally authorized to perform when necessary; usually set by state law or regulation and local medical direction.

Scrotum Loose layer of connective tissue that support the testes.

Sebaceous glands Found in the dermis; secrete oil (sebum) in the shaft of the hair follicle and the skin.

Sebum Oil secreted by the sebaceous glands in the shaft of the hair follicle and the skin; prevents excessive drying of the skin and hair; also protects from some forms of bacteria.

Second messenger A molecule that relays signals from a receptor on the surface of a cell to target molecules in the cell's nucleus or internal fluid where a physiologic action is to take place; also called a *biochemical messenger.*

Secondary apnea When asphyxia is prolonged, a period of deep, gasping respirations with a simultaneous fall in blood pressure and heart rate; gasping becomes weaker and slower and then ceases.

Secondary blast injury Injuries caused by shrapnel from the fragments of an explosive device and from things that have been attached to it.

Secondary contamination The risk of another person or health care provider becoming contaminated with a hazardous material by contact with a contaminated victim.

Secondary cord injury A spinal cord injury that develops over time after a traumatic injury to the spinal column or the blood vessels that supply the spinal cord with blood. Generally caused by ischemia, swelling, or compression.

Secondary device An explosive, chemical, or biologic device hidden at the scene of an emergency and set to detonate or release its agent after emergency response personnel are on scene.

Secondary hypertension High blood pressure that has an identifiable cause, such as medications or an underlying disease or condition.

Secondary injury prevention Preventing further injury from an event that has already occurred.

Secondary skin lesion Any lesion that has been altered by scratching, scrubbing, or other types of trauma.

Secondary triage Conducted after the primary search; determines the order of treatment and transport of the remaining patients.

Secondary tumor A tumor that has spread from its original location (e.g., lung tumor that spreads to brain); also called *metastasis.*

Secretion Release of water, acids, enzymes, and buffers that aid in the breakdown and digestion of food in the digestive tract.

Secretory phase Portion of the menstrual cycle in which the corpus luteum secretes progesterone to maintain the endometrial lining in case of fertilization.

Sedative-hypnotics Prescription central nervous system depressant drugs that cause powerful relaxation and euphoria when abused; typically barbiturates and benzodiazepines.

Segment Line between waveforms; named by the waveform that precedes and follows it.

Seizure A temporary alteration in behavior or consciousness caused by abnormal electrical activity of one or more groups of neurons in the brain.

Self-injury An unhealthy coping mechanism involving intentionally injuring one's own body, often through cutting or burning oneself to relieve emotional tension; also known as *self-mutilation.*

312

Sellick maneuver Technique used to compress the cricoid cartilage against the cervical vertebrae, causing occlusion of the esophagus, thereby reducing the risk of aspiration; cricoid pressure.

Semicircular canals Three bony fluid-filled loops in the internal ear; involved in balance of the body.

Semilunar (SL) valves Valves shaped like half moons that separate the ventricles from the aorta and pulmonary artery.

Seminal fluid Liquid produced in the seminal vesicles.

Seminal vesicles Ducts that produce seminal fluids.

Sensing Ability of a pacemaker to recognize and respond to intrinsic electrical activity.

Sensorineural hearing loss A type of deafness that occurs when the tiny hair cells in the cochlea are damaged or destroyed. In addition, damage to the auditory nerve prevents sounds from being transmitted from the cochlea to the brain.

Sensory cortex Area of brain tissue on the frontal lobe responsible for receiving sensory information from different parts of the body.

Sepsis Pathologic state, usually accompanied by fever, resulting from the presence of microorganisms or their poisonous products in the bloodstream; commonly called *blood poisoning.*

Septic abortion An abortion associated with intrauterine infection.

Septic arthritis Invasion of microorganisms into a joint space, causing infection of the joint.

Septic shock Sepsis with hypotension, despite adequate fluid resuscitation, along with the presence of perfusion abnormalities that may include lactic acidosis, decreased urine output, and a sudden change in mental status.

Septicemia A serious medical condition characterized by vasodilation that leads to hypotension, tissue hypoxia, and eventually shock; usually caused by gram-negative bacteria; diagnosed by blood tests called cultures.

Septum Tough piece of tissue that divides the left and right halves of the heart.

Serious apnea Cessation of breathing for longer than 20 seconds or any duration if accompanied by cyanosis and sinus bradycardia.

Serosanguineous discharge Blood and fluid discharged from the body.

Serous membrane Membrane that lines the thoracic, abdominal, and pelvic cavities; composed of the parietal membrane, which adheres to the cavity wall, and the visceral membrane, which adheres to the organ.

Serum base deficit Implies that the blood buffer, bicarbonate, is being used to combat a metabolic acidosis. Metabolic acidosis occurs in the setting of numerous shock states, such as burn shock. This number is reported on a standard blood gas assay and is detected in an arterial or venous blood sample.

Serum lactate Measure in the blood; a byproduct of anaerobic metabolism. As such, it is a good measure of end organ and cellular perfusion in shock states. Elevated serum lactate levels, or lactic acidemia, implies that cells, tissues, or organs are not receiving adequate oxygen to carry out their metabolic activities.

Sesamoid bones Specialized bones found within tendons where they cross a joint; designed to protect the joint (e.g., the patella [kneecap]).

Severe sepsis Sepsis associated with organ dysfunction, shock, or hypotension.

Sexual abuse Forced and/or coerced sex, violent sexual acts against the victim's will (rape), or withholding sex from the victim; includes fondling, intercourse, incest, rape, sodomy, exhibitionism, sexual exploitation, or exposure to pornography. According to the National Center on Child Abuse and Neglect, to be considered child abuse these acts must be committed by a person responsible for the care of a child (e.g., a babysitter, parent, or daycare provider) or related to the child. If a stranger commits these acts, it is considered sexual assault and handled solely by the police and criminal courts.

Sexual assault Sexually explicit conduct used as an expression of interpersonal violence against another individual; nonconsenting sexual acts achieved through power and control.

Shaft The length of a needle; the needle shaft connects to the hub. Also called the *cannula.*

Shear points Hazardous machinery locations created when the edges of two objects are moved toward or next to one another closely enough to cut a relatively soft material.

Shingles Infection of a nerve, often by the herpes zoster virus, causing severe pain and a rash along a unilateral dermatome.

Shock Inadequate systemic perfusion.

Short bones Specialized bones of the skeleton designed for compactness and strength, often with limited movement (e.g., bones of the wrist [carpals])

Short haul The transport of one or more people externally suspended below a helicopter.

Shoulder dystocia Impaction of a newborn's anterior shoulder underneath the mother's pubic bone, slowing or preventing delivery.

Shunt Insertion of catheters into an artery and a vein from outside the body. Most shunts are located on the forearm. When not in use to dialyze a patient, the catheters are connected to each other with clear tubing, allowing the continuous flow of blood from artery to vein, then covered with self-adhering roller gauze for protection.

Side effect An effect of a drug other than the one for which it was given; may or may not be harmful.

Side impact airbags Deployable airbags located inside any or all vehicle doors, front and rear outboard seatbacks, as well as along all or a portion of the roof line.

Sighing Involuntary and periodic slow, deep breath followed by a prolonged expiratory phase. Occurring approximately once per minute, the act of sighing is thought to open atelectatic (collapsed) alveoli.

Sigmoid colon Part of the large intestine.

Signs and symptoms Signs are a medical or trauma condition of the patient that can be seen, heard, smelled, measured, or felt during an examination. Symptoms are conditions described by the patient, such as shortness of breath, or pieces of information bystanders tell you about the patient's chief complaint.

Silo gas The gases produced from the fermentation of plant material inside a silo.

Simple asphyxiants Inert gases and vapors that displace oxygen in inspired air (e.g., carbon dioxide, nitrogen).

Simple partial seizure A seizure affecting only one part of the brain without an alteration in consciousness.

Simple pneumothorax Injury to the thoracic cavity in which a lung is ruptured, allowing air into the space between the chest wall and the lungs.

Simplex A system that allows only one-at-a-time communication. The transmission cannot be interrupted; both operators use the same frequency.

Singular command Command type involving one agency.

Sinoatrial node Pacemaker site of the heart; where impulse formation begins in the heart.

Sinus block (barosinusitis) A condition of acute or chronic inflammation of one or more of the paranasal sinuses; produced by a negative pressure difference between the air in the sinuses and the surrounding atmospheric air.

Sinus rhythm A normal heart rhythm.

Sinuses Cavities within the bones of the skull that connect to the nasal cavity.

Situational awareness The state of being aware of everything occurring in the surrounding environment and the relative importance of all these events.

Size-up The art of assessing conditions that exist or can potentially exist at an incident scene.

Skeletal muscles Muscles that affect movement of the skeleton, usually by voluntary contractions.

Skin grafting Transplantation of skin, either from the same person or from a cadaver, to the site of a wound, such as a burn.

Skin turgor The elasticity of the skin; good skin turgor returns the skin's natural shape within 2 seconds.

Slander False statements spoken about a person that blacken the person's character or injure his or her reputation.

Slipped capital femoral epiphysis A disease in which a posterior displacement of the growth plate of the femur occurs (the epiphysis).

SLUDGEM Mnemonic for *s*alivation, *l*acrimation, *u*rination, *d*efecation, *g*astrointestinal pain, *e*mesis, and *m*iosis.

Smallpox A disease caused by variola viruses, which are members of the Orthopoxvirus family; eradicated in the 1970s but still remains a threat as a bioterrorism agent.

Sneezing Occurs from nasal irritation and allows clearance of the nose.

Sniffing position Neck flexion at the fifth and sixth cervical vertebrae, with the head extended at the first and second cervical vertebrae. This position aligns the axes of the mouth, pharynx, and trachea, opening the airway and increasing airflow.

Snoring Noisy breathing through the mouth and nose during sleep; caused by air passing through a narrowed upper airway.

Social distance The acceptable distance between strangers used for impersonal business transactions. In the United States, social distance is 4 to 12 feet.

Sodium bicarbonate Neutralizes hydrochloric acid from the stomach.

Solid organ An organ (a part of the body or group of tissues that performs a specific function) without any channel or cavity within it; examples include the kidneys, pancreas, liver, and spleen.

Solubility Pertaining to the ease with which a drug can dissolve.

Solution A medication dissolved in a liquid, often water.

Soman A G nerve agent. The G agents tend to be nonpersistent, volatile agents.

Somatic Portion of the peripheral nervous system that carries impulses to and from the skin and musculature; responsible for voluntary muscle control.

Somatic delusions False perceptions of the appearance or functioning of one's own body.

Somatic nervous system Division of the peripheral nervous system whose motor nerves control movement of voluntary muscles.

Somatic pain Pain that arises from either the cutaneous tissues of the body's surface or deep tissues of the body, such as musculoskeletal tissue or the parietal peritoneum.

Somatoform disorders A group of disorders characterized by the manifestation of psychological problems as physical symptoms; this includes conversion disorder, hypochondriasis, somatization disorder, and body dysmorphic disorder.

Sore throat Any inflammation of the larynx, pharynx, or tonsils.

Space blanket A blanket resembling aluminum foil used to help the patient maintain body temperature.

Space-occupying lesion A mass, such as a tumor or blood collection, within a contained body space, such as the skull.

Spacer A hollow plastic tube that attaches to the metered-dose inhaler on one end and has a mouthpiece on the other; sometimes called a *holding chamber*.

Span of control The amount of resources that one person can effectively manage.

Special needs Conditions with the potential to interfere with usual growth and development; may involve physical disabilities, developmental disabilities, chronic illnesses, and forms of technologic support.

Specialty center A hospital that has met criteria to offer special care as a burn center, level I trauma center, stroke center, or pediatric center.

Specific gravity The ratio of a liquid's weight compared with an equal volume of water (which has a constant value of 1); materials with a specific gravity of less than 1.0 float on water and materials with a specific gravity greater than 1.0 sink.

Sperm Mucus-type secretion made of prostatic fluid and spermatozoa.

Spermatic cord Nerves, blood vessels, and smooth muscle that surround the vas (ductus) deferens.

Spermatocele Benign accumulation of sperm at the epididymis presenting as a firm mass.

Spermatogenesis Spermatozoa formation.

Spermatozoa Product of the male reproductive system.

Sphincters Smooth muscles that regulate flow through the capillary beds.

Spina bifida Malformation of the meninges and spinal cord in utero, often leading to permanent physical disabilities.

Spina bifida occulta Mildest form of spina bifida in which the spinal cord is intact but one or more vertebrae fail to close in the lumbosacral area.

Spinal cord Part of the central nervous system that connects the brain to the periphery of the body; contains the main reflex centers of the body.

Spinal cord injury (SCI) An injury to the spinal cord that results from trauma; usually a permanent injury.

Spinal cord injury without radiological abnormality A spinal cord injury not detected on a standard radiograph.

Spinal nerves Paired nerves that originate from the spinal cord and exit the spine on either side between vertebrae; each has a sensory root and a motor root.

Spinal shock Shock with hypotension caused by an injury to the spinal cord.

Spirit A medication that contains volatile aromatic substances.

Split-thickness skin graft A skin graft in which only a fraction of the thickness of the natural dermis is taken.

Spontaneous abortion See *Miscarriage*.

Spontaneous bacterial peritonitis (SBP) Infection of cirrhotic fluid in the abdominal cavity.

Spontaneous pneumothorax Pneumothorax occurring without trauma, usually by rupture of a pulmonary bleb.

Sprain An injury to a ligament that results when the ligament is overstretched, leading to tearing or complete disruption of the ligament.

Stagnant phase Vascular response in shock when precapillary sphincters open, allowing the capillary beds to engorge with fluid; follows the ischemic phase.

Stair chair A collapsible, portable chair with handles on the front and back used to carry patients in sitting position down stairs.

Standard of care Conduct exercising the degree of care, skill, and judgment that would be expected under like or similar circumstances by a similarly trained, reasonable paramedic in the same scenario.

Standard operating procedures (SOPs) An organized set of guidelines distributed across the organization.

Standing orders Written instructions that authorize EMS personnel to perform certain medical interventions before establishing direct communication with a physician.

Standard precautions Infection control practices in healthcare designed to be observed with every patient and procedure and prevent the exposure to bloodborne pathogens.

Stapes The stirrup-shaped bone that links the middle ear to the inner ear; connects to the malleus and incus.

Status asthmaticus Condition of severe asthma that is minimally responsive to therapy; a serious condition.

Status epilepticus A single seizure lasting longer than 30 minutes or repeated seizures without full recovery of responsiveness between seizures and lasting longer than 30 minutes.

Statute A law passed by a legislature.

Statute of limitations A law that sets the time limits within which parties must take action to enforce their rights.

Statutory law Statutes and ordinances enacted by Congress, state legislatures, and city councils.

Steady state An evenly distributed concentration of a drug in the plasma.

Stellate laceration A laceration with jagged margins.

Stem cells Formative cells whose daughter cells may give rise to other cell types.

Stenosis Abnormal constriction or narrowing of a structure.

Stereotyping The attribution of some trait or characteristic to one person on the basis of the interviewer's preconceived notions about a general class of people of similar characteristics.

Sterile Free of any living organism.

Sterilization Process that makes an object free of all forms of life (e.g., bacteria) by using extreme heat or certain chemicals.

Sterilize To kill all microorganisms.

Stimuli Anything that excites or incites an organism or part to function, become active, or respond.

Stomach Organ located at the inferior end of the esophagus; large storage vessel surrounded by multiple layers of smooth muscle; cells within it produce acid.

Stored energy Any energy (mechanical, electrical, hydraulic, compressed air, etc.) that has the potential of being released either intentionally or inadvertently, causing further injury or problems.

Strain An injury to a muscle that results when the muscle is overstretched, leading to tearing of the individual muscle fibers.

Strainer A water hazard formed by an object or structure in the current that allows water to flow but that strains out large objects, such as boats and people.

Strangulation Compression of the vessels that carry blood, leading to ischemia.

Stratum corneum Outer layer of the epidermis where skin cells are shed.

Stress Mental, emotional, or physical pressure, strain, or tension resulting from stimuli.

Stressor A stimulus that produces stress.

315

Stricture A specific form of narrowing, usually from scar tissue formation.

Stridor A harsh, high-pitched sound heard on inspiration associated with upper airway obstruction; often described as a high-pitched crowing or "seal-bark" sound.

Stroke volume Amount of blood ejected by either ventricle during one contraction; can be calculated as cardiac output divided by heart rate.

Struck-by A situation in which a responder, working in or near moving traffic, is struck, injured, or killed by traffic passing the incident scene.

Stye An external hordeolum.

Stylet A relatively stiff but flexible metal rod covered by plastic and inserted into an endotracheal tube; used for maintaining the shape of the relatively pliant tube and "steering" it into position.

Subarachnoid hemorrhage Bleeding from the arteries between the arachnoid membrane and the pia mater that occurs suddenly and often is fatal.

Subcutaneous (Sub-Q) Injection of medication in a liquid form underneath the skin into the subcutaneous tissue.

Subcutaneous emphysema Air entrapped beneath the skin, typically caused by rupture of a structure containing air; feels like crackling when palpated.

Subcutaneous tissue Thick layer of connective tissue found between the layers of the skin; composed of adipose tissue and areolar tissue; insulates, protects, and stores energy (in the form of fat).

Subdural hematoma A collection of blood in the subdural space, which is between the dura mater and arachnoid layer of the meninges.

Subdural space Area below the dura mater; contains large venous vessels, drains, and a small amount of serous fluid.

Subjective information Information told to the paramedic.

Sublingual Medication placed under the tongue.

Sucking chest wound Open thoracic injury characterized by air being pulled into and pushed out of the wound during respiration.

Sudden cardiac death (SCD) An unexpected death from a cardiac cause that either occurs immediately or within 1 hour of the onset of symptoms.

Suffix Added to the end of a root word to change the meaning; usually identifies the condition of the root word.

Suicide The act of ending one's own life.

Sulfur mustard The most well known and commonly used of the vesicants.

Summarization Briefly reviewing the interview and your conclusions.

Summation The combined effects of two or more drugs equaling the sum of each of their effects.

Superficial burn A burn with a pink appearance that does not exhibit blister formation; painful both with and without tactile stimulation (e.g., sunburn); also known as a *first-degree burn.*

Superficial fascia Connective tissue that contains the subcutaneous fat cells.

Superficial partial-thickness burn Burns involving the more superficial dermis. These burns have a moist, pink appearance, and when lightly touched, are painful and sensate. Blood vessels, hair shafts, nerves, and glands may be injured, but not to the extent that regeneration cannot take place.

Superior Situated above or higher than a point of reference in the anatomic position; top.

Superior vena cava Vessel that returns venous blood from the upper part of the body to the right atrium of the heart.

Supernormal period Period during the cardiac cycle when a weaker than normal stimulus can cause cardiac cells to depolarize; extends from the end of phase 3 to the beginning of phase 4 of the cardiac action potential.

Supine Position in which the patient is lying on his or her back (face up).

Supine hypotensive syndrome A fall in the pregnant patient's blood pressure when she is placed supine; caused by the developing fetus and uterus pressing against the inferior vena cava.

Suppository Medications combined to make them a solid at room temperature; when placed in a body opening such as the rectum, vagina, or urethra, they dissolve because of the increase in body temperature and are absorbed through the surrounding mucosa.

Supraglottic Any airway structure above the vocal cords (e.g., the epiglottis).

Suprasternal notch A depression easily felt at the base of the anterior aspect of the neck, just above the angle of Louis.

Supraventricular Originating from a site above the bifurcation of the bundle of His, such as the sinoatrial node, atria, or atrioventricular junction.

Supraventricular dysrhythmias Rhythms that begin in the sinoatrial node, atrial tissue, or the atrioventricular junction.

Surfactant Specialized cells within each alveolus that keep it from collapsing when little or no air is inside.

Surge capacity The ability to expand care based on a sudden mass casualty incident developed in the emergency management plan.

Susceptibility Vulnerability or weakness; the opposite of resistance.

Suspension Medication suspended in a liquid, such as an oral antibiotic.

Sutures Seams between flat bones.

Sweat glands Odor-forming glands in the body; two types are merocrine and apocrine.

Swimmer's ear See *Otitis externa.*

Sympathetic division of the autonomic nervous system Division of the autonomic nervous system that, when stimulated, provides a fight-or-flight response, including increased heart rate, pupil dilation, bronchodilation, and the shunting of blood to the muscles.

Sympathetic nervous system Division of the autonomic nervous system that prepares the body for stress or the classic fight-or-flight response.

Sympatholytics Drugs that block or inhibit adrenergic receptors.

Sympathomimetics Drugs that mimic the sympathetic division of the autonomic nervous system.

Sympathy Sharing the patient's feelings or emotional state in relation to an illness.

Symphysis Cartilaginous joint; unites two bones by means of fibrocartilage.

Synapse Microscopic space at the neuroeffector junction that neurotransmitters cross to stimulate target tissues.

Synaptic communication Method of intercellular communication in which neural cells communicate to adjacent neural cells by using neurotransmitters.

Synaptic junction The open space in which neurotransmitters traverse to reach a receptor.

Synchondroses Cartilaginous joint; unites the bones by means of hyaline cartilage.

Synchronized intermittent mandatory ventilation (SIMV) A ventilator setting.

Syncope A brief loss of consciousness caused by a temporary decrease in blood flow to the brain.

Syndesmosis Joint in which the bones are united by fibrous, connective tissue forming an intraosseous membrane or ligament.

Synergism The interaction of drugs such that the total effect is greater than the sum of the individual effects.

Synonym A root word, prefix, or suffix that has the same or almost the same meaning as another word, prefix, or suffix.

Synovial fluid Fluid located within the joint capsules of synovial joints; provides lubrication and cushioning during manipulation of the joint.

Synovial joint Freely movable; enclosed by a capsule and synovial membrane.

Synovium Soft tissue that lines the noncartilaginous surfaces of a joint.

Synthetic drugs Drugs chemically developed in a laboratory; also called *manufactured drugs.*

Syrup A medication dissolved in water with sugar or a sugar substitute to disguise taste.

System At least two kinds of organs organized to perform a more complex task than can a single organ.

System Status Management The dynamic process of staffing, stationing, and moving ambulances based on projected call volumes; also called *flexible deployment.*

Systemic damage Damage remote to the site of exposure or absorption.

Systemic effect Drug action throughout the body.

Systemic inflammatory response syndrome A response to infection manifested by a change in two or more of the following: temperature, heart rate, respiratory rate, and white blood cell count.

Systole Contraction of the heart (usually referring to ventricular contraction) during which blood is propelled into the pulmonary artery and aorta; when the term is used without reference to a specific chamber of the heart, the term implies ventricular systole.

Systolic blood pressure The pressure exerted against the walls of the large arteries at the peak of ventricular contraction.

T lymphocytes Cells present in the lymphatic system that mediate cell-mediated immunity (also known as *T cells*).

Tablets Medications that have been pressed into a small form that is easy to swallow. They are a specific shape, color, and may have engraving for identification.

Tachycardia A heart rate grater than 100 beats/min.

Tachyphylaxis The rapidly decreasing response to a drug or physiologically active agent after administration of a few doses; rapid cross-tolerance.

Tachypnea A respiratory rate persistently faster than normal for age; in adults, a rate faster than 20 breaths/min.

Tactical EMS EMS personnel specially trained and equipped to provide prehospital emergency care in tactical environments.

Tactical patient care Patient care activities that occur inside the scene perimeter or hot zone.

Tangential thinking A progression of thoughts related to each other but that become less and less related to the original topic.

Tardive dyskinesia A neurologic syndrome caused by the long-term or high-dose use of dopamine antagonists, usually antipsychotic medications, characterized by repetitive, involuntary, and purposeless movements. The patient may appear to be grimacing. Rapid movements of the face, tongue, and extremities occur. Lip smacking, puckering, and rapid eye blinking may also be seen. No standard treatment is available. Symptoms may last for a significant period after removal of the offending agent.

Teachable moment The time just after an injury has occurred when the patient and observers remain acutely aware of what has happened and may be more receptive to learning how the event or illness could have been prevented.

Teamwork The ability to work with others to achieve a common goal.

Teeth Provide mastication of food products in preparation for entry into the stomach.

Telemetric A system set up as mayday call reporting, such as On-Star and Tele-aid. This system can send information from an automobile that has been involved in an accident directly to an emergency dispatch center with the exact location and the amount of damage that may have occurred.

Telephone aid Ad-libbed instructions most often used in emergency dispatch centers by dispatchers who have had previous training as paramedics, EMTs, or cardiopulmonary resuscitation providers; strictly relies on the dispatcher's experience and prior knowledge of a particular situation or medical condition and is considered an ineffective form of telephone treatment.

317

Telson Venom-containing portion of a scorpion's abdomen that is capable of venomous injection into human beings.

Temporal demand Measurement of call demand by hour of the day.

Temporal lobe Section of the cerebrum that receives and evaluates smell and auditory input; plays a key role in memories.

Temporal modeling Predicting the times when calls occur.

Tendonitis Inflammation of a tendon, often caused by overuse.

Tendons Tough, fibrous bands of connective tissue that connect muscle to muscle and muscle to bones.

Tension-building phase Period when tension in the relationship is high and heightened anger, blaming, and arguing may occur between the victim and the abuser.

Tension pneumothorax Life-threatening injury in which air enters the space between the lungs and the chest wall but cannot exit. With each breath, the pressure increases until it prevents ventilation and causes death.

Teratogen A drug or agent that is harmful to the development of an embryo or fetus.

Term gestation A gestation equal to or longer than 37 weeks.

Terminal drop A theory that holds that mental and physical functioning decline drastically only in the few years immediately preceding death.

Terminal illness Advanced stage of illness or disease with an unfavorable prognosis and no known cure.

Tertiary blast injury Injuries caused by the patient being thrown like a projectile.

Testes Male reproductive organs suspended within the scrotum.

Testicular torsion Twisting of the spermatic cord inside the scrotum that cuts off the blood supply to the testis.

Testosterone Male hormone secreted within the testes.

Tetany Repeated, prolonged contraction of muscles, especially of the face and limbs.

Tetraplegia Paralysis to all four extremities as a result of a spinal cord injury high in the spine. The injury can either be complete (a complete loss of muscle control and sensation below the injury site) or incomplete (a partial loss of muscle control or sensation below the injury site).

Thalamus Structure located within the limbic system that is the switchboard of the brain, through which almost all signals travel on their way in or out of the brain.

Therapeutic abortion Planned surgical or medical evacuation of the uterus.

Therapeutic dose The dose required to produce a beneficial effect in 50% of the drug-tested population; also called *effective dose.*

Therapeutic index The ratio between the amount of drug required to produce a therapeutic dose and a lethal dose of the same drug. A narrow therapeutic index is dangerous because the possibility of underdosing or overdosing is higher.

Therapeutic threshold The level of a drug that elicits a beneficial physiologic response.

Thermogenesis The process of heat generation.

Thermolysis A chemical process by which heat is dissipated from the body; sometimes results in chemical decomposition.

Thermoreceptor A sensory receptor that responds to heat and cold.

Third space Extravascular and extracellular milieu; also known as the *interstitium.*

Thirst mechanism Sensation activated by cells in the hypothalamus when cells called osmoreceptors detect an imbalance in body water; as the body is replenished by drinking fluid, the osmoreceptors sense a return to baseline and turn off this mechanism.

Thoracic vertebrae A group of 12 vertebrae in the middle of the spinal column that connect to ribs.

Thought blocking A symptom of thought disorder in which a patient is speaking and then stops mid-sentence, unable to remember what he or she was saying and unable to continue.

Thought content The dominant themes and ideas of a patient; may include delusions, hallucinations, and preoccupations.

Threatened abortion Vaginal bleeding or uterine cramping during the first half of pregnancy without cervical dilation.

Threshold limit value The airborne concentrations of a substance; represents conditions under which nearly all workers are believed to be repeatedly exposed day after day without adverse effects.

Thrombocytes One of three formed elements in the blood; also known as *platelets.*

Thrombocytopenia A lower than normal number of platelets circulating in the blood.

Thromboembolism Movement of a clot within the vascular system.

Thrombophlebitis Development of a clot in a vein in which inflammation is present.

Thromboplastin Blood coagulation factor.

Thrombus Blood clot.

Thrush A fungal infection of the mouth.

Thyroid storm Severe form of hyperthyroidism characterized by tachypnea, tachycardia, shock, hyperthermia, and delirium.

Thyrotoxicosis A condition in which the thyroid gland produces excess thyroid hormone; also called *hyperthyroidism* or *Graves' disease.*

Tidal volume The volume of air moved into or out of the lungs during a normal breath; can be indirectly evaluated by observing the rise and fall of the patient's chest and abdomen.

Time on task The average time a unit is committed to manage an incident.

Tincture A medicine consisting of an extract in an alcohol solution (e.g., tincture of iodine, tincture of mercurochrome).

Tinea capitis Located on the head and scalp; appears as a round, scaly area where no hair is growing; diffuse scaling.

Tinea corporis Located on the body; appears annular (e.g. ringworm).

Tinea cruris Located on the groin and genitalia; appears as a sharply demarcated area with elevated scaling, geographic borders.

Tinea manuum Located on the hands; appears as dry, diffuse scaling, usually on the palm.

Tinea pedis Located on the feet; appears as maceration between the toes, scaling on soles or sides of the foot, sometimes vesicles and/or pustules.

Tinea unguium Located on or under fingernails or toenails; appears as dark debris under the nails.

Tinea versicolor Located on the trunk; appears as pink, tan, or white patches with fine, desquamating scale.

Tinnitus A ringing, roaring sound or hissing in the ears that is usually caused by certain medicines or exposure to loud noise.

Tissue A group of cells that are similar in structure and function.

Tocolytic A medication used to slow uterine contractions.

Tolerance Decreasing responsiveness to the effects of a drug; increasingly larger doses are necessary to achieve the effect originally obtained by a smaller dose.

Tongue Muscular organ that provides for the sensation of taste; also directs food material toward the esophagus.

Tonic-clonic seizure Form of generalized seizure with a tonic phase (muscle rigidity) and a clonic phase (muscle tremors).

Topical Medication administered by applying it directly to the skin or mucous membrane.

Tort A wrong committed on the person or property of another.

Total body surface area burned (TBSAB) Used to describe the amount of the body injured by a burn and expressed as a percentage of the entire body surface area.

Total body water (TBW) The total amount of fluid in the body at any given time.

Totally blind Description of someone who has no vision and uses nonvisual media or reads Braille.

Toxic organic dust syndrome A flulike illness caused by the inhalation of grain dust, with symptoms including fever, chest tightness, cough, and muscle aches; inhalation may occur in an agricultural setting or from covering a floor with straw.

Toxicology The study of poisons.

Toxidrome A classification system of toxic syndromes by signs and symptoms.

Toxin A poisonous substance of plant or animal origin.

TP segment Interval on the ECG between two successive PQRST complexes during which electrical activity of the heart is absent; begins with the end of the T wave through the onset of the following P wave and represents the period from the end of ventricular repolarization to the onset of atrial depolarization.

Trachea Air passage that connects the larynx to the lungs.

Tracheal stoma A surgical opening in the anterior neck that extends from the skin surface into the trachea, opening the trachea to the atmosphere.

Tracheitis Inflammation of the mucous membranes of the trachea.

Tracheostomy The surgical creation of an opening into the trachea.

Trade name The name given a chemical compound by the company that makes it; also called the *brand name* or *proprietary name.*

Transcellular compartment Compartment classified as extracellular but distinct because it is formed from the transport activities of cells; cerebrospinal fluid, bladder urine, the aqueous humor, and the synovial fluid of the joints are considered transcellular.

Transdermal Through the skin.

Transection A complete cutting (severing) across the spinal cord.

Transient ischemic attack (TIA) Neurologic dysfunction caused by a temporary blockage in blood flow; by definition the symptoms resolve within 24 hours but usually within 1 or 2 hours.

Transient synovitis A nonspecific inflammation of a joint, usually the hip, that affects the synovium and synovial fluid in children.

Transverse colon Part of the large intestine.

Transverse plane Imaginary straight line that divides the body into top (superior) and bottom (inferior) sections; also known as the *horizontal plane.*

Traumatic asphyxia Life-threatening injury in which the thorax is severely crushed, preventing ventilation; typically results in death.

Traumatic iritis An inflammation of the iris caused by blunt trauma to the eye.

Triage Classifying patients based on the severity of illness or injury.

Tricuspid valve Right atrioventricular valve of the heart.

Trigeminal neuralgia Irritation of the seventh cranial nerve (trigeminal nerve), causing episodes of severe, stabbing pain in the face.

Trip audit The review of a prehospital care report written by a paramedic to a peer or a third party.

Tripod position Position used to maintain an open airway that involves sitting upright and learning forward with the neck slightly extended, chin projected, and mouth open and supported by the arms.

Trismus Spasm of the muscles used for chewing, resulting in limited movement of the mouth because of pain.

Trunking system A system that uses multiple repeaters (five or more) so that the computer can search for an open channel to transmit by.

Tube trailers Trailers that carry multiple cylinders of pressurized gases.

Tuberculosis (TB) A highly contagious bacterial infection known for causing pneumonia and infecting other parts of the body.

Tularemia A disease resulting from infection of *Francisella tularensis;* normally transmitted through handling infected small mammals such as rabbits or rodents or through the bites of ticks, deerflies, or mosquitoes that have fed on infected animals; also known as *rabbit fever* or *deer fly fever*.

Tumor, benign A cancer that is not malignant (i.e., is not known for spreading and growing aggressively).

Tumor, malignant A cancer that is known for being aggressive and spreading to other parts of the body.

Tumor necrosis factor-alpha An inflammatory cytokine released in response to a variety of physical trauma, including burns. In burn injuries, massive quantities are produced by the liver; has been implicated as the causative agent in myocardial depression seen in burns.

Tumor, primary A tumor in the location where it originates (e.g., a primary lung tumor is in the lung).

Tumor, secondary A tumor that has spread from its original location (e.g., lung tumor that spreads to the brain); also called *metastasis*.

Tunica adventitia Outermost layer of the blood vessel; made of mainly elastic connective tissue; allows the vessel to expand to great pressure or volume.

Tunica intima Innermost layer of the blood vessel; composed of a single layer of epithelial cells; provides almost no resistance to blood flow.

Tunica media Middle layer of the blood vessel; mainly composed of smooth muscle; functions to alter the diameter of the lumen of the vessel and is under autonomic control, which enables the body to adjust blood flow quickly to meet immediate needs.

Tunics Layers of an elastic tissue and smooth muscle in the blood vessels.

Tunnel vision Focusing on or considering only one aspect of a situation without first taking into account all possibilities.

Turbinates Large folds found in the nasal cavity; highly vascular area in the nose that warms and humidifies inhaled air.

Turgor Normal tension of a cell or tissue.

Tympanic membrane A thin, translucent, pearly gray oval disk that protects the middle and conducts sound vibrations; eardrum.

Type and crossmatch Mixing a sample of a recipient's and donor's blood to evaluate for incompatibility.

Type I ambulance Regular truck cab and frame with a modular ambulance box mounted on the back.

Type II ambulance Van-style ambulance.

Type III ambulance A van chassis with a modified modular back.

Type IV (quaternary) blast injuries All other miscellaneous injuries caused by an explosive device.

Ulcer A full-thickness crater that involves the dermis and epidermis, with loss of the surface epithelium; this lesion is depressed and may bleed; it usually heals with scarring.

Umbilical An administration route that may be used on a newborn infant; because the umbilical cord was the primary source of nutrient and waster exchange, it provides an immediate source of drug exchange.

Umbilical cord The cord, containing two arteries and a vein, that connects the fetus to the placenta.

Umbilical cord prolapse Appearance of the umbilical cord in front of the presenting part, usually with compression of the cord and interruption of blood supply to the fetus.

Umbilical vein route Route of administration that achieves access through the one umbilical vein set between the two umbilical arteries.

Unethical Conduct that does not conform to moral standards of social or professional behavior.

Unified command Command type involving multiple agencies.

Unintentional injury Injuries and deaths not self-inflicted or perpetrated by another person (accidents).

Unintentional tort A wrong that the defendant did not mean to commit; a case in which a bad outcome occurred because of the failure to exercise reasonable care.

Unipolar lead Lead that consists of a single positive electrode and a reference point; a pacing lead with a single electrical pole at the distal tip of the pacing lead (negative pole) through which the stimulating pulse is delivered. In a permanent pacemaker with a unipolar lead, the positive pole is the pulse generator case.

Unit hour utilization (UhU) A measure of ambulance service productivity and staff workload.

United Nations (UN) number The four-digit number assigned to chemicals during transit by the U.S. Department of Transportation; the *2004 Emergency Guidebook* lists useful information about these chemicals.

Upper airway Portion of the respiratory tract above the glottis.

Upper flammable limit The concentration of fuel in the air above which the vapors cannot be ignited; above this point too much fuel and not enough oxygen are present to burn (too rich); also called the *upper explosive limit*.

Upper respiratory tract infection (URI) Viral syndrome causing nasal congestion, coughing, fever, and runny nose.

Upregulation The process by which a cell increases the number of receptors exposed to a given substance to improve its sensitivity to that substance.

Upstream A term describing the approaching traffic side of the damaged vehicles and the crash scene.

Uremia A term used to describe the signs and symptoms that accompany chronic renal failure.

Uremic frost Dried crystals of urea excreted through the skin that appear to be a frosting on the patient's body.

Ureter Tube that drains urine from the kidney to the bladder.

Urethra Passageway for both urine and male reproductive fluids; opening at the end of the bladder.

Urethral meatus Opening of the urethra between the clitoris and vagina.

Urinary bladder Hollow organ that stores urine; surrounded by smooth muscle.

Urinary retention The inability to empty the bladder or completely empty the bladder when urinating.

Urinary system Eliminates dissolved organic waste products by urine production and elimination.

Urticaria Also known as *hives*; a skin condition in which a wheal on the skin forms from edema; often caused by a reactions to a drug or through contact with substances (skin contact or even inhaled), causing hypersensitivity in the patient.

Uterine cavity Innermost region of the uterus.

Uterine prolapse Protrusion of part or all of the uterus out of the vagina.

Uterine tubes Tubular structures that extend from each side of the superior end of the body of the uterus to the lateral pelvic wall; they pick up the egg released by the ovary and transport it to the uterus; also known as *fallopian tubes.*

Uterus Muscular organ approximately the size of a pear; grows with the developing fetus.

Uvula Fleshy tissue resembling a grape that hangs down from the soft palate.

Vagina Female organ of copulation, the lower part of the birth canal, extending from the uterus to the outside of the body; extends from the cervix to the outside of the body.

Vaginal orifice Opening of the vagina.

Vaginitis An inflammation of the vaginal tissues.

Vallecula The depression or pocket between the base of the tongue and the epiglottis.

Vancomycin-resistant *Enterococcus* Bacteria resistant to vancomycin (a potent antibiotic); commonly acquired by patients in the hospital or patients who have indwelling catheters.

Vapor density The weight of a volume of pure gas compared with the weight of an equal volume of pure dry air (which has a constant value of 1); materials with a vapor density less than 1.0 are lighter than air and rise when released; materials with a vapor density greater than 1.0 are heavier than air and sink when released.

Vapor pressure The pressure exerted by a vapor against the sides of a closed container; a measure of volatility — high vapor pressure means it is a volatile substance.

Varicella An acute contagious vesicular skin eruption caused by the varicella zoster virus (chickenpox).

Varices Distended veins.

Varicocele Dilation of the venous plexus and internal spermatic vein, presenting as a lump in the scrotum.

Variola major A member of the *orthopoxvirus* family that causes the most common form of smallpox; the most likely form of the organism to be used as a weapon.

Vas deferens Tubes that extend from the end of the epididymis and through the seminal vesicles; also known as the *ductus deferens.*

Vascular access device Type of intravenous device used to deliver fluids, medications, blood, or nutritional therapy; usually inserted in patients who require long-term intravenous therapy.

Vascular headaches Headaches that involve changes in the diameter or size and chemistry of blood vessels that supply the brain.

Vascular resistance Amount of opposition that the blood vessels give to the flow of blood.

Vascular tunic Layer of the eye that contains most of the vasculature of the eye.

Vector A mode of transmission of a disease, typically from an insect or animal.

Vegetative functions Autonomic functions the body requires to survive.

Vehicle hazards Hazards directly related to the vehicle itself, including undeployed airbags; fuel system concerns; electrical system and battery electricity; stability of the vehicle; sharp glass and metal; leaking hot antifreeze; and engine oil, transmission oil, or antifreeze spills. Even the contents inside a vehicle's trunk or cargo area are typical vehicle hazards that can be encountered.

Vehicle stabilization Immediate action taken to prevent any unwanted movement of a crash-damaged vehicle.

Vena cava One of two large veins returning blood from the peripheral circulation to the right atrium of the heart.

Venipuncture Piercing of a vein.

Venom The poison injected by venomous animals such as snakes, insects, and marine creatures.

Venous return Amount of blood flowing into the right atrium each minute from the systemic circulation.

Ventilation The mechanical process of moving air into and out of the lungs.

Ventral Referring to the front of the body; anterior.

Ventricles Two pumping chambers in the heart.

Ventricular fibrillation Disorganized electrical activity of the ventricular conduction system of the heart, resulting in inefficient contractile force. This is the main cause of sudden cardiac death in electrical injuries.

Venules Small venous vessels that return blood to the capillaries.

Verbal apraxia Speech disorder in which the person has difficulty saying what he or she wants to say in a correct and consistent manner.

Verbal stimulus Any noise that elicits some sort of response from the patient.

Vertebrae Specialized bones comprising the spinal column.

Vertebral foramen Open space in the middle of vertebra.

Vertigo An out-of-control spinning sensation not relieved by lying down that may get worse when the eyes are closed.

Very high frequency A type of radio signal used to make two-way radio contact between the communications center and the responders. Now considered old technology compared with more contemporary 800-MHz radio systems.

Vesicants Agents named from the most obvious injury they inflict on a person; will burn and blister the skin or any other part of the body they touch; also known as *blister agents* or *mustard agents.*

Vesicles The shipping containers of the cell. They are very simple in structure, consisting of a single membrane filled with liquid; they transport a wide variety of substances both inside and outside the cell.

Vestibule Space or cavity that serves as the entrance to the inner ear.

Veterinary medical assistance team Teams designed to provide animal care and assistance during disasters.

Vials Glass containers with rubber stoppers at the top.

Viral hemorrhagic fevers A group of viral diseases of diverse etiology (arenaviruses, filoviruses, bunyaviruses, and flaviviruses) having many similar characteristics, including increased capillary permeability, leukopenia, and thrombocytopenia, resulting in a severe multisystem syndrome.

Viral shedding Release of viruses from an infected host through some vector (e.g., sneezing, coughing, bleeding).

Virions Small particles of viruses.

Virulence A term to describe the relative pathogenicity or the relative ability to do damage to the host of an infectious agent.

Virus Microorganism that invades cells and uses their machinery to live and replicate; cannot survive without a host, does not have a cell wall of its own, and consists of a strand of DNA or RNA surrounded by a capsid.

Visceral Portion of the peripheral nervous system that processes motor and sensory information from the internal organs, includes the autonomic nervous system.

Visceral pain Deep pain that arises from internal areas of the body that are enclosed within a cavity.

Visceral pleura Lining of the pleural cavity that adheres tightly to the lung surface.

Viscosity The thickness of a liquid; a high-viscosity liquid does not flow easily (e.g., oils and tar); a low-viscosity liquid flows easily (e.g., gasoline) and poses a greater risk for aspiration and consequent pulmonary damage.

Visual acuity card A standardized board used to test vision.

Vitreous chamber The most posterior chamber of the eyeball.

Vitreous humor Thick, jellylike substance that fills the vitreous chamber of the eyeball.

Voice over Internet protocol Telephone technology that gives Internet users the ability to make voice telephone calls.

Volatility A measure of how quickly a material passes into the vapor or gas state; the greater the volatility, the greater its rate of evaporation.

Volkmann contracture A deformity of the hand, fingers, and wrist caused by injury to the muscles of the forearm; also known as *ischemic contracture.*

Voltage Difference in electrical charge between two points.

Voluntary guarding Conscious contraction of the abdominal muscles in an attempt to prevent painful palpation.

Volvulus Intestinal obstruction caused by a knotting and twisting of the bowel.

Vomiting Forceful ejection of stomach contents through the mouth.

Vowel The letters *a, e, i, o, u,* and sometimes *y.*

Vulva External female genitalia.

Vulvovaginitis Inflammation of the external female genitalia and vagina.

VX Most toxic of the nerve agent class of military warfare agents.

Warm zone Area surrounding the hot zone that functions as a safety buffer area, decontamination area, and as an access and egress point to and from the hot zone; also called the *contamination reduction zone.*

Warts Benign lesions caused by the papillomavirus.

Washout phase Vascular response in shock when postcapillary sphincters open, allowing fluid in the capillary beds to be pushed into systemic circulation; follows the stagnant phase.

Water solubility The degree to which a material or its vapors are soluble in water.

Water-reactive materials Materials that violently decompose and/or burn vigorously when they come in contact with moisture.

Waveform Movement away from the baseline in either a positive or negative direction.

Wernicke-Korsakoff syndrome Neurologic disorder caused by a thiamine deficiency; most often seen in chronic alcoholics; characterized by ataxia, nystagmus, weakness, and mental derangement in the early stages. In later stages, the condition is much more likely to become permanent and is characterized by amnesia, disorientation, delirium, and hallucinations.

Wheal A firm, rounded, flat-topped elevation of skin that is evanescent and pruritic (itches); also known as a *hive.*

Wheeze A musical, whistling sound heard on inspiration and/or expiration resulting from constriction or obstruction of the pharynx, trachea, or bronchi. Wheezing is commonly associated with asthma.

Wilderness command physician A physician who has received additional training by a Wilderness Emergency Medical Services Institute–endorsed course in wilderness medical care and medical direction of wilderness EMS providers and operations.

Wilderness emergency medical technician An emergency medical technician who has obtained EMT certification by Department of Transportation criteria and has completed additional modules in wilderness care; sometimes abbreviated as WEMT, W-EMT, or EMT-W.

Wilderness EMS An individual or group that preplans to administer care in an austere environment and then is called on to perform these duties when needed.

Wilderness EMS system A formally structured organization integrated into or part of the standard EMS system and configured to provide wilderness medical care to a discrete region.

Wilderness first aid A level of certification indicating a provider has been trained in traditional first aid with added training in wilderness care and first aid administration in austere environments.

Wilderness first responder A first responder who has obtained certification by Department of Transportation criteria and has completed additional modules in wilderness care.

Wilderness medicine Medical management in situations where care and prevention are limited by environmental considerations, prolonged extrication, or resource availability.

Window phase The period after infection during which the antigen is present but no antibody is detectable.

Withdrawal Physical and/or psychological signs and symptoms that result from discontinuing regular administration of a drug; effects are usually the opposite of the effects of the drug itself because the body has changed itself to maintain homeostasis.

Wolff-Parkinson-White syndrome Type of preexcitation syndrome characterized by a slurred upstroke of the QRS complex (delta wave) and wide QRS.

Word root The foundation of a word; establishes the basic meaning of a word.

Word salad The most severe form of looseness of associations in which the topic shifts so rapidly that it interrupts the flow of sentences themselves, producing a jumble of words.

Workload management Planning resources and support services around demand.

Wrap point A machinery entanglement hazard formed when any machine component rotates.

Xenografting Transplanting tissue from a member of a different species (e.g., porcine heart valves harvested from pigs).

Years of potential life lost (YPLL) A method that assumes that, on average, most people will live a productive life until the age of 65 years.

Yeast A unicellular type of fungus that reproduces by budding.

Yersinia pestis The anaerobic, gram-negative bacterium that causes plague disease in human beings and rodents.

Zone of coagulation In a full-thickness burn wound, the central area of the burn devoid of blood flow. This tissue is not salvageable and becomes visibly necrotic days after the injury.

Zone of stasis or ischemia Outside the zone of coagulation, where blood supply is tenuous. The capillaries may be damaged but oxygenated blood can still pass through them to perfuse the surrounding tissues.

Illustration Credits

CHAPTER 37

All images from Aehlert B. (2006). *ECGs made easy* (3rd ed.). St Louis: Mosby.

CHAPTER 38

All images from Aehlert B. (2006). *ECGs made easy* (3rd ed.). St Louis: Mosby.